THE STIMULATED MIND

THE STIMULATED MIND

Future-Proof Your Brain from Dementia and Stay Sharp at Any Age

DR TOMMY WOOD

Illustrations by Alex Stewart

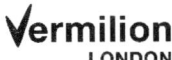

VERMILION

UK | USA | Canada | Ireland | Australia
India | New Zealand | South Africa

Vermilion is part of the Penguin Random House group of companies whose addresses can be found at global.penguinrandomhouse.com

Penguin Random House UK
One Embassy Gardens, 8 Viaduct Gardens, London SW11 7BW

penguin.co.uk

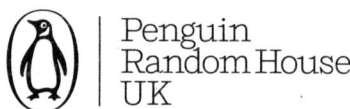

First published in the United States of America by Harmony Books in 2026
First published in Great Britain by Vermilion in 2026

3

Copyright © Thomas R. Wood, BM BCh, PhD 2026
The moral right of the author has been asserted.

Penguin Random House values and supports copyright. Copyright fuels creativity, encourages diverse voices, promotes freedom of expression and supports a vibrant culture. Thank you for purchasing an authorised edition of this book and for respecting intellectual property laws by not reproducing, scanning or distributing any part of it by any means without permission. You are supporting authors and enabling Penguin Random House to continue to publish books for everyone. No part of this book may be used or reproduced in any manner for the purpose of training artificial intelligence technologies or systems. In accordance with Article 4(3) of the DSM Directive 2019/790, Penguin Random House expressly reserves this work from the text and data mining exception.

Typeset by Six Red Marbles UK, Thetford, Norfolk

Printed and bound in Great Britain by Clays Ltd, Elcograf S.p.A.

The authorised representative in the EEA is Penguin Random House Ireland, Morrison Chambers, 32 Nassau Street, Dublin D02 YH68

A CIP catalogue record for this book is available from the British Library

Hardback ISBN 9781785045141
Trade paperback ISBN 9781785046858

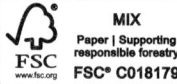

Penguin Random House is committed to a sustainable future for our business, our readers and our planet. This book is made from Forest Stewardship Council® certified paper.

In memory of Simon Marshall, who taught me that the brain is so much more than its component parts

PREFACE

Most neuroscience books begin with a grand statement about the awesome power and wisdom of the human brain. This one begins with owls, who are nearly as wise but look way more fetching in a pair of spectacles.

Back in the 1980s and '90s, a group of neuroscientists at Stanford University studied the way the brain adapts to new information by doing exactly that: fitting barn owls with glasses. These glasses weren't just stylish avian accessories, though; the lenses of these glasses contained prisms. Because prisms redirect light, the glasses made the viewer (the owl) think that everything around it was in a different place from where it actually was.

Imagine for a second that you're an owl. Your eyes are fixed in your skull so the only way to look around is to move your whole head. An enterprising neuroscientist has attached some prism glasses to your face, so now everything you see is shifted slightly to one side. You hear what you think is a tasty mouse rustling in the leaves, but when you turn your head, there's nothing there. Because of the glasses there's suddenly a mismatch in your brain between your ears and eyes. Much to your consternation, where you hear something is not where you see it.

Just like humans, owls have to know where they are in the world in order to survive. So, their brains build internal maps of how they expect the world to be arranged. The Stanford group found that owls wearing prism glasses could rewire their internal maps of the world so that everything eventually aligned again. Once this realignment happened, the owls were able to account for the visual discrepancy. This is all thanks to the phenomenon of neuroplasticity—the brain's ability to change its structure and functioning in response to new information.

Initially, this team of owl optometrists found something that probably won't surprise you: while young owls adapted very quickly to the glasses, *adult owls did not*.[1] Even months later, adult animals would still miss that pesky mouse even if it was right under their beak. If I stopped right there, my arcane owl story would support a pervasive notion of how we think about our brains—that at some point we become the proverbial old dogs unable to learn new tricks. That, at a certain age, we lack the ability to meaningfully change or improve our brains. After all, neuroplasticity is for kids (or baby owls), right? And the only thing the rest of us can look forward to is an unstoppable process of decline as we increasingly forget names, faces, and where our tasty mouse dinner is. But luckily, the story *doesn't* end there.

Another decade of work by these nocturnal raptor enthusiasts sets the stage for us to completely change the way we think about the adult brain. While the blank canvas of a young brain continuously absorbs new information and wires itself accordingly, it wasn't that adult owl brains *couldn't* adapt—they just needed a good reason to.

This was beautifully demonstrated in a series of experiments that I think every brain buff should know about. In the initial experiments the owls were fed dead mice, meaning that they could sit in their cages wondering why the world looked a bit weird but otherwise happily snacking on a dinner that came without any effort. If this isn't a perfect metaphor for modern human life, I don't know what is. But then the scientists switched things up. In one follow-up experiment, owls wearing glasses were forced to hunt *live* mice for dinner.[2] Surprisingly, their adult brains proved able to adapt to the visual shift just fine. Yet another experiment showed that adaptation could occur much later in life when owls were housed with other birds rather than being on their own in a cage with no social interaction. The takeaway is that adult brains are able to adapt and rewire themselves regardless of age, but to do so requires us to actually engage with the world—either socially or with challenges (like finding dinner) that tell our brains they need to change.

Having dropped this owl-shaped bombshell, it's probably important to let you know that adult neuroplasticity isn't just for birds. It turns out that neuroscientists have been performing similar experiments with humans for more than a hundred years.³ For example, in the early twentieth century, researchers at the University of Innsbruck in Austria made adult study participants continuously wear goggles that flipped their vision upside down. Impressively, their brains adapted to this new orientation within just a few days:

> Between the first and third day, the world was upside down for the participant . . . the participant held a cup upside down when it was about to be filled, or they tried to step over things on the ceiling. Swift reactions, such as parrying an attack during fencing, were in the wrong direction. By the fifth day, the participant's clumsiness and vision started to change. Things that had been seen upside down suddenly were upright once the participant traced the shapes they saw with their hands—*an immense effort of the brain* [emphasis mine]. From the sixth day of uninterruptedly wearing reversing spectacles, permanent upright vision ensued, and behaviour was perfectly correct. For example, a participant drew a picture in a quality as if drawn without wearing reversing spectacles.⁴

I'm still amazed every time I read this passage, because it provides such a vivid example of how incredibly adaptable the brain is—even the adult brain. In this experiment, the participant's brain rewired itself as they interacted with the world in various engaging ways—fencing, drawing, walking around—getting constant feedback and making mistakes. Luckily, you don't have to wear world-altering glasses to stimulate neuroplasticity. As you'll see, learning new skills or taking on new challenges that stimulate new connections is one of the most important ways we can change our brains as adults. And these changes are possible at any time in our adult lives.

As an adult, you've already spent years or decades engaging your brain with your own individual environment, and your brain has responded and developed accordingly. This is a good thing. We want our brains to be optimised for our environment, which allows us to hone our skills at work and to develop relationships with people who are important to us. The accumulated shaping of our brains over time is also partly what drives beneficial characteristics such as wisdom—the ability to see larger patterns and integrate experience and information—which increases as we get older. But one consequence of having already shaped our brains in adulthood is that in order to make new pathways and further engage the process of neuroplasticity, we need to give our brains a compelling reason to do so. This generally involves time and focus as well as effort, all of which are ways that we convince the brain that these new connections or skills are important to us. Though not always easy, the recipe for changing and improving the adult brain may be relatively simple. As Michael S. Brainard and Eric I. Knudsen of the famed owl experiments put it, if we want to drive neuroplasticity and adaptation in the human brain, "a rich environment is required to reveal the full capacity for adjustment."

In short, what we thought we knew about the adult brain being fixed and then inevitably declining over time is almost certainly wrong. And the good news is: if we change the way we think about our brains and what we expect of our lives as we age, we're capable of so much more than we previously imagined.

CONTENTS

Introduction   xiii

PART ONE
Can a Neuroscientist Understand the Brain?

CHAPTER 1	Baby Neuroscientist's First Reality Check	3
CHAPTER 2	How Do Neuroscientists Study the Brain?	13
CHAPTER 3	In Search of the Bigger Picture	24
CHAPTER 4	Dominance of the Environment	34
CHAPTER 5	The Game of Brain Health	53

PART TWO
Winning the Brain Game

CHAPTER 6	The Rules of the Game	65
CHAPTER 7	Move	79
CHAPTER 8	Nourish	115
CHAPTER 9	Stimulate	160
CHAPTER 10	Connect	204
CHAPTER 11	Adapt	222

| CHAPTER 12 | Recover | 261 |
| CHAPTER 13 | Sex, Drugs, and Environmental Toll | 299 |

PART THREE
A Brain for Today and the Future

| CHAPTER 14 | The 3-S Model of Brain Health | 345 |
| CHAPTER 15 | Future-Proofing Your Brain | 379 |

References 419

Acknowledgments 421

Index 427

INTRODUCTION
VISIONS OF A FUTURE-PROOF BRAIN

The ultimate goal of this book is to help you develop a healthy brain that has better function not only now but also in the future, while being resilient to the everyday stressors we all face (figure 1). In other words, I hope to help you make your brain future-proof. This process is largely grounded in factors such as nutrition, sleep, physical exercise, and stimulating our brains by engaging with others and the world around us. By appropriately using and supporting our brains we can increase our cognitive function today, thrive in a complex and unknowable future environment, and dramatically decrease our long-term risk of Alzheimer's disease and dementia.[1]

In my mind, a future-proof brain is one that is able to deal with the current and future challenges that our brains face:

1. Staying sharp and focused in a world of information overload that demands instant response times and 24/7 workloads, which cause us to feel increasingly fatigued, stressed, and distracted.
2. Avoiding or minimising the risk of long-term cognitive decline and Alzheimer's disease, which are becoming more common as the population ages.
3. Being prepared to perform well and develop new skills as technology and other advances in the modern world change the way we interact with our workplaces and environments.

In the short term, having a future-proof brain might help you to think better and perform under pressure, or when sleep-deprived. Not that this is necessarily *encouraged*—I can be pretty cranky when I'm

A FUTURE-PROOF BRAIN

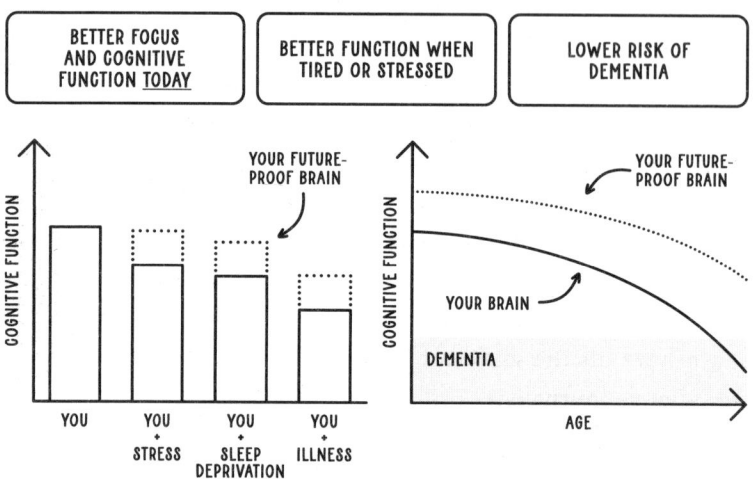

FIGURE 1. What to expect from a future-proof brain. Left: this graph shows your cognitive function at any given moment in time. When you then add stress or illness or sleep deprivation, cognitive function drops. With the future-proofing methods described in this book, your brain is more resilient and capable of maintaining higher levels of function even under these types of stress. Right: here you can see changes in cognitive function with age. As you might expect, on average, cognitive function decreases over time (solid lines). Different people have different trajectories, and some will end up with enough loss of function that they are diagnosed with dementia such as Alzheimer's disease (shaded area). In a future-proofed brain (dotted lines), cognitive function is increased at every age, and though the effect of age cannot be completely prevented, this higher line means that the likelihood of ever being diagnosed with dementia is decreased.

short on sleep, no matter how many tips and tricks I employ. But stress and lost sleep are going to happen, and we should be able to handle them when they do. In the long term, a future-proof brain can maintain more of its function with age, hopefully avoiding the significant loss of day-to-day cognitive function we call dementia.

If this all sounds too good to be true, you're not alone. My own path to realising we have huge capacity to alter our cognitive fortunes was a decades-long journey that began with some (hopefully) unforgettable words from my father: "Remember, this doesn't mean you actually *know* anything."

It was the summer of 2003, and I had just learned my A-level results would allow me to attend Cambridge University for my undergraduate degree. My initial youthful pride was quickly tempered by these words from my dad—a world-renowned scientist in his own right—and they have remained indelibly burned into my mind ever since. And though it felt a little like an affront at the time, I now know that this was sage and important advice. Not only did I go on to discover that getting an A on a biology exam as a teenager requires only a limited understanding of the true complexities of biology, there is also a much more important lesson in these words that relates to the nature of knowledge itself; that no matter how successful we are or how smart we think we are, we shouldn't delude ourselves into thinking that we have all the answers. While today's social media environment, science journalists, and celebrity health podcasters often have us believing otherwise, we can never be certain of very much when it comes to human biology. In fact, one well-used phrase suggests that "there is no such thing as proof in biology." We can build evidence and use that evidence to develop a framework to help us understand the world, but at any given moment we're just one well-designed experiment (or one well-phrased question) away from having to completely reevaluate the way we see the world.

AN EARLY CAREER OF TWISTS AND TURNS

As an undergraduate at Cambridge, my time outside of lectures was split evenly between writing essays and rowing. I spent countless hours each morning training before sunrise in every type of weather imaginable, followed by long afternoons and evenings at my desk writing thousands of words about the regulation of biological pathways. And while I promise not to make you read thousands of words about the regulation of biological pathways (or make you get up early to go rowing in the rain), these experiences were particularly formative for me in at least two ways.

The first is that the endless essay writing changed the way I thought about accumulating knowledge. And yes, I know that sounds a bit haughty and intellectual. But what I mean is that we often think and learn about science, especially in biology and medicine, as a large collection of facts to be memorised. But when you have to write three thousand words about a single enzyme, you're forced to think about how that enzyme is regulated, its inputs and outputs, and how it fits into the bigger picture of a cell and a whole organism. Some of the tensions we experience as a society when we talk about science, health, and indeed our brains, come from losing sight of that interconnected bigger picture.

Outside of the purely academic pursuit of knowledge, my experiences in rowing, first as an athlete and then as a coach, were equally transformative. Rowing is such a cultural phenomenon at Oxford and Cambridge (lovingly contracted to *Oxbridge*) that something like 50 percent of students who attend either institution get in a rowing boat at least once. At Oxbridge, rowing is also a way of life. Most of the rowing competitions are internal (both universities are split into multiple small universities who compete against one another), yet the top crews will train for twenty hours a week. These are some of the best rowers in the world, with crews often featuring numerous former and future Olympians and World Champions.

In my second year at Cambridge, I joined the university's development squad, which was a programme that took inexperienced rowers like me to see if they could be trained up to join one of the top crews. For two years, I was lucky enough to have some of the best rowing coaches invest huge amounts of time trying to teach me how to row better. I got to train with (and watch) some of the best rowers of my generation. And while this didn't turn me into a top rower myself— not through a lack of effort on their part or mine—it allowed me to develop a large tool kit of potential ways to help others improve their technique and fitness.

Seeing how some of the best coaches and rowers in the world approached performance allowed me to begin developing my own framework as a coach, which I have continued to develop as a consultant to professional athletes. It's not just a matter of thinking about all the minutiae of health and fitness, but understanding that they interact and have to be addressed in an approachable and practical manner tailored to the individual. When I was head coach of the Oxford medical school boat club, one of our best rowers, who had regularly competed internationally, told me that I was the only amateur coach she'd ever had whose coaching she "didn't hate." To this day I think that's one of the nicest compliments I've ever received.

Even before I became a coach, the influence of my rowing experiences as an undergraduate played a large role in my decision to go to medical school. In particular, I was motivated by the desire to apply the complex biochemistry and physiology I had learned in a practical manner. When asked why I wanted to be a doctor, I told my interviewers that I had developed a deep personal interest in how lifestyle factors such as exercise could dramatically improve health, and I wanted to bring that information to my future patients. While this answer was good enough to earn me a place as a medical student, I later learned that most doctors don't have the time or space to impact their patients in this way. Not that they don't want to; it's just not how the system is set up.

Doctors do, of course, have a massive impact, and I saw that every day as a resident doctor in central London. I spent two years mending broken bones, treating drug overdoses, and experiencing the final moments of patients suffering from dementia. Sometimes I still miss night shifts as a doctor on the medical wards. On those shifts you are an integral part of a small team, and all your time is spent doing what you're trained for—keeping people alive. As humans, one of our core needs is to feel useful. In those moments, I felt confident that what I was doing really mattered.

But as my two-year training period in London came to an end, I was faced with a dilemma. I didn't really know what type of medicine I wanted to specialise in, and I also felt disconnected from my interests in lifestyle and disease prevention that had gotten me interested in medicine in the first place. While I struggled to decide what to do next, a former mentor offered me the opportunity to do a PhD in neonatal neuroscience in Norway. Though it was a fairly substantial detour from where I thought I was heading at the time, this unexpected offer provided me the opportunity to develop my skills as a scientist, gave me the time and tools to build my career as a coach and educator, and informed my perspective about how the brain can be shaped and supported across the entire lifespan. All of those experiences are critical to the information in this book. (Though, if I'm completely honest, I moved to Norway because it sounded interesting and I wasn't sure what I should do instead.)

NEUROSCIENCE UNDER THE MACROSCOPE

Because I come from an academic family, many people have said that I was always destined to be a professor of some kind. But as you can maybe see, I never planned to be a neuroscientist. And having come to neuroscience the long way, in many ways I'm not a very *typical* neuroscientist.

Like any decent neuroscientist, I was trained to dissect cells and pathways in order to better understand the inner workings of the brain. I can reel off the biochemistry of neurotransmitters and the esoteric names of the regions in the brain where those neurotransmitters act. I can tell you how those neurotransmitters drive signaling processes that are linked to whether you feel motivated or focused. And I can do it in such an authoritative way that you'd believe I'm an expert in a field with a complete grasp of how the brain works. But you won't often find me doing that. Not because this information isn't important but because it can be easy to get stuck in the weeds, when it's the bigger picture of how we use our brains and live our lives that determines our long-term cognitive function.

To date, generations of diligent neuroscientists have cataloged huge volumes of information by delving deeper and deeper into the brain— first its cells, then the proteins and organelles of the cells, and later how individual cells control gene expression and function. But despite this, we're sadly not much closer to understanding, curing, or preventing the wide range of brain-related conditions that affect nearly half of the world's population.[2] As a result, I'm increasingly convinced that our current approach isn't working as well as we'd hope.

I'm not here to tell you that I have solved this problem and miraculously discovered the hidden secrets of neuroscience. But I *am* confident that we (both individually and as a species) can have much more of an impact on brain health and disease than perhaps we realise. The difference is mainly in perspective—and, more importantly, in where we choose to intervene.

Like most scientific fields, modern neuroscience has an ever-increasing suite of amazing tools with which to perform experiments and gather information. These have allowed us to zoom deeper and deeper into the inner workings of the brain to try to understand its components in elaborate detail. However, despite all these tools at my disposal, and having now spent two decades as a (neuro)scientist, doctor, and performance coach to athletes, there is still only one thing about the brain that I am completely certain of: its function is more than the sum of its parts.

If we want to truly understand the brain and how to keep it healthy for decades to come, we need to zoom out rather than in. When you do that, one consistent theme that underpins everything in this book becomes clear: *The brain is a product of the environment.*

This is good news. If the brain is a product of your environment and your environment is something that can be changed, that means that your long-term cognitive function is ultimately malleable. Even better, by zooming out we can often bypass a large amount of conflicting, and oftentimes confusing, information about the brain's inner workings to find a framework that helps us understand where best to act when it comes to our own individual brain health. And even if the model of how I think about the brain turns out to be wrong someday, I'm confident that the evidence-based approaches I will provide aren't going to change anytime soon. This is largely because they've been battle-tested for decades by me and others and are grounded in the very basics of biology, some of which we've known for centuries.

APPLYING SCIENCE IN THE REAL WORLD

When I say that the approaches and ideas outlined in this book are battle-tested, I mean that they were built using a combination of rigorous science and years of application that included a lot of failure, growth, and learning. While a good grounding in the theory of biochemistry and physiology is important for anybody working in the fields related to human health, you don't really know what you know until those ideas have either succeeded or failed in the real world.

For my entire career, I've spent half my time performing carefully controlled experiments in the lab as a scientist—I'm currently an associate professor of paediatrics and neuroscience at the University of Washington, where my research focuses on brain health across the lifespan—and the other half applying knowledge and theories in the much messier arena of the real world as a doctor and a coach.

During my PhD studies, I remained committed to the idea that simple lifestyle changes could have a big impact on health, so I started a blog and a podcast. I know everybody has a podcast now, but back then it was still relatively novel. My goal was to provide practical, evidence-based approaches for improving health, with less of the mudslinging and tribalism that has only seemed to increase over time. Somewhere on a dusty hard drive there's a series of podcasts I recorded called *Everybody's Right About...*, in which I talked about the evidence for multiple sides of nutrition topics. The premise was that it's hard to say that something is "good" or "bad" because people on either side of the argument each have evidence to support their opinion. These discussions are interesting to a professional nerd like me but can be confusing and frustrating to most other people. Though we often have to accept that there will be some nuance, and each person's path will look a little different, my goal has always been to provide some clarity for people navigating contentious or complex topics to better support their health and well-being.

Soon after starting this foray into science communication, I connected with the founder of a start-up company working with athletes to support their long-term performance. Many of these athletes were trying to train and compete while managing chronic health issues. With a new outlet for my enthusiasm for these topics, I bombarded the company's doctor and health coaches with multiple daily emails on a variety of topics related to biochemistry, physiology, nutrition, and health and performance in general. Eventually, they invited me to join the company as their chief scientist, which, looking back, might have just been an attempt to stop me from sending so many emails.

I continued my work as a health and performance coach during my PhD studies in Norway and then my early years as an academic in the United States. Nowadays, most of my performance-related work is as head scientist for motorsport for a company called Hintsa Performance that provides medical and coaching services to Formula 1 drivers. For those not familiar with it, Formula 1 is considered by many to be the pinnacle of car racing, where the best engineers, tacticians, and drivers in the world come together to point multimillion-dollar cars at brick walls at two hundred miles an hour.

In Formula 1, as well as other work I do outside the lab like consulting with large digital health companies, my primary role is to be a translator and integrator of scientific research. Take, for instance, one of my standout memories in Formula 1, when a driver asked to meet me for dinner during the U.S. Grand Prix in Austin. He had recently watched a nutrition "documentary" (a word I use very loosely in this context) and had some questions. Like, a *lot* of questions. He showed up with a small pad full of notes and proceeded to grill me for the best part of three hours while we enjoyed a delicious meal. My job was to help him separate fact from fiction and figure out what (if anything) was relevant to him. This is the core of my work as a coach and consultant: helping athletes decide whether a new supplement or piece of technology is worth integrating into their routine, as well as working with companies to develop health frameworks that are relevant to thousands of people.

As a result, over the past two decades, I've done everything under the vast umbrella of coaching. With my own athletes, that includes writing training plans, running training sessions, and preparing post-workout protein shakes. As a health coach to people struggling with a variety of chronic health conditions, I've written diet and sleep plans and interpreted vast reams of complex health data they've sent me from laboratory tests and wearables (while disregarding low-quality data and tests that are often sold to people desperately looking to improve their health). As a performance consultant in professional sports, I've been responsible for tweaks to diet, lifestyle, and supplementation strategies in a world where fractions of a second can literally cost millions of dollars. In most of these scenarios, I worked as part of a (sometimes very large) team. But in each case, I had to put my money where my mouth was and take responsibility when my idea failed. And every time that happened, I've had to adapt and expand my thinking in order to incorporate this new piece of information. As a result, I've been lucky to have experiences that many typical scientists are missing. That's definitely not through any fault of their own, though. I meandered through multiple potential careers and had a much slower career progression because of it. To this day, when people read my CV, the first thing they tell me is that it's "eclectic."

But in my opinion, the practical experience of applying scientific knowledge to the lives of real people is where my greatest learning has happened. As proud as I am of my formal academic accomplishments, it is the chances to fail, learn, and solve problems that have ultimately shaped the stories and ideas in this book. These experiences helped me turn a lot of theory and science into an overarching idea for how we can think about the complex underpinnings of brain function while keeping things simple enough for us to intervene and change it in a beneficial and practical way.

In part 1 of *The Stimulated Mind*, I will draw heavily from my experiences as a professor and neuroscientist. These are the lessons that come from decades spent performing experiments in the lab and analysing data. I will cover some of the history behind how and why we think about the brain the way we do, and how that's holding us back in the face of an ever-increasing burden of cognitive and mental health disorders. These issues include the downsides of trying to break the brain down into its individual components, as well as critical assumptions we've made about the brain in order to tell a simple story about cognitive decline that doesn't completely fit the data. I will then cover some of my favourite science that shows just how much the brain is capable of if we broaden our scope and move away from traditional ways of thinking about neuroscience.

In part 2, I will outline all the major modifiable components of the environment that contribute to brain health and cognitive function. Though still grounded in the latest cutting-edge science, part 2 will draw heavily from my experiences as a coach in the world of sports helping individuals navigate the multiple daily choices they face when thinking about ways to improve their health and performance. In this part, I will provide simple but powerful frameworks to help you support your short- and long-term brain health and function through skill learning, social connection, stress management, sleep, exercise, and nutrition.

In part 3, I will zoom out to show you how the components in part 2 fit together and interact in my model for brain health and function, leveraging some of the problem-solving approaches I learned working with engineers as a trainee physician and academic. This model will then provide the basis for understanding how to improve focus and learn better on a day-to-day basis, as well as for thinking about how to approach our brains as we age. By appreciating that the brain is much more than the sum of its parts, and can only be understood based on its environment, you can emerge empowered with the knowledge to future-proof your brain for decades to come.

PART ONE

Can a Neuroscientist Understand the Brain?

CHAPTER 1
BABY NEUROSCIENTIST'S FIRST REALITY CHECK

I can still vividly remember the first time I had to completely reevaluate the landscape of my work in neuroscience. This happened just over a decade after first hearing my dad's reminder of how little we all truly *know*. My journey in between involved a fair amount of luck and indecision, but also an ever-increasing curiosity about how to understand and impact human health.

It was now the summer of 2014. I was just nine months into my PhD studies when I attended a scientific conference with some of the biggest names in my new field. While I'd made early inroads into at least two other careers (medicine and athletic performance coaching), I knew very little about cutting-edge neuroscience.

On the first day of the conference, we heard a talk that referenced a scientific paper with the catchy title "1,026 Experimental Treatments in Acute Stroke."[1] The essence of the paper is this: At the time it was written (now more than twenty years ago), there were over a thousand treatments that could dramatically decrease the injury caused by a stroke. In rats. But none of these treatments, with the exception of thrombolysis (clot busting), which has been used in humans since the 1950s, have improved outcomes in human stroke patients.

For days afterwards, I couldn't get this study out of my head. If decades of research and billions of dollars had been invested in the search for better stroke treatments, and literally nothing that worked in the lab had successfully worked in humans, why should we expect the next decades and next billion dollars to have a different result?

This situation is unfortunately not unique to strokes. When it comes to almost every brain injury or neurodegenerative condition, the last major breakthrough in treatment occurred several decades ago. Or, in the case of age-related cognitive decline and dementias such as Alzheimer's disease, no breakthrough has occurred at all. During the conference, I couldn't shake the feeling that there was something missing in how we research the brain as we look for ways to treat or support it. And since that day, there is one question that I have continued to reflect on as I've built my career as a professor and neuroscientist: What if we're thinking about the brain all wrong?

THE CURRENT STATE OF THE BRAIN

Before we delve into a little neuroscience to understand what we do and don't know about the brain, and how that applies to our own brains, I think it would be useful to start with a discussion of brain health. Because ultimately, that's what we are all striving to improve.

Most simply, *a healthy brain is one that performs the (cognitive) functions you want, at the time you want it to perform them.*

Obviously, my simple definition of brain health has to be applied within the reality of our individual experiences. For example, as much as I would love for my brain to suddenly allow me to clear a dance floor with jaw-dropping breakdancing moves, that's not going to happen. Anyone who has seen me strut my stuff at an after-hours neuroscience conference disco will gladly attest as much. But, as somebody who has lived and worked in many countries, I might reasonably expect my brain to understand and speak one of the languages I've learned, even when I'm under pressure or haven't slept well.

Brain health, therefore, is incredibly personal. What I want my brain to do could be very different from what you want yours to do, especially as we age. As we'll see later, this information can help us tailor the skills and tasks we engage our brains in. Of course, there are also common functions that we all want our brains to perform: remember day-to-day occurrences and conversations, sustain focus on specific tasks that are important to us, process a wide range of information, and make decisions in a calm and timely manner. Luckily, the factors that help us achieve our individual goals of brain health and cognition also support these more general components of daily brain function.

There's one final piece to my definition of a healthy brain that's critically important—the element of time. In addition to supporting our cognitive function right now, I believe a healthy brain should be as *future-proof* as possible. This means minimising the effects of ageing on the brain and making sure we're able to function in, and adapt to, unknown future situations for decades to come. Unfortunately, at least right now, that's not necessarily the future that our brains can expect.

It's undeniable that we as a society appear to be at a critical moment when it comes to our collective mental and cognitive health. Everywhere we look, it seems that our brains are increasingly under duress. The sheer volume of information we're expected to handle—unthinkable to previous generations—keeps increasing, and we're fracturing our attention by moving from one cognitive task to another much more frequently than we did even twenty years ago.[2] Among the generations who grew up with smartphones and social media as part of their daily lives, more women are receiving prescriptions of antidepressant medications than ever before, and men have a higher-than-ever risk of dying by suicide.[3] At the same time, one in nine American adults over forty-five says they've noticed worsening cognitive function, and more than one in ten adults over sixty-five has dementia.[4] In the next fifteen to twenty years, the burden of dementia is expected to at least double, if not triple, worldwide, becoming either the first or second most common cause of death in most high-income countries by 2040.[5]

Phew. Deep breath.

When contemplating statistics like these, it's not surprising that the default feeling is one of helplessness. In the face of this palpable sense that our brains are collectively struggling, we then layer on a coating of inevitability. We assume that there's nothing we can do to change the state or trajectory of our brain health, and that decline is unavoidable. But, while not all these issues have simple solutions, and we should never pretend that's the case, there's plenty of evidence to suggest that these statistics can be a call to action rather than a reason to despair.

Perhaps because we believe there's nothing we can do to help or change its fate, the brain often doesn't get the attention it should. Even those of us who are interested in reading books about health tend to focus externally, and mostly below the neck. This is partly because we've been taught to think that the way we look in the mirror is a direct expression of our overall health (which is often not true at all), and partly because the brain remains a mystery, its skills and functionality hard to decipher and measure.

The story of how our brains function (or not) as they age is a familiar one. Early in life, our cognitive potential seems limitless. We marvel at the ability of children to learn languages and the remarkable capacity of the adolescent brain to effortlessly master an ever-increasing suite of complex modern technology. Looking back at your own young brain, you'll no doubt fondly remember a time when *you* were blessed with sharp wits and instant recall. Back then, you were the proverbial young owl from the preface—able to immediately adapt to the strange new world you saw through prism glasses.

Fast-forward to the present day, though, and you tell yourself that you just can't learn or focus like you used to. Everything "upstairs" feels like much more of a struggle. It may even seem like you're doomed to experience an unending, unstoppable, unforgiving road to cognitive decline and dementia. And if you ever take time to ponder what you can do about all this, it's usually to worry about how you're making it worse—a few more brain cells killed every time you have a bad night of sleep or drink a few too many cocktails (figure 1).

It amazes and saddens me to think that we've passed the first quarter of the twenty-first century and still have this fixed (and slightly morbid) view of how our brain function will change over time. On almost a daily basis I talk to scientists, physicians, science journalists, clients, and members of the public who believe we have very little control over our cognitive faculties, especially later in life. But what if I told you that this story we tell ourselves is more fiction than fact? The truth is that, while cognitive function does tend to change over time, and we can't prevent the ageing process entirely, our brains are able to adapt and improve at almost any age, as long as we give them the tools and the environment to do so.

But if we're going to have the lofty yet achievable goal of developing and maintaining a future-proof brain, we need a strategy for how to achieve that. My personal strategy is to think about building what economist Art De Vany calls *headroom*. Simply defined, headroom is the total amount of function that we have available to us when we really need it. It's the buffer that we rely on to help us resist the forces of ageing over time.

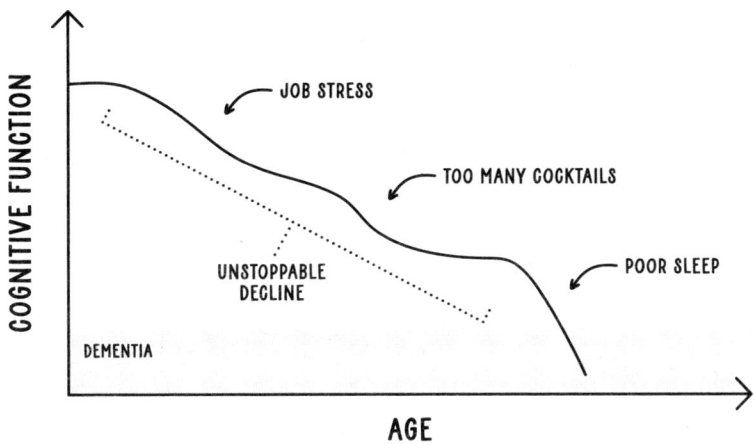

FIGURE 1. How we *think* brain function changes with age.

Take, for example, strength. On any given day, most of us might need to be able to pick up ten to twenty-five pounds in each hand—for instance, to carry shopping from the car. But if a total of fifty pounds was the most you ever picked up, trying to lift more than that when your friend asks you to help move some furniture might cause issues. At best, it would be very hard, and at worst, you might experience an injury. Perhaps, though, after reading this book, you start lifting weights at the gym and work your way up to being able to pick one hundred pounds up off the floor (with good form, of course). Unsurprisingly, the shopping now feels lighter, and you have no problem helping that same friend move their furniture.

That difference between the function you need on a day-to-day basis and the maximum that you're truly capable of is your headroom. By building headroom, we're able to function better during those inevitable times when we need to tap into extra reserves, such as when we're stressed or sleep-deprived. And even if we lose some function later in life, we still have more capacity left over because we had a bigger buffer to start with.

When it comes to the brain, there are several scientific concepts that make up what I think of as cognitive headroom. These include cognitive reserve, brain reserve (sometimes called brain maintenance), and cognitive resilience.[6] Cognitive reserve is a measure of our total cognitive capacity—how well our brains can function when performing at their best—as well as how much function we can lose as we age before we suffer from significant cognitive impairment or get diagnosed with dementia. Brain reserve is the same idea, but more related to the structure of the brain itself and how much brain you have in your skull—more is usually better, and as we age, we want to preserve as much brain size as possible. Cognitive resilience is your brain's ability to tolerate the accumulation of damage over time without function being affected.

Some people have likened cognitive reserve to the software of the brain—the quality of the computer programs that our brains are trying to run.[7] Brain reserve is the hardware—the number of processors and the amount of memory we have to run the software. Cognitive resilience is the redundancy in our computer system—the additional circuit boards and processors that allow the software to run even if the hardware gets a little dusty with age. While these are all distinct theoretical properties of the brain, and people can have very different levels of each,[8] they all contribute to the bigger idea of headroom—an overarching neurobiological buffer that can help counter the natural processes of ageing, allowing the brain to adapt and maintain optimal cognitive function for as long as possible.

One of the main reasons that I think we can distill multiple concepts of reserve and resilience into the idea of headroom is that the lifestyle factors that improve one tend to improve the others as well. For example, as you'll see in part 2, cognitive and physical activities can improve both the structure and functioning of the brain (reserve), while increasing resilience to processes of ageing. So, while a scientist might measure different properties of the brain and call them resilience or reserve, when it comes to what we care about—our brain "computer" switching on and performing quickly and efficiently—ensuring we have the right inputs to the system is what really matters. Maintaining these critical inputs requires my third "R" of headroom, *resolve*: shedding the expectation of cognitive decline with age and instead committing to lifelong engagement in activities that produce resilience and reserve.

By building headroom, we can ensure that significant cognitive decline and dementia are not inevitable. Better yet, every one of us has the ability to dramatically improve our brain health and cognitive function *today* by doing things that are simple and enjoyable. And most importantly, it's never too late to start (figure 2). However, there's a fair

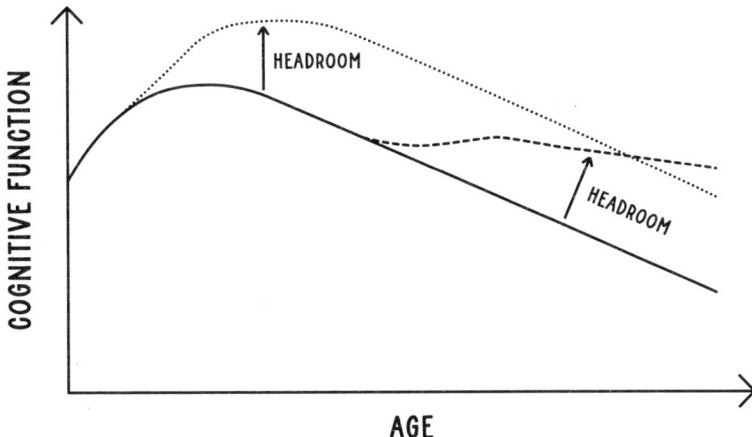

FIGURE 2. The many paths of brain function. Whatever trajectory we're currently on and whatever age we currently are, the brain is able to increase function and slow the rate of change over time. This is done by building headroom, for instance, through cognitive activity (early life education is one way to build headroom when we're younger) or physical activity (which improves cognitive function and slows decline even when we're older).

amount of work to be done to develop that brain buffer. Not just the individual work of engaging with activities that support brain health, but also the collective work of undoing the idea that the ageing brain will inevitably decline over time—an idea that has been baked into our consciousness for more than a century.

HUMANS DON'T HAVE AN EXPIRATION DATE

As we all face an increasing uncertainty about how our brains will function in the future, it is more critical than ever to understand how we can improve and support our brain health and cognition. Our environment and the way we live our lives has changed so rapidly that our brains and our physiology have sometimes struggled to keep up. As a result, there is often a big difference between how the human brain has evolved to function and the ways we currently live our lives. This is a phenomenon that biologists call *mismatch*, and it underlies many of the issues that our brains experience today.

One of the best examples of a mismatch is retirement. Since the days of the Roman Empire, many civilizations have had pensions to support people who had served in the military.[9] But only since the late nineteenth century has retirement become a consistent feature of working life. This shift is often credited to the world-renowned physician Sir William Osler, whose ideas helped to make retirement acceptable to society in the early twentieth century.[10] Because he was a professor of medicine at Oxford University until his death in 1919, many of my memories at medical school are Osler-themed. Osler House is both a physical building specifically for Oxford medical students and the name of the society that oversees their extracurricular activities. I studied for medical school exams in Osler House, played for the Osler House football and rugby clubs, and was head coach of the Osler House Boat Club. Having this connection to Osler makes me feel a bit better about blaming him for one of the *worst* ideas the human brain ever encountered.

In a 1905 valedictorian address at Johns Hopkins University, Osler said that retirement was necessary because workers were "useless" after the age of sixty. While the health of the average industrialised sixty-year-old probably wasn't great in 1905 (average life expectancy in the United States at this time was around fifty years),[11] Osler's proclamation has permeated so deeply into society that we still believe it more than a century later.

Even if we think we deserve a nice break after a long career, the human body and brain were never meant to retire. This doesn't mean you should have to work forever, though, because there are lots of other fantastic things for your brain to do. But the idea that older people are no longer useful goes completely against our evolutionary history.

Humans are one of the few species who live for several decades after their reproductive years. For a long time, this was thought to be a quirk of biology, but studies of less industrialised populations show that older members of society have incredibly active roles—and are generally very healthy—right up until their deaths in their seventies and eighties.[12] In fact, it's very likely that evolution selected for genes associated with living a long time because healthy grandparents can support the survival of their children, grandchildren, and community by acting as teachers and providers. For example, a group of scientists from Harvard analysed data from modern hunter-gatherer groups and found that grandparents were at least as active as parents, often hunting and gathering for several hours per day. Older adults in those societies who were in their seventies and eighties were still three times more physically active every day than the average U.S. adult is at *any* age.

When we place a body and brain that evolved to be extremely active for several decades into the modern (work) environment, we encounter a problem. Our biology *expects* activity—engagement of both our brains and our bodies with the people and world around us—as a signal to maintain health and function. When we remove that activity, for instance by retiring, function declines as a result. In fact, the loss of the cognitive and social stimulus our brains get from the work environment is probably why retirement is often the point at which cognitive decline accelerates.[13]

In addition to the idea of retirement, potential mismatches exist across many aspects of our daily lives, from our food and physical activity to our sleep, social environment, and interaction with modern technology. Despite all this, however, there is cause for significant hope. A huge amount of research, including my own, shows that simple changes to our daily lives can be leveraged to decrease these mismatches. The downstream effects of decreasing mismatch include reduced dementia risk, which in some cases might be prevented entirely, as well as improvements in daily focus, cognitive function, and mood.

To do that, though, we must rewrite Osler's story about our inevitable decline into uselessness as we get older. Because one big driver of cognitive decline seems to be our own expectations. Over time, we expect less and less of ourselves because we think our ageing brains are no longer capable of what they once were. We therefore use our brains less or offload difficult tasks to technology or other people. As we do less, the brain responds by decreasing its own capacity. After all, why would the body invest energy and resources into something that isn't being used? As a result, cognitive function starts to decrease, and the cycle of decline starts. The brain, though, is exactly like a muscle; the more we exercise it, the stronger it becomes and the better it works, regardless of how old we are. Reframing what we expect from our brains therefore sets the scene for them to be healthy and happy in the long term.

I'll admit that I don't expect you to take my word for it right away. If you're like most people, you will have thought to yourself—maybe even very recently—that your brain doesn't work as well as it used to, that you're "too old" to try to do a certain activity, or that you just can't learn or take in information like you did when you were younger. Those statements may very well be true *right now*, but that doesn't have to be the end of the story. In reality, each one of us can improve our brain health at any age.

At this point, you might be wondering where the disconnect is. If we're experiencing an ever-increasing burden of issues with our cognitive function but there's a significant body of evidence to suggest that this doesn't need to be the case, why aren't we more aware of it? As we'll see, a lot of this seems to stem from the way that scientists have historically studied the brain, as well as the struggles we've faced when trying to fully understand our brains in all their complex, unique, and slightly unpredictable glory.

CHAPTER 2

HOW DO NEUROSCIENTISTS STUDY THE BRAIN?

If the promise of this book is improved cognitive function and decreased long-term risk of dementia, the first question we need to ask is "What do we *really* know about how the brain works?"

The short answer to that question is: not that much. To be fair, researching and understanding the brain is *exceptionally hard*. While significant advances will continue for decades to come, rapidly accelerated by advances in computing and AI, it's very likely that we'll never fully understand the mysteries of the human brain.

At the time of writing, scientists have only just fully mapped the fly brain and begun to figure out how many *thousands* of different types of cells there are in rodent brains.[1] For example, a huge recent project led by the Allen Institute for Brain Science in Seattle, in partnership with Princeton and Baylor—involving more than a hundred scientists and costing over $100 million—fully mapped out all the connections in just one small part (about 0.2 percent) of the mouse brain. This map included more than two hundred thousand cells and 0.5 billion connections between those cells, requiring two million gigabytes of hard drive space to store the data.[2] Scaling this kind of work up to the entire human brain, which is a thousand times larger and much more complex, is currently unfathomable. And that's just mapping the cells of the brain, let alone figuring out what all those cells are actually *doing*.

There's a famous poem by physicist Emerson Pugh that seems appropriate here:

If the human brain were so simple
That we could understand it,

We would be so simple
That we couldn't.

In other words, the human brain is essentially so complex that even such a complex organ cannot fully understand itself. And it's the sheer scale of the problem of trying to understand the human brain that has created a big gap between what we expect of our brains and the reality of our ability to influence our own cognitive function as we age. Much of this boils down to the approach that scientists have historically taken when they've studied the brain. While important in many ways, this approach has left us focusing on cells and proteins while underestimating the magic that happens when a brain exists in an environment that challenges and supports it.

REDUCTIONISM

To counteract the vast complexity of human biology and health, we have become increasingly focused on isolating individual components of the system to understand the whole. This approach is called *reductionism* and is common across scientific fields, from physics to neuroscience. In the lab, we isolate, inhibit, or remove individual components of a biochemical pathway or function of a cell to see what happens. And because that's not something we can readily do in humans, we do it in animals such as rodents or worms. But while lots of interesting information has been gleaned using this approach, the failure rate when it comes to using that information to improve human health is incredibly high.

During my PhD, I studied cooling as a treatment for babies with a type of brain injury called hypoxic-ischemic encephalopathy (HIE). HIE is caused when a problem during birth results in too little blood flow and oxygen reaching the baby's brain. Sometimes we know the cause—such as the umbilical cord being wrapped around the baby's neck—but most of the time we don't know exactly what happened. After birth, these babies are immediately cooled down for three days, which increases the likelihood that they will survive and live without a significant disability. Cooling for babies with HIE was a major breakthrough when it became the standard of care in 2010 and, as of right now, is perhaps the most recent significant breakthrough in treatment for any neurological condition.[3]

Despite its success, cooling works much better in the lab than it does in babies. To try to understand why, I once did a study looking at data from three years of experiments in a rat model of HIE. With this large dataset, I could explore factors that are hard to study in a single experiment. For example, we found that male animals experienced less benefit from cooling treatment. This result was not necessarily surprising. Biological sex can change how brain cells respond to injury, and we know there are sex differences in the risk for multiple neurological conditions—including Alzheimer's disease, where around twice as many women are affected as men.[4]

What worried me, though, was that there were people who read my study and suggested that human male babies with HIE would not benefit from cooling. While I'm confident this finding was real in rats, it felt like a stretch to suggest that around half of all patients wouldn't benefit from a therapy that had been successful in multiple clinical trials. So I gathered all the patient data from every large hypothermia trial to date to see whether males and females had different outcomes from cooling treatment. They did not.[5]

This doesn't mean that the biology of sex isn't important—or that related issues, such as hormone levels, don't affect our long-term brain health. It is, and they do. But in this particular example, my own reductionist studies in the lab weren't relevant to humans and just generated confusion, even amongst experts. This is frequently the case when it comes to neuroscience research. It's also why almost every article published in the news about a mouse study will probably never be useful to you personally, and why we have to be incredibly careful when trying to extrapolate what we see in the lab to people out in the real world.

CAN A BIOLOGIST FIX A BROKEN RADIO?

One of my favourite papers is an essay that perfectly summarises the problems with a reductionist approach to biology. In this essay, Professor Yuri Lazebnik imagines scientists using these same principles to fix a broken radio:[6]

First, we would obtain a large supply of functioning radios to dissect. We would open the radios and find objects of various shape, colour, and size. Because the objects would vary in colour, we would investigate whether changing the colours affects the radio's performance. We would then remove components one at a time and catalogue them. Once all the components are cataloged, the connections between them described, and the consequences of removing each component or their combinations documented, this will be the time to ask: "Can the information that we accumulated help us to repair the radio?" If the radio has tunable components, such as those in all live cells and organisms, the outcome will not be promising. Indeed, the radio may not work because several components are not tuned properly, which is not reflected in their appearance or their connections. [Lightly edited for clarity and brevity.][7]

This essay still makes me chuckle because I can absolutely imagine neuroscientists gleefully changing the colours of neurons to see if it changes their function. But the broader message really speaks to the downside of a component-based approach to studying disease, particularly when we become overly focused on the metaphorical transistors and capacitors. It leads us to think that the accumulation of one type of protein in the brain causes most cases of dementia, a deficiency in one neurotransmitter causes depression, or that we can isolate some of the metabolites released during exercise and turn them into a pill so that we never have to go jogging again. Sadly (or not, depending on your feelings about jogging), none of these things are ever likely to be true. When it comes to the brain, at least, the full picture is always going to be a lot more complicated than that.[8]

Reading Professor Lazebnik's essay made me think back to my experiences of neuroscience in medical school, which mainly involved feelings of intense boredom as I stared down a microscope at slides of brains taken from people with different neurological diseases. I think my general lack of excitement stemmed from the fact that it was hard for me to connect these thin slices of long-dead brain to the fabulously complex (and very alive) organ and person they came from. I know this is an issue that many neuroscientists struggle with, but a lot of it stems from how the field came to be in the first place.

A (VERY) BRIEF HISTORY OF THE BIRTH OF NEUROSCIENCE

Many consider Santiago Ramón y Cajal to be the first neuroscientist. In the late 1880s, new methods for processing brain tissue allowed Cajal to look into a microscope and discover that the nervous system was not one homogeneous mass, as was previously thought, but was in fact made up of individual cells—later called neurons.[9] The human brain has something approaching one hundred billion neurons, which communicate via nearly one quadrillion (1,000,000,000,000,000) connections called synapses to control your muscles and allow you to think and sense the world around you.[10] Cajal's discovery led to an explosion of research focused on understanding the components of the brain, primarily by looking at them under a microscope. In 1906, Cajal shared a Nobel Prize with Camillo Golgi "in recognition of their work on the structure of the nervous system." By interesting coincidence, 1906 is also the year Alzheimer's disease was first described.

A SLIGHTLY LESS BRIEF HISTORY OF ALZHEIMER'S DISEASE

Because Alzheimer's disease is the most common cause of dementia, most of us have heard of it and likely have a feeling of anxiety just reading about it. However, I think it will be helpful to pause and dig into what we mean when we talk about it. Dementia has many causes but generally involves a chronic, irreversible decline in cognitive function that ends up significantly impacting an individual's ability to perform routine tasks and care for themselves. Of the more than 150 million people worldwide projected to have dementia by 2050, around two-thirds will be diagnosed with Alzheimer's disease.[11] This is why Alzheimer's has become such a large focus of research and source of fear.

Alois Alzheimer was a German psychiatrist and neuropathologist who, alongside his mentor Emil Kraepelin, helped to establish the field of biological psychiatry in the early 1900s. At the time, psychiatry focused largely on psychoanalysis. But whereas Freud wanted to delve into your sexual fantasies to figure out what was wrong with you, Alzheimer felt that mental health disorders originated from specific biological processes in the brain that could be identified and studied. In 1906, the main tool he had to do this with was the microscope. What

Alzheimer saw the first time he examined the brain of a dementia patient after death—a woman named Auguste Deter—started a century-long reductionist approach to dementia that has completely dominated the way we think about the brain as it gets older.

Auguste Deter was a German housewife admitted to an asylum in Frankfurt by her husband at the age of fifty-one after she became increasingly forgetful and paranoid. Alzheimer was her psychiatrist for five years before she passed away. Though the cause was unknown at the time, and is in fact still hotly debated,[12] Auguste Deter suffered from some form of early-onset dementia. Dementia is considered early-onset (sometimes called young-onset or *presenile* dementia) when the individual is under sixty-five years old at the time of diagnosis. In the absence of clear causes like long-term excessive alcohol intake or repeated head injury, the most common cause of early-onset dementia is Alzheimer's disease.

I must admit that Alzheimer's disease itself can quickly become confusing, even for those of us with intact cognitive function. This is because there are *two* versions of Alzheimer's disease, which I would argue are quite different. Early-onset Alzheimer's disease is usually caused by one of a handful of genetic mutations but only accounts for around 1 percent of all cases.[13] Those affected by early-onset Alzheimer's due to one of these genetic mutations can start to be affected as early as their thirties and experience a fairly predictable decline in cognitive function.

The remaining 99 percent of cases of Alzheimer's disease are what we now call either *late-onset* (because it happens after sixty-five years old) or *sporadic* (because it isn't caused by a single genetic mutation). This is what most of us picture when we think about Alzheimer's disease. The late-onset version of the disease usually occurs in adults in their seventies and older, is much less predictable, and—though genes do play a role—appears to be tightly linked to modifiable factors in our lifestyles and the environment.

Though two forms of the disease are now recognised, early-onset dementia, like that experienced by Auguste Deter, is what Alzheimer studied. When examining sections of her brain under the microscope after she died, Alzheimer noted "tangles that eventually replace the perished cells" and abundant "miliary foci."[14] These miliary foci (called that because they look like a small pile of millet seeds under the microscope) were what we now know to be amyloid plaques. Amyloid plaques are deposits of a protein called amyloid beta (Aβ), which accumulates in small clumps throughout the brains of individuals with Alzheimer's disease, but also those with other neurological conditions. In fact, amyloid plaques were first described in the brains of patients with epilepsy.[15] Amyloid plaques are still a bit of a mystery but tend to accumulate when neurons age or get stressed or injured.

The tangles that Alzheimer described were abnormal strands of *tau*, a protein that helps to maintain the structure of cells. As neurons have long arms (called axons) that extend out to communicate with other neurons, proteins like tau are important to hold the shape and stability of those arms. Just like the bicep muscles on your arms help you lift and pull objects, tau protein helps stabilise and guide the arms of the neuron. However, when neurons become injured, these tau proteins can become tangled up, looking like long strands of frayed rope inside the cell. Alzheimer's disease is one of several *tauopathies* where some kind of injury or disease process causes tau to become tangled up. Another tauopathy you might have heard of is chronic traumatic encephalopathy (CTE), which results from repeated head impacts or concussions.[16]

The combination of amyloid plaques and tau tangles seen by Alzheimer set the scene for the dominant idea of what causes Alzheimer's disease—the amyloid cascade hypothesis (ACH). The proposed mechanism of the ACH is relatively simple: triggered by genetics, the environment, or some other unknown factor, amyloid beta builds up in the brain and clumps together to form plaques. The brain responds by activating inflammation and stress pathways that help to clear the offender, just like the body would for an infection or a splinter. But because these amyloid plaques can't be killed by the immune system or removed with a pair of tweezers, they start to cause even more problems. In this case, the ACH suggests that neurons become even more stressed and injured by the plaques and inflammation around them, causing the tau inside the neuron to become tangled up. As a result, the neurons eventually die, with the patient experiencing increasing cognitive decline as this happens.[17] However, though it provides an elegant explanation that helps us to understand two complex diseases, it's still not clear that reducing all of Alzheimer's disease down to just amyloid and tau will provide the insight and treatment breakthroughs we hope for.

A CASE BECOMES A DISEASE

After his work with Auguste Deter, Alzheimer described three additional patients who suffered from similar symptoms and whose brains looked similar under the microscope. Despite this, recent retellings of the story suggest that Alzheimer himself wasn't particularly convinced that these patients all suffered from the same disease. Instead, it was his mentor Kraepelin who grouped the cases together to define "Alzheimer's disease" in a textbook, describing it as a "peculiar" and severe form of dementia that begins early in life.[18]

It's interesting to note that, after some extensive detective work, it was determined that Auguste Deter may not have suffered from Alzheimer's disease at all. In 2013, a group took tissue from some of Alzheimer's original slides of Deter's brain and reported that she had a mutation in the presenilin 1 gene, which is one of the gene mutations known to cause early-onset Alzheimer's.[19] However, a second group tried to confirm the results a year later and couldn't detect any mutations related to early-onset Alzheimer's disease at all.[20] Deter also didn't carry the apolipoprotein E4 gene, which is the most important genetic risk factor for late-onset Alzheimer's disease.[21] While the cause of her dementia therefore isn't known, some have suggested that she might have suffered from syphilis, which can cause accumulation of amyloid plaques in the brain in a pattern that looks a lot like Alzheimer's disease.[22] It's even possible that Deter instead suffered from depression or some other mental health condition caused by the effects of the stress and isolation associated with the life she lived as a downtrodden housewife, which were then made much worse by being placed in an asylum.[23]

Regardless of its origins, you might be wondering how Alzheimer's work with a small collection of unusual dementia cases led to his name being used to refer to the common form of dementia that we all fear today. For decades after the publication of Kraepelin's textbook, Alzheimer's disease referred only to early-onset dementia and was relatively rare. Back then, what we now call late-onset Alzheimer's disease was called age-related or senile dementia. The word *senile* originally meant a process related to the general declines in function associated with ageing but eventually became code for dementia itself—I'm sure you've heard or said that somebody is "going senile" as a reference to their declining cognitive function.

Around 1960, some classic reductionism started to take hold of dementia research. Under the microscope, the brains of patients with early-onset Alzheimer's disease and age-related dementia look very similar, with both tending to have accumulation of amyloid plaques and tau tangles. This gave researchers a target—amyloid—that could drive research funding and drug development. Though there were many other differences, the connection to amyloid resulted in the two diseases both being grouped under the umbrella of Alzheimer's disease.

In 2011, the scope of amyloid research was expanded even further with the concept of *preclinical* Alzheimer's disease. Saying something is preclinical means that the disease process has started, but the patient doesn't have symptoms yet. A good example is heart disease, where atherosclerotic plaque builds up in the walls of the arteries years before a heart attack (when those arteries become completely blocked) occurs.

The idea of preclinical Alzheimer's disease was almost identical to the idea of heart disease, with the accumulation of amyloid in the brain over decades thought to eventually trigger dementia. However, while damage to the walls of coronary arteries is associated with only one condition, many other conditions can cause amyloid to accumulate in the brain, such as epilepsy, syphilis (thankfully now relatively rare), and brain trauma. It's also possible to have a large amount of amyloid in the brain without having dementia. A large study by a group in Austria that used data from nearly four thousand patients across the United States, the UK, Europe, and Japan found that, on average, 30 percent of people who were cognitively normal when they died had a level of pathology in their brains that made it look as if they had Alzheimer's disease, despite having no evidence of cognitive decline.[24] A similar study spearheaded by a team at the University of Washington found that 70 percent of older adults in their late seventies to early nineties will have some Alzheimer's-type pathology in their brains, even if they have normal cognitive function.[25]

In addition to this discrepancy between how brains look and how they perform, some of the original research studies that were used to support the ACH have since been discredited or withdrawn due to manipulation or fabrication of data.[26] This doesn't mean that amyloid isn't an important part of the biology of Alzheimer's disease, but an increasing number of studies show that most people with dementia—even those diagnosed with Alzheimer's disease—have multiple pathologies that don't fit the amyloid cascade hypothesis. This suggests that Alzheimer's is not a disease we can tie to a single protein.[27] And though amyloid and tau are clearly related to ageing and cognitive decline in some way, there's more to it than how the brain looks under a microscope. Much of this discrepancy is potentially explained by the factors, such as resilience, that come together in my idea of headroom and are potentially modifiable with lifestyle factors.

While early-onset Alzheimer's disease *is* driven by genetic mutations that increase the accumulation of amyloid plaques, late-onset Alzheimer's disease has a huge number of interacting genetic, environmental, and modifiable lifestyle-related risk factors that may or may not have anything to do with amyloid.[28] As a result, each patient experiences different cognitive issues over time—so much so that there is a common phrase amongst neurologists who work with individuals with Alzheimer's disease:

"If you've seen one patient with Alzheimer's, you've seen *one* patient with Alzheimer's."

THE RADIO IS STILL BROKEN

At this point, you might be wondering whether all this talk of amyloid is getting us anywhere, either in the search for a treatment for Alzheimer's disease or in terms of a practical takeaway from this chapter. If I'm completely honest, I'm not yet sure about either. But if we're interested in brain health and cognitive function, I think it's useful to know about the history of the field to help us think about an alternative approach that *does* give me a lot of hope.

Thousands of scientific papers and hundreds of books could be filled—and have been—with discussions around whether or not a reductionist approach is going to help us make significant inroads into the prevention or treatment of late-onset Alzheimer's disease. Though it does play a role, amyloid is likely just one part of a much bigger picture. For example, a 2023 analysis of data from the Alzheimer's Disease Neuroimaging Initiative (ADNI) in the United States showed that there is no amount of amyloid that distinguishes the brain of somebody who does or does not have cognitive impairment;[29] you can have a lot of amyloid in your brain and normal cognitive function, or dementia with only a small amount of amyloid. For that reason, only 20 percent of a composite cognitive function score was predicted by the amount of amyloid that somebody had on a brain scan. The upshot of this is that at least 80 percent of cognitive function must be related to other factors.

Until recently, decades of clinical trials of drugs targeting amyloid have also failed to show any benefit in either form of Alzheimer's disease, despite clearing large amounts of amyloid from the brain.[30] More recent therapies show evidence of slowing the rate of cognitive decline by just over 25 percent in individuals with Alzheimer's disease, but they come with a high risk of side effects and it's unclear whether they benefit patients in a way that will change their lives meaningfully on a day-to-day basis.[31] It's not my job to adjudicate whether these therapies are worthwhile for a given individual, and this book is not about the *treatment* of dementia. I also sincerely hope that these therapies continue to improve over time so that more treatment options are available to those suffering from dementia. However, when thinking about the long-term trajectory of cognitive function, the main takeaway is this: multiple lines of evidence show that the amount of amyloid in our brains might only determine 20–25 percent of our cognitive function and rate of cognitive decline.

If the brain of an individual with Alzheimer's disease is Lazebnik's metaphorical broken radio, a reductionist focus on amyloid has maybe brought back some of the sound, but the volume is still low, and it's hard to enjoy the music because there's still a lot of static. Luckily, as we'll see, most factors related to age-related dementia and cognitive decline—regardless of whether they increase amyloid accumulation in the brain—appear to be modifiable, and many of these are driven by variables that we have control over.[32]

CHAPTER 3
IN SEARCH OF THE BIGGER PICTURE

If the story of amyloid and Alzheimer's disease leaves you feeling a little dissatisfied, you're not alone. I sometimes feel that way too. The truth is that when we take out our microscopes to look at the brains of people who had dementia, we still don't really know exactly how much the different cells and proteins we see are related to the symptoms and function that person experienced. But that doesn't mean that we don't know how to support improving brain function for people lucky enough to still be alive.

To continue our comparison of the brain to inanimate objects, I'm going to switch gears from radios to cars. Unlike a radio, but just like a car, your brain has a lot of moving parts. As you drive your car to and from work, to and from the supermarket, and to and from kids' soccer games and dogs' vet appointments, various parts of your car accumulate wear and tear. And to minimise the long-term effects of that wear and tear, you need to regularly do some basic vehicle maintenance. The brain is the same.

Imagine that amyloid is rust, and your brain is your car. Rust doesn't just suddenly appear—it's usually a sign that environmental conditions or lack of maintenance have started to take their toll. So, if you wanted to prevent rust, you might think about ways to make sure your car is protected from the elements and serviced regularly. Poor sleep, diet, and environmental exposures like air pollution all seem to be associated with the amount of amyloid in the brain.[1] At the same time, if you drive your car enough, a little rust is inevitable, without necessarily affecting the overall driving performance. Without proper maintenance, though, there are lots of ways that a car can stop working that have nothing to do with rust—fluid pumps can fail, electrical wiring can become disconnected, and tyres can become misaligned. Again, the brain is the same. There are lots of factors that improve cognitive function and are associated with a lower risk of dementia but don't seem to consistently affect amyloid levels in the brain, like exercise and cognitive activity.[2] So if we only worry about rust, we might miss the bigger picture of what's needed to keep our car on the road.

The twist here is that your brain is its own mechanic, and the way we use our brains directs the processes of maintenance. At the cellular level, stimulating our brains through exercise and engaging with the environment activates the basic housekeeping pathways that keep the brain functioning at its best.[3] This includes processes such as *autophagy*, in which junky proteins and other cell components that get damaged are broken down and recycled. Impaired autophagy is one of the hallmarks of ageing—the collection of biological mechanisms that seem to drive the ageing process in all animals.[4] Other hallmarks of ageing include chronic inflammation, impaired energy production, and DNA damage, many of which are related to a loss of maintenance or function that can be offset by continuing to stimulate our bodies and brains.

Though we need to infer some of this information from animal studies because it's hard to measure in humans, cognitive and physical activity help to keep your brain's mechanics motivated, directing their maintenance efforts toward the areas of the brain you need for everyday functions as well as any unique abilities you want to develop and keep. By activating a brain area or network for a specific task—for instance, learning a musical instrument—our cellular mechanics then work on the parts of the brain that were actively used, doing their repairs accordingly to keep those areas in tip-top shape.

In many ways, it's not just that using our brains has an anti-ageing effect; it's that *not* using them seems to be *pro-ageing*. The hallmarks of ageing are essentially different ways in which the processes that support the function of our organs and cells stop working. The fact that these processes are tied to activity makes a lot of sense because our daily engagement in the world is what tells our brain that it still has a role to play and that it is worth investing the time and effort to maintain itself. If, on the other hand, we stop giving the brain those inputs, it thinks those functions aren't needed anymore. Our brains then stop maintaining themselves, and their function deteriorates.[5] We see this idea clearly reflected in the mismatch of retirement, which several studies suggest can accelerate cognitive decline.[6] Collecting your gold watch and enjoying long days in your favourite chair doesn't suddenly result in a huge accumulation of amyloid in the brain. Instead, it's the removal of the complex cognitive stimuli we get from our work and interacting with our colleagues that stops our brain continuing to make regular repairs. And as a result, our brains become less and less roadworthy.

WHAT BRAINS ARE MADE OF

Understanding now that we need to move beyond overly simplistic ideas of reductionism to understand how to build and maintain the best possible brain, we need to think about what brains are designed to do. But before we get to that, I have a little more neuroscience for you. To know what brains can do, we have to know what they're made of. And so far, we—this book as well as most neuroscientists—have tended to ignore many of the critical components that make up our brains. However, each of these components will become important as we begin to understand how we can change our brain function, today and in the future.

If you're in the habit of thinking about neuroscience (and maybe also if you aren't), the word itself might conjure up thoughts of neurons. After all, *neuro* is right there in the name. Often referred to as the fundamental units of the nervous system, neurons are responsible for transmitting information throughout the body as electrical and chemical signals. As I mentioned briefly before, each neuron has an axon— a long arm-like projection that carries signals to communicate with other neurons, muscles, or organs. Each neuron has many dendrites— branched extensions like fingers that send and receive signals. This communication happens at synapses, where neurotransmitters are released from one neuron and bind to receptors on the next neuron to continue the flow of information. At any given time, every neuron in your brain is integrating multiple signals from a large number of other neurons in order to decide what to do. These neurons then contribute their decisions and actions to brain-wide networks that allow you to perform complex tasks like seeing, speaking, and making decisions.

Even if you're only loosely familiar with the very basics of neuroscience, the idea of how neurons function may be familiar. But ever since Cajal first described the neuron, there have been those who felt that neuroscience is too neuron-centric. As both amyloid and tau are produced by or accumulate in neurons, the reductionist focus on these specific proteins has also made us think that cognitive function and dementia are specifically related to neurons. But, as you're already starting to appreciate, this is probably not the complete picture.

I already mentioned that Cajal shared his Nobel Prize with another scientist named Camillo Golgi. Cajal and Golgi were such fierce scientific rivals that they refused to give their Nobel acceptance speeches on the same day (neuroscience feuds are no joke). The main disagreement between them revolved around how the nervous system was organised. In contrast to Cajal's focus on neurons, Golgi felt that the brain should be considered a *reticulum*—an interconnected network of cells that functions as one. Golgi also felt that more prominence should be given to the other cells in the brain: the glia.

In the epic battle of Cajal versus Golgi, Cajal largely won out. This is why you might never have heard the word *glia*. Cajal's dominance over the early development of the field is also why glia have only recently become more of a focus in neuroscience research. Though the exact estimates have changed over time, we now know that there are nearly as many glia in the human brain as there are neurons.[7] Named after the Greek word for "glue," glial cells include many different cell types whose only real similarity to one another is the fact that they are *not* neurons. And as the name suggests, it was originally thought that glia just formed the glue of the nervous system that allowed the neurons to do all the hard work.

Broadly speaking, there are three main types of glial cells: astroglia (more commonly called astrocytes), microglia, and oligodendroglia (also called oligodendrocytes). When you consider all the glia and then add the extensive network of blood vessels in the brain, neurons make up, at most, 50 percent of the cells in the brain. So, while Cajal was correct about the nature of neurons, later research has confirmed that the brain functions much more similarly to Golgi's model of an interconnected network, where glia should be considered at least as important as neurons.

Have you ever been part of a team where you did a ton of hard work, only for somebody else to take all the credit? That's how I imagine glial cells feel pretty much all the time.

ASTROCYTES

In our car analogy where neurons are the engine, astrocytes are the lines and pumps that bring in fuel, cool the engine, and wash the windows. Named after the huge number of projections that make them look like stars (*astro* coming from the Ancient Greek for star, and *cyte* meaning cell), astrocytes regulate fluid flow through the brain, coordinate sleep and responses to injury, and direct the supply of energy to neurons.[8] Astrocytes are also directly involved in the brain's electrical signaling, including responses to external inputs and regulating attention and memory formation.[9] In humans, a single astrocyte can communicate with up to two million neuronal synapses at a time![10]

The flow of fluid regulated by astrocytes is critically important for waste clearance during sleep, constantly making sure there isn't a build-up of proteins or other molecules that might negatively affect brain function. In fact, one reason brain trauma (like a concussion) is thought to increase the risk of dementia is because of impaired astrocyte function. This decreases waste clearance and impairs sleep, memory formation, and the brain's energy supply. Therefore, when we think about brain health, cognitive function, and the risk and onset of dementia, astrocytes play a critical role.

OLIGODENDROCYTES

As you may have noticed, Greek has a bit of a monopoly on the naming of cells in the brain. In this case, *oligo* means "few" and *dendro* means "branch." So oligodendrocytes are cells with a few branches. Oligodendrocytes are your car's wiring. If you want an electrical signal to go from one place to another—turning on the lights, tuning the radio to blast nineties hip-hop (maybe that's just me), or even turning the car on in the first place—this is the job of oligodendrocytes. They do this by forming a sheath (called myelin) that surrounds the axons of certain neurons. This sheath allows electrical signals to be transmitted long distances quickly and efficiently.

Though you probably didn't realise it, it's oligodendrocytes that gave us one of the phrases we frequently use to describe the brain—*grey matter*. If you were to cut a brain open in cross-section, the wrinkly outer portion (and some of the bit right in the middle) is the "grey matter." In reality, it's more of a fleshy pinkish-grey sludge-like colour, but that's a lot less catchy. The grey matter is grey because of the *absence* of the fatty myelin sheath, which, due to its very high fat content, is white. As you might expect, the part of the brain that contains lots of oligodendrocytes and myelin is therefore called the *white matter*. The white matter, which sits right underneath the outer grey matter, is like the most complex junction box in existence—quickly directing information back and forth across the brain and from the brain to the body. Almost all the thoughts and actions that make us human rely on the electrical connections in the white matter, and the critical importance of oligodendrocytes and white matter is one reason human brains are much more complex than the brains of other species.

In addition to ensuring fast, reliable information transfer through the brain, oligodendrocytes are directly involved in the brain's overall energy metabolism and are one of the cell types that is most vulnerable to injury or stress.[11] Many neurological diseases that only affect humans often involve injury to the white matter, including multiple sclerosis, cerebral palsy, and Alzheimer's disease. In fact, several studies have suggested that cognitive decline as we get older tracks much more closely with injury to oligodendrocytes and the loss of white matter than with the accumulation of amyloid.[12]

While we can model some white matter disease processes in animals—usually rodents—one reason that brain-related scientific discoveries in rodents usually fail to give the same results in humans is that only around 10 percent of the brains of rodents is white matter, compared to more than 60 percent in humans.[13] Importantly, as you'll see later, there are specific activities that can help to boost and maintain our white matter as we age, such as exercise. No mice required.

MICROGLIA

This whistle-stop tour of the glia now brings us to microglia, and our last bit of Greek for a while—*mikros* is Greek for "small." Microglia are the brain's immune system, activating inflammation and repair in response to infection or injury. However, a huge amount of recent work has shown that microglia are perhaps the single most complex cell type in the body, with a vast array of other functions, including regulating the connections of neurons at synapses, the formation and removal of myelin by oligodendrocytes, and the production and function of blood vessels.[14] Microglia also influence day-to-day cognitive functions by overseeing how the brain regulates and responds to exercise and sleep.[15]

If I'm honest, I struggled to find a part of the car to compare microglia to because they do so many things. At this point, it would be safe to estimate that the human brain has thousands of different kinds of microglia, depending on the function and the region of the brain we're looking at. Maybe the microglia are like a large toolbox that can be used to modify, repair, and improve the workings of the car. Except, in this analogy, the tools are alive and the car does the repairs itself, like a Transformer. That's how cool microglia are.

While the generation of an inflammatory response by microglia is important for recovery after brain injury, inflammation also needs to be switched off at the right time. Many, if not all, chronic neurological disorders include some aspect of ongoing microglial inflammation that is not always beneficial.[16] And microglia can have very long memories. For example, a group at Imperial College London did a study where they scanned the brains of patients who had experienced brain trauma. Using a special tracer taken up by proinflammatory microglia in the brain, they found that ongoing microglial inflammation was associated with worse cognitive function up to seventeen *years* after the initial injury.[17]

The influence of microglia on cognitive function is also relevant to anybody who wants to have a future-proof brain. The Allen Institute in Seattle recently developed an "atlas" of cells in the brain over time and found that in those experiencing late-onset Alzheimer's disease, changes in microglia were seen *before* any significant accumulation of amyloid or tau.[18] This means that the "glue" of the brain might be changing in dementia well before the neurons really get involved. Most importantly, microglia can be directly affected by our own actions. For example, one study that was part of the Memory and Ageing Project at Rush University explored how physical activity during late life was related to cognitive function, brain pathology, and microglial inflammation. Participants had their cognitive function tested and wore monitors that tracked their activity. Later, once a participant passed away, the researchers looked at their brain under a microscope. What they found was that physical activity late in life modulated the function of microglia, making them less inflammatory, even in the face of accumulating damage. This appeared to help those individuals maintain cognitive function as they aged—many of them into their nineties—suggesting that physical activity can help to build headroom even late in life regardless of how much wear and tear our brains have accumulated, in this case by making microglia more resilient.[19]

THE NETWORK THAT RUNS THE BRAIN

In addition to neurons and glia, there's a critical component of the brain that neither Cajal nor Golgi gave enough credit: the blood supply.

As you now know, most modern neuroscience is based on what can be seen under the microscope after death. Clumps of amyloid, which in the most severe cases can be seen with the naked eye, are easy to focus on. Detecting more subtle changes in the numbers or function of microglia, astrocytes, and oligodendrocytes is much harder, even if they're just as important. And when looking at slices of brain, it's harder still to appreciate the importance of a structure that has been destroyed in the process of preparing the brain slice you're looking at.

For brains to be examined under a microscope, they are preserved and dehydrated, then cut into very thin slices and placed on glass slides. During this process, the blood vessels collapse entirely and become little more than small holes where blood used to flow. As a result, these vessels are easy to ignore.

But in life, around 3–5 percent of brain volume is blood, and each neuron is generally only ten to twenty micrometres—about one tenth the width of a human hair—from a blood vessel.[20] In fact, in the brain, there are around four hundred miles of capillaries, the smallest blood vessels that supply oxygen and nutrients to cells throughout the body. So, while the blood vessels were easy to miss when they first described the structure of the nervous system, we have to realise that Cajal's neurons and Golgi's glia are actually suspended inside an incredibly complex vascular network that allows the whole system to function in the first place. In fact, the ability of the brain to continuously adapt to the environment and develop the wide range of skills that each of us benefits from every day is only possible because the blood supply is just as adaptable.

Around the same time that Cajal and Golgi were arguing about the nature of the brain, Charles Roy, Charles Sherrington, and Angelo Mosso were discovering that the metabolites produced by brain activity could direct blood flow to those regions in a stimulus-dependent manner.[21] Angelo Mosso also developed the first ever technique used to take images of the brain, showing that local brain blood flow changed in response to mental activity.[22] Modern versions of this technique, such as functional magnetic resonance imaging (fMRI), are used to track brain activity in response to specific stimuli or cognitive tasks by measuring changes in blood flow. A century of work in this field eventually led to the intimate and inseparable connection between brain cells and their blood supply being named the *neurovascular unit*. This is because the blood supply in your brain isn't just a bunch of pipes—it's an integrated part of the brain tissue. The endothelial cells and pericytes that make up the blood vessels are in direct contact and constant communication with other brain cells, constantly monitoring activity and responding accordingly. When a region of the brain becomes more active, the electrical and metabolic activity of neurons and astrocytes releases metabolites like potassium and nitric oxide that cause the local blood vessels to dilate.[23] This directly drives increases in blood supply through a process called *neurovascular coupling*—directing oxygen, energy, and nutrients to exactly where they're needed. Therefore, a critical part of long-term brain health is maintaining happy blood vessels that can rapidly adapt to our brain's needs and provide our neurons and glia with everything they need to do their jobs. Recent studies in both humans and animal models even suggest that our blood vessels may be the part of the body that is most susceptible to ageing, triggering inflammation and loss of white matter as the brain struggles to get enough blood flow.[24]

This trip down the austere and moustache-filled hallways of neuroscience history does serve a purpose, aside from satisfying my inner nerd. As we start to realise the complexity of all the different types of cells in the brain and their functions, it becomes clear that the brain is a box of infinitely complex and tunable components. The highly coordinated way that all the different cells and structures of the brain function in response to activity also shows the limitations of a reductionist approach that isolates each of these components in an attempt to understand them. Because they only work when they're working together. This brings Pugh's poem back to mind, and reminds us that we may never fully understand everything happening at the cellular or biochemical level to allow a human brain to do what it does. The good news is that we might not need to.

CHAPTER 4
DOMINANCE OF THE ENVIRONMENT

Now that we know a bit about what the brain is made of, we need to consider what a brain is really *for*. Because that will finally start to give us some insight into the primary drivers of brain health and function. Some of the most important functions of the brain are consistent across species and are primarily related to *survival*—navigating the environment, finding food, and reproducing. But beyond those basics, there's a lot more that we want our brains to do, which leads to the question: What makes the human brain so special?

Maybe that's a loaded question, because it implies up front that the human brain is in some way unique—which, depending on your viewpoint, may or may not be true. For instance, based on the overall structure and number of neurons and glia we have, the human brain is just a scaled-up version of other primate brains.[1] And like humans, many other species—including mammals, birds, and cephalopods like octopuses—display emotions and complex cognitive functions, including learning, problem-solving, and play.

But while other lines can be hard to draw, some features of the human brain do stand out. For example, some scientists suggest that the evolution of the human brain was driven by the increasing complexity of our social relationship structures, as compared to other animals.[2] We could probably also say that the human brain is the only one that has shown a clear interest and investment in trying to understand its own function.

GUIDED BY WRONGNESS

During the decade I spent as a student, and another decade spent as a clinician and scientist, two broad ideas defined how I thought about the brain, both of which turned out to be wrong. But from my wrongness came the ideas that underpin the critical components of this book. As we step away from reductionism in search of a more practical approach to thinking about the brain and supporting long-term cognitive function, I wanted to highlight some of the research that forced me to rethink my core ideas about the brain. This also gives me an opportunity to demonstrate how amazing the brain really is.

The first idea was that, for a wide range of neurodegenerative disorders, a breakthrough drug is just around the corner. Whenever I learned or read about neurological disorders, there was a constant suggestion that the next blockbuster drug was on the horizon. Of course, this optimism makes sense considering the vast amount of information we have accumulated about the brain, and the huge burden that neurological diseases have on our society. However, while drug therapies will always play an important role, the complex and varied nature of the factors that contribute to cognitive function and cognitive decline means that any meaningful approach to disease prevention or treatment is going to have to be multipronged. And as a result, the hope that one day a single drug or drug type will cure all of Alzheimer's disease is increasingly looking like it's not going to happen.

The desire for curative pharmaceutical therapies is one that I understand well because it has been a major part of my work in neuroscience. However, that work has also taught me something critically important: when it comes to brain growth, development, and long-term function, the impact of drug treatments pales in comparison to the impact of the environment. By environment I mean the world around us and the way we engage with it.

One of my favourite examples of the dominant effect of the environment on our brains is a collection of studies done with taxi drivers—more specifically, London taxi drivers. For decades, if you wanted to take a taxi in London, the only option was a licensed cab—one of those bulbous black cars with the iconic orange light on top that you've seen driving past Big Ben in the movies. When I was a junior doctor in London, Big Ben was just a few hundred gardens away from the hospital I worked at, so this image was a part of my daily life.

To be a black cab driver in London, you have to pass something called the Knowledge of London exam. The Knowledge, as it is also known, involves memorising a map of twenty-five thousand streets in a six-mile radius around Charing Cross train station. This is a herculean feat of learning that leaves an indelible mark on the brains of London cabbies. In one classic study, researchers followed individuals in their thirties and forties who were studying the Knowledge, as well as a control group.[3] Learning the Knowledge takes three to four years, and the prospective drivers had their brains scanned before and after studying for the exam. In those who passed the exam, changes to the structure of the posterior hippocampus—a part of the brain that is critical to remembering where you are in the world (also known as spatial memory)—were seen. Those who failed the test saw no changes to their brains, and neither did the control group. A similar study showed that this same brain region is bigger in London taxi drivers compared to bus drivers who have fixed routes and therefore don't rely on their navigational skills as much.[4]

Now, that's all very interesting, but what might it mean for our own long-term brain health and function? Being intimately involved in memory function, the hippocampus is usually affected in Alzheimer's disease. And amazingly, recent evidence suggests that the constant workout taxi drivers give their hippocampi (plural of hippocampus—you have one on each side of the brain) might protect them from Alzheimer's disease. In a large study exploring dementia rates in the United States, taxi drivers and ambulance drivers—two professions that both require frequent navigation—had a lower risk of death due to Alzheimer's disease than all other occupations, even after accounting for age and socioeconomic status. And while we can never do a study in which people are randomised to be taxi drivers for a whole career to see if that really *does* decrease their risk of Alzheimer's, the studies of taxi drivers give us a pretty cool idea of how the brain might respond to the environment—even in adulthood—and the long-term effect that can have.

THE HUMAN BRAIN IS BUILT TO ADAPT TO THE ENVIRONMENT

A large body of recent work has found that the human brain places a much greater emphasis on the ability to respond to the environment than those of other species. This may help to explain why humans are particularly good at finding ways to thrive in an incredibly wide range of environments, providing both a significant survival advantage over other species as well as an excellent ability to navigate the streets of London.

The ability of the human brain to adapt to its environment is baked into our evolutionary history. In 2010, a group from Washington University in St. Louis compared the trajectories of human brain development and human brain evolution. What they found was that the parts of the human brain that display the greatest amount of development after birth are the prefrontal cortex, the lateral parietal lobe, and the lateral temporal lobe. These also happen to be the same parts of the human brain that have shown the greatest amount of evolutionary change compared to other primates.[5]

The prefrontal cortex sits right inside your forehead. The upper- and outermost part of it—the dorsolateral prefrontal cortex—is sometimes referred to as the *deliberative* prefrontal cortex because it plays a critical role in making decisions.[6] If you've ever had an impulse to do or say something stupid but stopped yourself at the last moment, that's your dorsolateral prefrontal cortex at work. The lateral temporal lobe is in the area right by your ears and is involved with language comprehension, hearing, visual processing, and facial recognition.[7] The lateral parietal lobe sits behind the prefrontal cortex and above the temporal cortex and is similarly multitalented, with functions including attention, working memory, movement planning, and social cognition.[8]

The main finding of the study comparing human brain development and human brain evolution was that these three parts of the brain—areas that evolved most recently and are responsible for our most complex cognitive functions—are the parts of the brain that are the *least* developed at birth. It's almost like the parts of our brain that make us distinctly human are just waiting to see what world they're going to exist in before developing accordingly.

Even beyond those specific brain regions, the human brain is very immature at birth compared to other primates. For example, a newborn chimpanzee is able to complete a number of basic movements from birth, immediately clinging to its mother for protection. A newborn human, by comparison, is almost completely immobile, not to mention generally inept at just about everything except sleeping, eating, and crying. Human brains also mature much more slowly than the brains of other species, taking thirty years or more to reach full maturity.[9] This means that human brains take 40–50 percent of the average human lifespan (which is around seventy years) to finish developing. By comparison, mouse brains only develop for the first 5 percent of their lifespan.

What starts as a human weakness (and general ineptitude) at birth becomes a massive strength later in life. The slow-growing and slow-maturing nature of the human brain gives a decades-long window for the environment to shape how our brains function as they soak in and respond to a wide range of environmental inputs in order to optimise their function. And as we've seen from the taxi drivers, this window doesn't close after the initial period of development is finished—the human brain is always ready to adapt to the challenges and environment it is faced with.

THE ENVIRONMENT DETERMINES THE OUTCOME OF EVEN THE MOST FRAGILE BRAINS

In order to test the limits of the idea that the environment is the primary driver of brain function, I think it's useful to see what happens when the brain is forced to start out under less-than-optimal circumstances. One of the main areas of focus in my lab is finding ways to support the brains of babies who are born prematurely, or *preterm*. About 10 percent of all births in the United States are preterm, and the more prematurely a baby is born, the greater their risk of some kind of neurological disorder, such as cerebral palsy or cognitive impairment.[10] This risk is particularly high in extremely preterm infants, who are born at around 60–70 percent of the length of a normal pregnancy (before twenty-eight weeks). Currently, there are no drugs available specifically to improve the neurological outcomes of these babies. Even promising therapies that I myself have found to work in the lab have failed to show benefit in human trials.[11]

While this lack of real-world efficacy is frustrating, it also illuminates alternate paths we might take toward success. One way to do this is to consider those who navigate being born preterm without experiencing significant cognitive consequences. In fact, a large number of these babies go on to have normal—or even exceptionally high—cognitive function later in life. While it is essentially impossible to accurately predict how babies will develop, an interesting question to ask is what factors increase the likelihood that an infant will do very well despite having a difficult start in life.

Right as I was joining the faculty at the University of Washington in 2018, my mentor, Sunny Juul, was completing the largest and most complex neuroprotection drug trial ever done with extremely preterm infants—the Preterm Erythropoietin Neuroprotection Trial (PENUT). A total of 941 babies were recruited at thirty hospitals across the United States, and these babies were followed until they were two years old, when their emotional, language, motor, and cognitive skills were assessed.[12] I was enlisted to build a variety of machine-learning models to see what we could discover about factors related to cognitive function in these babies as they grew up.[13]

To me, at least, the results were fairly eye-opening. Preterm babies regularly experience severe injury to their guts, eyes, lungs, and brains, and spend months in the hospital being exposed to painful and stressful procedures as well as drugs including opioids, steroids, and antibiotics that can negatively impact the brain. But in PENUT, it wasn't any of these exposures that had the biggest effect on a baby's later cognitive function. Of the thousands of variables we started with, the strongest predictor of an infant's cognition at two years of age was the number of years of schooling that their mother had. Maternal education was more important than whether the baby had a significant brain injury on a brain scan, and it also beat out all the fancy (reductionist) markers of inflammation or injury that had been measured.

As with all studies like this one, we have to think carefully about what this result means. All we could do was look at the large body of data and see which variables were related to cognition, which is not the same as being able to explain those relationships. But this study is now one of dozens showing that the effect of a newborn's experience in the hospital, even if that experience is lengthy and difficult, pales in comparison to the influence of the environment that the baby goes home to.[14]

The ways in which maternal education can affect brain development are many and complex, and some are beyond the scope of this book. But you can probably imagine the impact parental education can have on the environment in which a baby is raised. This includes the type of food and schooling children can access and the financial or other stressors that children and families have to navigate. As one example, mothers who have graduate degrees may be more likely to have the time and resources needed to read to their children, which is one of the most impactful ways to improve a child's cognitive development.[15] The idea here is not to make a judgment about somebody's economic circumstances or level of education; parents around the world are doing a phenomenal job raising healthy children regardless of their background. The relationship between education and the home environment is also often driven by societal factors that are outside the parent's control. However, multiple studies show the incredible and decisive impact that the environment can have on the brain. And knowing how the environment can impact the brains of both babies and adults—including those with healthy brains and those with some kind of brain injury—opens up endless possibilities for how we can help our own cognitive function, as well as the cognitive function of those near and dear to us.

BRAIN DEVELOPMENT AND AGEING ARE INTRICATELY LINKED

The outsized influence of the home environment on the developing brain maybe shouldn't have been so surprising to me. After all, anybody who has seen kids grow up knows how adaptable they are. Watch closely, and you can almost *see* their brains figure out the world in real time. We've also all watched kids excel despite difficult circumstances. At the same time, it's a humbling and important reminder that no amount of biochemistry, physiology, or neuroscience knowledge I could accrue or use to develop new therapies is going to outcompete the evolutionary hardwiring that drives the developing brain to adapt and thrive.

But what about adults? Even if the human brain takes thirty years to fully develop, many of us either are nearing the end of that process or saw the back of it some time ago. This brings me to the second idea that was used to shape how I thought about the brain, and which has proven to be completely wrong: that the adult brain is largely fixed and resistant to change. Though the taxi drivers gave us an inkling of what might be possible, I long assumed any learning or adaptation as an adult would be a slow and arduous process that just gets harder and harder with age.

It's not uncommon for people to tell me they just don't remember things like they used to, or that they can't learn new skills or languages like they could when they were younger. If you're reading this, I bet you've thought something like that as well. In the past few decades, however, it's become increasingly clear that the brain is amazingly *plastic*— a fancy neuroscience word for adaptable and changeable—even in old age. We just have to give it the right inputs and tools to make it adapt.

Mirroring the study showing that the most evolutionarily recent parts of our brains are the ones that develop after birth and help us adapt to our environment, another group looked at the regions of the brain that are most susceptible to the processes of ageing.[16] What they found was surprisingly similar—the regions of the brain that evolved most recently are those that decline most rapidly when we age. This supports an idea called the "last-in first-out" hypothesis, where both evolutionarily and developmentally, the areas of the brain that are most recent and most unique to humans are those that are most vulnerable to age-related decline.

While potentially compelling in many ways, the last-in first-out hypothesis doesn't *quite* fit the pattern of decline we see in the ageing brain. In addition to the prefrontal cortex and temporal lobes, ageing seems to particularly affect parts of the medial parietal cortex, which sits near the middle of your head and just behind the top of it. The structures of the medial parietal cortex that are susceptible to ageing combine with certain parts of the prefrontal cortex (and a few other regions, depending on the scenario) to form the *default mode network* (DMN). The DMN increases in activity when we're not focused on a specific task and is also activated when we think about ourselves and plan for the future.

Other species do have evidence of DMN-like activity, but some of the functions of the DMN are likely to be uniquely human. So, when looking at the connection between the human brain's susceptibility to ageing and its evolutionary history, we have to include structures like the DMN.[17] It might be less a case of "last-in first-out" and more a case of "last-in first-out, plus the bits of the brain that those bits are connected to."

Thinking more broadly about the brain regions most affected by ageing is important because, outside of significant gene mutations or injury, age is the single most important risk factor for cognitive decline and dementia. In fact, two things have to be true for somebody to experience late-onset Alzheimer's disease: they have to be human, and they have to be old.[18] Our closest evolutionary cousins—the great apes, including chimpanzees and gorillas—do experience cognitive decline and develop some evidence of Alzheimer's-like pathology in the brain with age, but it's largely agreed that they don't get dementia.[19] This means that both the process of ageing and the unique properties of the human brain are critical for Alzheimer's disease to occur. Humans do live longer, which may explain part of the difference, but the main reason behind Alzheimer's being a human disease seems to be tied to the dynamic nature of the human brain, which makes it more vulnerable to both the influence of the environment *and* the processes of ageing. In fact, the regions of the human brain that are responsible for adaptation to the environment and most susceptible to ageing are also the areas that have the greatest capacity for neuroplasticity. Several researchers have therefore suggested that dementia and Alzheimer's disease are fundamentally driven by the loss of neuroplasticity.[20] As one of the hallmarks of ageing cells is loss of the capacity to adapt to the environment,[21] this could be one way that ageing, loss of neuroplasticity, and dementia are directly related.

The neuroplasticity we can experience as adults is in many ways just a continuation of the neuroplasticity that occurs during brain development. In fact, there is one theory of ageing that suggests that ageing is just the decades-long continuation of the processes that drive development. For example, when I say that the cortex—the outer grey matter of the brain—*develops* in the years after birth, you might imagine that I mean that part of the brain is *growing*. But for most of our brain's development, that's not the case.

The thickness of your cortex peaks when you're a toddler, and the total grey matter in your brain peaks around the time you're in year 1 at school.[22] After that, development of grey matter involves selectively *remov-*

ing neurons and synapses that aren't needed, and this process is directed by the inputs the brain is receiving from the environment—for instance, when practicing motor, language, and social skills. As we get older, the brain continues to refine itself in response to environmental inputs in the same way, only building and maintaining the structures and functions that it needs. So a decrease in cognitive function at retirement, which we experience as accelerated ageing, could instead be thought of as the brain and body responding normally to the removal of an input. At the same time, studies show that learning new skills or engaging in creative activities (art, languages, music, and even video games) can slow or reverse changes in brain networks that are susceptible to ageing.[23]

Therefore, we know that both ageing and the capacity for neuroplasticity are themselves modifiable by changing the inputs that the brain receives. Understanding these inputs and the influence we have over them is, in essence, the goal of *The Stimulated Mind*. Exercise is another perfect example of this—it is the only intervention that seems to either slow or reverse every biochemical hallmark of ageing.[24] And, amazingly, exercise can also measurably improve the brain's neuroplasticity.[25]

TRAIN THE FUNCTIONS YOU WANT TO KEEP

One of my favourite studies on ageing and plasticity measured neither of those things, but I think it nicely demonstrates a practical concept that each of us can apply to our own brains. What the study found was that our ability to perform complex skills is much more related to how we use our brains than it is to how old our brains are.[26]

In this study, researchers recruited younger and older amateur pianists and compared them to younger and older *expert* pianists from internationally renowned music academies. The younger pianists were mainly in their twenties, and the older pianists ranged from their early fifties to their late sixties. Between each of these four groups (young or old, amateur or expert), they compared performance in two types of tasks: (1) a nonspecific cognitive task related to how fast the brain processes information; and (2) tasks related to piano skills, such as the ability to perform coordinated movements and patterns with the fingers.

The nonspecific task was a cognitive test called the *digit symbol substitution test* (DSST, figure 1). The DSST involves filling in numbered

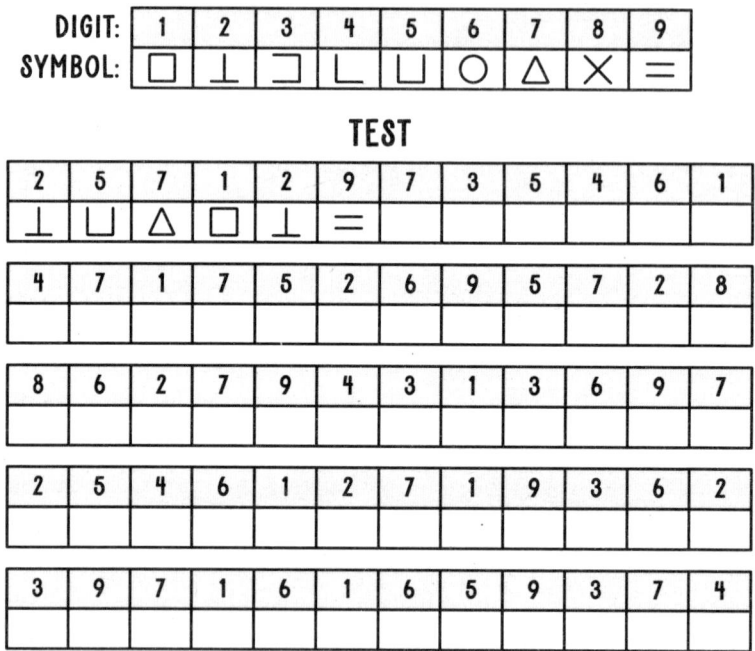

FIGURE 1. Example of a digit symbol substitution test (DSST). Based on the examples at the top, you have to rapidly write the correct symbol in the empty numbered boxes. This involves memorising the symbols and quickly remembering them. A perfect score (such as 100 symbols in 90 seconds) requires you to fill in more than one symbol per second.

boxes with a corresponding symbol in a short time frame—more than one symbol per second to achieve a perfect score. The DSST is considered a measure of brain processing speed that can be easily applied to a wide range of individuals to provide information about a person's ability to focus and quickly process and remember information. If you were born in the twentieth century, you might remember that there was once a time when you would have to remember a phone number for a few seconds before you could find a pen and paper to write it down. The DSST would be a good test of your ability to do that. Scores on the DSST generally decrease with age but are also influenced by short-term factors like sleep that can influence your memory.[27]

Whereas it's hard to really train for the DSST unless you are familiar with the evil tendencies of cognitive neuroscientists, the piano skill test was designed to assess skills that the participants were actively practic-

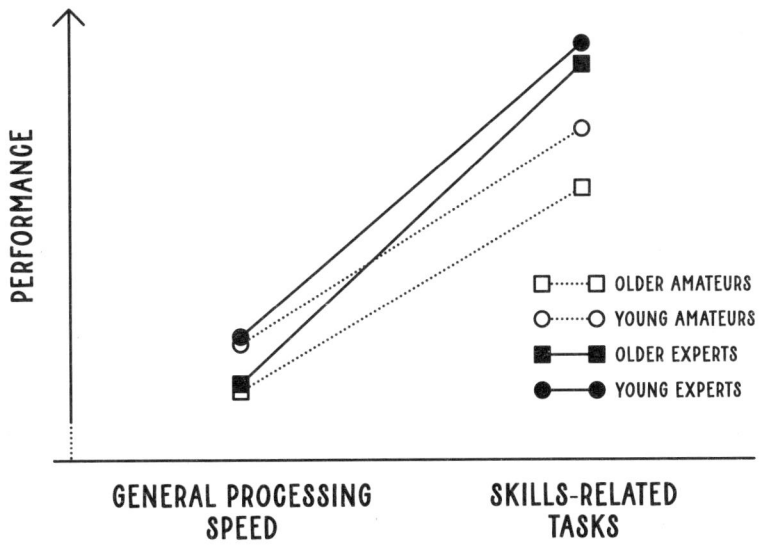

FIGURE 2. Comparing performance in non-specific cognitive tasks (general processing speed) and skills-related tasks in younger (20–30 years old, circles) and older (50–60, squares) expert (black symbols) and amateur (white symbols) pianists. In the expert groups, skill-specific performance was not affected by age, and instead was most associated with amount of recent piano practice. Modified from Krampe and Ericsson, *Journal of Experimental Psychology* 1996.

ing. Testing piano skills in pianists also provides information relevant to all of us because it's just like any other complex skill that we might regularly perform as a hobby or as part of our work, such as neurosurgery, speaking a second language, riding a skateboard, or juggling swords.

Perhaps unsurprisingly, the scientists found that younger participants performed better at the DSST—the nonspecific processing-speed test—regardless of their piano skills. However, when they did piano-skill-related tasks, expert pianists outperformed the amateurs (also maybe not a surprise), with no difference between the older and younger pianists (figure 2).

When the researchers then tried to determine which factors were most associated with performance in the piano-related tasks, practice was consistently the most important factor—especially the total amount of piano practice an individual had undertaken in the last ten years. This was most pronounced in the older expert group, suggesting that deliberate practice in your fifties and sixties can almost completely offset any decrease in performance that you might otherwise expect with increasing age.

IS AGE JUST A NUMBER?

At this point, we've seen a lot of evidence that the adult brain is perfectly capable of learning and maintaining complex skills and information. And while people should absolutely benefit from the fruits of their labours and be able to retire, there isn't necessarily an expiry date on the brain (or body) that means we have to be put out to pasture at a certain age. Nobody told the older pianists they needed to give up the keys, and with some practice they still had the necessary skills to play at an expert level in their late sixties.

With all that said, I am still a realist. With age and ageing does come some inevitable decrease in function. However, by working smarter rather than harder (though sometimes a little harder as well), we can leverage the benefits of age and still maintain peak performance for much longer than we previously thought. The sports enthusiasts among us have seen a number of examples of this in the athletic world very recently.

It seems increasingly common that athletes can continue to perform with the best in the world well into their forties. LeBron James and Diana Taurasi in basketball, Tom Brady in American football, Christie Pearce and Cristiano Ronaldo in what I would call football (and you might call soccer). In Formula 1, there are also two drivers in their forties who are still highly competitive, both former world champions and both still considered good enough to win another championship— Fernando Alonso and Sir Lewis Hamilton. While part of this new era of athletic longevity is the result of better training and recovery strategies, it also reflects what we can do as mere mortals to keep ourselves performing at a high level in whatever it is we choose to perform at.

One aspect of cognitive function that doesn't automatically decline over time and may even peak at some point in our sixth or seventh decade of life is *crystallised intelligence*. This is a fancy neuroscience term for the different components of cognition that combine to form the concept of wisdom. As we get older, we tend to be less impulsive and better at integrating multiple strands of information to see the bigger picture. In recent F1 history, there are many examples of an older driver consistently outdriving his much younger teammate because they make fewer mistakes and their tactics and "race craft" are better.

But for an athlete to be able to maximally express their accumulated wisdom does require some focused effort. All those mentioned above remained singularly focused and dedicated to their sport. There's no getting around the fact that you still have to really want it; as with pianists, engagement in the task is what drives performance. Of course, in some cases athletes adapt their game over time, which is another benefit of wisdom. Ronaldo doesn't run nearly as much as he used to, but he can still get himself in the right position to score a goal—which is why he's scored more goals than anybody else, ever. LeBron has maintained most of his impressive physical prowess, but he excels by focusing on getting the best out of his (often much younger) teammates.

On top of the need for sport-specific skills, longevity in a sport requires a lot of background work to keep the basic machinery of the brain and body in a position to support performance. If you look at any athlete who performs at the top of their sport for multiple decades, you'll almost always find somebody who has taken great care with their diet, sleep, and training schedule to support their needs and goals. Anybody who has worked with young athletes knows that they can (and do) eat almost anything and do almost any kind of training and still manage to keep getting fitter, faster, and stronger. But successful older athletes are much more targeted—they know *why* they're doing what they're doing. And being targeted in their approach usually means they have more time for rest and recovery. As we'll see, this is where the magic happens.

Though I don't think we all need to live like athletes—and, let's be honest, most of us don't have the time to—our general physical health does contribute to core aspects of brain function that are difficult to train. An example of this is a study that some colleagues and I performed using data from the National Health and Nutrition Examination Survey (NHANES), a U.S. initiative that collects data from several thousand average Americans in yearly waves to explore how a variety of lifestyle and other factors affect our health. In some of the waves of NHANES, older adults were asked to do the DSST—the same nonspecific brain processing-speed task that the pianists did. In our study, using the results from this test, we looked at how different factors related to fitness, nutrition, and physical health were associated with processing speed in nearly 1,500 adults who were sixty to eighty-five years old.[28]

In this particular study, we were interested in physical activity and brain function, but we also included several other risk factors for cognitive decline. Though older individuals did have slower processing speed on average, higher levels of leg strength and physical activity were associated with faster processing speed, suggesting that physical activity might offset some of the effects of age on the brain. At the same time, poor physical health (e.g., higher blood sugar, higher blood pressure, and increased levels of inflammation) and worse nutrient status (e.g., being deficient in B vitamins or iron) were associated with slower processing speed. Some follow-up work we did in a different NHANES cohort found something similar: strength, nutrient status, physical health, and sleep were all associated with brain processing speed. And these factors are known to be modifiable—we can make changes to improve them.

The usual caveats to this kind of research still apply: as we're just looking at current lifestyle and brain processing speed, we can't *prove* that changing these factors will improve how our brains work. But our studies align with a huge amount of research showing that, regardless of age, there are a number of modifiable factors that can improve the basic level at which our brain functions and processes information. These factors will be the focus of part 2.

THE BRAIN CAN CHANGE ITSELF

So far, we've focused largely on the importance of the external and the physical, like skill learning and exercise. But I've also alluded to the importance of the internal—the stories we tell ourselves. And what's fascinating to me is that what we *think* doesn't just hold us back psychologically and philosophically; our thoughts can directly change our health and physiology.

While the other studies in this chapter provide some practical examples of why the function of the ageing brain might not necessarily be fixed, there's another fascinating body of work that suggests that ageing is, at least in part, a state of mind. A lot of this work comes from Ellen Langer, a professor of psychology at Harvard who has consistently performed and published some of the most mind-blowing studies on the effect of the mind on physiology. In one of her classic studies, Langer showed that hotel cleaners who didn't have time to exercise outside of work saw significant improvements in body composition and blood pressure if they were simply told that all the cleaning and moving they did as part of their jobs counted as exercise.[29] Though we don't know exactly why this happened, it's clear that just *thinking* they were supporting their health through regular movement at work was enough to trigger processes that resulted in some health benefits.

Studies like this, I think, might be the final nail in the coffin of reductionist approaches to the brain. No matter how good the technology or how diligent the scientist, there's just no way we can isolate the effect of our thoughts on how our bodies function and study that in mice or under the microscope. We need a much bigger picture and an open-minded approach to the messiness of human health and biology.

Perhaps Langer's most famous work is the *Counterclockwise* study, which was done in 1979 and documented in a book of the same name.[30] In the study, eight older men lived together for five days as if they were living in 1959 (twenty years back in time). The environment was filled with props, magazines, music, radio programmes, and movies that were popular twenty years earlier. Twice a day, participants held discussions about "current events" during the Cold War in 1959 as if they were happening right then. Men in a comparison group lived in the same environment for a week and discussed the same topics but spent the week *reminiscing* about those events from the past. Compared to the men in the comparison group, the "counterclockwise" group saw greater improvements in measures of vision, flexibility, manual dexterity, IQ, gait, and posture. It was as if they had *thought* themselves younger in less than a week!

Luckily, we don't need to live in the past to slow our trajectory of ageing and cognitive function. In 1976, Ellen Langer and Judith Rodin performed a study that set the stage for Counterclockwise, where residents at a nursing home were randomly assigned to one of two groups. One group was told they could do whatever they wanted and that they had complete control over their own lives within the home. The other group was told that the staff were there to take care of them and help do everything for them. This second group was essentially told that their care and control of their lives had been given over to other people. During the study and eighteen months afterwards, residents who were given personal control and responsibility were more active, more social, and had improvements in their health. By having greater engagement in the world around them, they gave their brains and bodies a reason to maintain function, and their health benefited as a result. Though it wasn't the goal of this small study, a follow-up analysis even found that those in the active group lived significantly longer than the passive control group.[31]

When describing the original Counterclockwise study and planning a follow-up study in order to confirm the results using modern scientific techniques, Langer wrote about the *stereotype-embodiment theory*, which describes how people age by following their underlying stereotypes about older people.[32] This includes the risk of cognitive decline and dementia. Though it's not the only factor, the stereotype-embodiment theory suggests that if we *expect* to lose cognitive function as we get older, we will see greater cognitive decline with age as a result. Some of this is due to the subconscious effects of expectation, but some of it is also a direct result of the activities we choose to engage in, or not, as we get older.

DECREASING ENGAGEMENT WITH AGE IS THE ULTIMATE MISMATCH

I think it's easiest to understand the impact of activity and engagement by considering the brain over the entire lifespan. Imagine for a moment that I could measure how hard you're working your brain at any given moment—something that is surprisingly difficult to do. From infancy through to young adulthood, the brain is a learning machine. It actively *seeks* new knowledge and inputs across all of its senses.

A young toddler learning to walk is the perfect example. They expend a huge amount of time and effort trying first to stand, and then to coordinate the movements of taking their first steps. They are singularly focused on this task, and they fail. A lot. They also spend a lot of time sleeping, recovering from those efforts as their brains build and rewire based on the new information that has been acquired.

As children get older, the tasks become more complex—and often the stakes get a little higher—as the brain continues its quest for learning and engagement. Climbing trees, learning to drive, asking a classmate to prom, or learning biochemistry at university. These experiences of gaining knowledge and skills and interacting socially are exactly what drives development of the parts of the brain that make us uniquely human.

But ask yourself when you last did something like this—went out on a limb or tried to learn a new skill where the risk of falling on your metaphorical (or literal) butt was high. I'd wager that for most of us, it was a while ago. Taking multiple years to learn a huge amount of new information as an adult, like those prospective London cab drivers did, is surprisingly rare.

This change in approach with age isn't anybody's fault—most of us experience a fairly standard life trajectory dictated by the structure of society in the modern world. As we exit the period of formal learning and leave school to enter the workforce, routine takes over. We might become very specialised in a specific job—which can be incredibly important—and we're certainly very *busy*. But when it comes to the signals we send to our brains to increase and maintain function, our daily activities as adults pale in comparison to what we did when we were younger. And not only do we stop actively learning, but other inputs drop off as well. We don't have time to exercise, and we lose touch with friends. If we do find some spare time, especially as we enter retirement, we think that we're too old to learn or that exercise is only going to cause pain and injury.

The idea of changing engagement with age was highlighted in the pianist study. The authors acknowledged that as expert pianists got older, other life goals and commitments started to take priority. This naturally decreased the amount of time they had to practise, and it was those who practised less—rather than the oldest—whose performance was impacted. This is a pattern that most of us are familiar with—getting older comes with more responsibilities that result in us having less time to spend on periods of focused learning and development.

But what if we need to do the exact opposite? What if age doesn't make us slower and worse at learning new things? What if it's just the fact that, as we get older, we simply don't spend the same amount of time engaging with brain-boosting skills and activities as we did earlier in life? There's a gigantic difference between something being impossible (i.e., thinking that the brain cannot change as we age) and merely challenging (i.e., finding the time to prioritise learning). One is a matter of biology, and the other is more about resources, accessibility, and belief in what might be possible. And, as we've now started to see, the biology probably isn't holding us back as much as we might think.

As we've now learned, the evolutionary history of the human brain made it particularly adaptable and responsive to the environment. These recently evolved areas of the brain spend decades after birth optimising their function, and if the conditions are right, they can display significant neuroplasticity even late in life. However, we also know that these areas of the brain and the regions they're connected to are particularly susceptible to the process of ageing and loss of function that comes with it.

So, if complex social interaction, skill development, and physical activity are what drive the function of the most complex parts of our brain, and those same parts of the brain are the most susceptible to the process of ageing, what we need to do is keep providing the kinds of inputs that drove the development of the brain in the first place. In this way, we can see that many aspects of modern adult life create a mismatch between what the brain needs to maintain function and the inputs it actually receives. We stop learning, we stop moving, we stop sleeping enough, and we spend less time socializing with good friends.

As Langer and others have showed, our behaviour is probably a large part of what drives the ageing of our brains. If we expect to lose function as we get older and, as a consequence, stop exposing our brains to the conditions and environment that drove their development in the first place, it's the removal of those stimuli that drives the loss of function with age rather than the other way around. Thankfully, we can use this concept of mismatch between the developing brain and the ageing one to identify intervention points and maximise the likelihood that the standard adult experience of cognitive decline is something we avoid.

CHAPTER 5
THE GAME OF BRAIN HEALTH

By this point, it's hopefully becoming clear that the stories we tell ourselves about our brains and the stereotypes we embody as we age aren't true. Or at least they don't have to be. While cognitive function does tend to decrease with age on average, our brains are able to adapt and improve at almost any age as long as we provide the environment to do so.

In my work, I study ways to keep the brain as healthy as possible and performing at its best for as long as possible. What has been most interesting to me is the fact that the ingredients that are important for developing a healthy brain in the first place are also the ingredients that your brain needs to stay healthy decades later. As adults, though, we tend to stop paying attention to those elements of our lives—partly because life gets in the way, and partly because we don't know how critical they are.

Though I would never pretend to have all the answers, I was motivated to write this book because a large body of research, including my own work, clearly shows that there are multiple ways to support and change our cognitive function through simple daily actions. It is increasingly clear that through these actions, both cognitive decline and many forms of dementia can be slowed or maybe even prevented entirely.

Before we get into the details of what we can do to future-proof our brains, it's important to cover some of the reasoning behind why I think there's so much scope to improve our long-term cognitive health. Earlier, I outlined some statistics that suggest our brains are increasingly struggling with the burden of mental health issues and dementia, both of which are projected to increase in the coming decades. We may recognise these brain changes happening both collectively and in ourselves or people we know, and it can be all too easy to feel like there's nothing that can be done about them. We assume that we're destined to feel stressed or unfocused, that cognitive decline or Alzheimer's disease is somehow fixed in our destinies, and we are powerless to prevent it. I hope you're starting to realise that this isn't necessarily the case. We each have it within our power to build a resilient brain that keeps firing on all cylinders for decades to come—in other words, to build more headroom.

While you've probably come across multiple negative-sounding statistics about our brain health in the media, there are signs of hope within the same data that tend to get less airtime. This is because the human brain is evolutionarily wired to focus on information that is negative or emotive, primarily to help us avoid impending threats.[1] Negative or worrying news stories about plummeting mental and cognitive health, therefore, tend to get more clicks and more engagement, cementing themselves in our culture and psyche.

It's also fair to say that it can be hard to present a nuanced picture from complex data. And focusing on the negative can be a good way of creating a call to action; if the number of people with dementia is going to triple in our lifetimes, *what are you going to do to decrease the likelihood that you'll be one of them?* This framing makes sense, but in order to change your trajectory of brain health, you also need to believe that avoiding conditions such as dementia in the future is even possible.

One place to look for evidence that dementia is not predetermined might be within other cultures whose lives look a little different from ours and who don't necessarily suffer from the same types of mismatch that we tend to. A good example is the Tsimané, an Indigenous population of around seventeen thousand individuals in the tropical forests of lowland Bolivia. Their lifestyle includes a heavy reliance on physically demanding labour in the form of hunting, fishing, gathering, and farming without the assistance of motorised equipment or animals.[2] The Tsimané spend several hours every day working to provide for themselves and their families, with activity levels remaining high into their seventies and eighties.[3] Though the number of individuals in these societies is relatively small, the dementia rates of the Tsimané and other Amazonian Amerindians are estimated to be the lowest in the world.[4] Their brains also seem to age much more slowly than average American and European adults' brains, which has been attributed to their lifelong physical activity, nutrient-rich diet of vegetables, fish, and lean meat, and low risk of heart and metabolic disease—both high blood pressure and diabetes are very rare.[5]

If we look closer to home for some good news about dementia and our ability to change the trajectory of brain health, there is plenty to be found. For instance, the primary reason the global dementia burden is expected to expand so dramatically in the coming decades is because life expectancy continues to increase worldwide.[6] This is an impressive feat that is worth celebrating in its own right. After all, to get dementia you need to live long enough without dying of something else first. One of the reasons life expectancy is increasing is that we have become very good at treating infectious diseases and are getting increasingly good at treating and preventing heart disease, which for many countries has been the number one cause of death for decades.

Similar trends already appear to be happening with respect to dementia prevention. For example, a recent longitudinal study in the UK examining two cohorts of older adults twenty years apart (1989–1994 and 2008–2011) found that age-specific incidence of dementia had decreased.[7] A later meta-analysis (study of many studies) combined these data with other cohorts, including individuals in France, Sweden, Iceland, the Netherlands, the UK, and several communities across the United States as part of the Alzheimer Cohorts Consortium.[8] What the researchers found was very similar across the cohorts: the likelihood of having dementia at any particular age is actually *decreasing*.[9] This means that the likelihood you will be diagnosed with dementia at the age of seventy is now lower than it was twenty years ago. As a result, the authors suggest that some of the projections about the increase in dementia in the coming decades may be too pessimistic. However, as the population as a whole is living longer, the likelihood of *ever* getting dementia is still expected to increase—it will just happen later in life than it did previously.

Though it's hard to decipher why age-specific dementia is decreasing over time, the authors suggest it may be related to the recent public health focus on preventing heart disease, which has overlapping risk factors with Alzheimer's disease and dementia. Most individuals with Alzheimer's disease have diseased blood vessels in their brains, which probably mirrors a disease process that is happening in their hearts at the same time.[10] We've seen that a critical component of brain function is a blood supply that responds to activity by directing oxygen and nutrients to where they are most needed. But when blood vessels become diseased or age, they stiffen and are no longer able to provide the dynamic changes in blood supply that the brain needs, which can impair function.

We know efforts to decrease the burden of heart disease are working because hospitalizations and deaths from heart disease in the United States have been steadily declining over the past few decades. Interventions that have worked include a focus on stopping smoking as well as treating high blood pressure, high blood sugar, and "high cholesterol" (a terribly inaccurate phrase, but it does the job here), which the authors of the dementia study think have similarly translated to decreased dementia risk. Not only do these risk factors affect the health of the blood vessels in the heart and the brain, but smoking and diabetes also directly impact the brain to increase the risk of cognitive decline and dementia. The authors of the study did warn, though, that the rising rates of diabetes and high blood pressure in countries like the United States might reverse some of the improving trends. Nevertheless, their study provides evidence that focusing on specific health issues at a national scale can potentially decrease the likelihood of developing dementia, which gives us some optimism about our ability to improve brain health in the future. And luckily, the tools I'll cover in part 2 will include some of the most evidence-based ways to prevent issues like high blood pressure and diabetes, directly improving your brain as well as your overall health.

INTERNATIONAL EXPERTS AGREE—DEMENTIA IS PREVENTABLE

In 2024, a commission of world experts led by professor Gill Livingston estimated that at least 45 percent of dementia is preventable.[11] Using some statistical models, the team predicted what percentage of dementia cases might never occur if a given risk factor was completely eliminated, like if everybody in the world suddenly gave up smoking. Of this 45 percent of dementia cases that might be preventable, about half were explained by factors that we ourselves have significant control over, including physical activity, smoking, and alcohol. Some risk factors we have less control over, such as the 3 percent caused by traumatic brain injury, but we could certainly decrease the number of activities we do that have a high risk of brain trauma. For instance, maintaining strength and balance with training can reduce the risk of falls, which are the most common cause of head trauma in adults over sixty-five.[12] You might also consider skipping your weekly underground bare-knuckle boxing club and attend a Zumba class instead . . .

There are some significant contributors to dementia risk in the Livingston report that we may have less direct control over, such as the 7 percent associated with shorter periods of childhood education. This might be because we're now past the period of formal education, or because there are societal and socioeconomic factors that affect our ability to access education—all of which are themselves associated with increased dementia risk. However, as the later chapters will show, engaging in learning activities outside of formal education can enhance brain health and cognitive function at any age, regardless of how many years you spent at school. So this factor is also potentially modifiable.

There's even evidence to suggest that *more* than 45 percent of dementia cases may be preventable if we are able to take the full range of risk factors into account. For example, later-life cognitive activity was not included as a protective factor in the Livingston report despite good evidence to support its importance in dementia prevention, and neither were other important protective factors such as nutrient status and sleep. In line with this, a more recent analysis of data from nearly 350,000 people in the UK Biobank—a detailed database of medical and health-related data from half a million adults in the United Kingdom—suggested that over 70 percent of dementia cases may be preventable, though some risk factors, such as socioeconomic status, would require intervention at the societal rather than the individual level.[13] All of this is to say that an ever-increasing body of research gives significant hope that we can individually and collectively decrease dementia risk in a meaningful way.

PLAY THE GAME

At this point, you might appreciate that in many ways, the science behind long-term brain health can be simultaneously too simple and too complex. We've seen how the reductionist approach to neuroscience and dementia that stems from the very foundations of the field has resulted in a smaller impact on dementia treatment than we originally hoped. This is probably because brain function is the output of a collection of infinitely tunable parts, and there's only so much you can learn by staring at inanimate slices of brain that are completely disconnected from the person or animal they were a part of.

As soon as we start to think beyond neurons and proteins, however, the picture of how a brain works quickly becomes almost impossible to fathom because of all the different cells and their functions and interactions. Then add on the fact that our brains can affect their own health and physiology based on thoughts and expectations, and the amount of information can become overwhelming. But some elements of clarity start to emerge when we think about what brains need to develop and function at their best, the risk factors for dementia that we have some control over, and how the average modern life introduces mismatches between what our brains thrive on and what they get exposed to. To illustrate how I think we can deal with all this complexity, I will steal an analogy from my friend and colleague, neurologist Josh Turknett.

Imagine that an extraterrestrial race travels across space to arrive on Earth. While searching the area, they find a pair of (unlocked) smartphones that both contain a game. In Josh's original telling it is the game *Angry Birds,* which tells you something about either Josh's maturity or the age of the anecdote.

In order to better understand this alien (to them) device, the visitors split into two teams and plan a competition to see who can "win" *Angry Birds.* Team One decides that the best option is to play the game as much as possible, training hours every day until they've completed the game multiple times. Team Two decides that the only way to truly understand and master the game is to hack into the phone and manipulate the game's source code.

On competition day, Team One crushes it. They know the tricks and skills required for every level and complete the game in record time despite having no understanding of computer code or how the game actually works. By comparison, Team Two still can't beat a single level. They've dissected the phone and analysed thousands of lines of code, but every time they try to change the code while the game is running, it crashes. What they don't realise is that even the people who designed the game would probably find it impossible to beat the game by manipulating its code in real time.

Team Two's approach to playing *Angry Birds* is much like the biologist's approach to fixing a broken radio. This method works brilliantly when there is one single broken component in your radio and it's easy to identify the problem. Fixing a broken limb or treating an infection is like replacing a burned-out transistor or editing a single faulty section of game code. Using this approach, we can even identify and treat diseases caused by single genes. But trying to understand cognitive decline and dementia by breaking the phone and its code into constituent parts and then trying to manipulate them has so far resulted in a lot more failure than success.

It's worth highlighting that some of the most impactful tools we have for improving human health are ones that—much like Team One's successful *Angry Birds* strategy—we use without fully understanding how they work. They impact multiple components across multiple circuit boards in our metaphorical car or radio, often requiring a whole game's worth of code in order to run.

One of the best examples is exercise. We know exercise works to improve multiple aspects of health, and we have some idea of the parametres required to achieve that (much more on that later). We also know that exercise acts via a multitude of overlapping and complementary mechanisms in multiple pathways, many of which we're still discovering. In fact, at least once per year there is a breakthrough study in a major scientific journal describing yet another mechanism by which exercise improves the health of the body or brain. But the fact that we still don't know exactly how exercise works hasn't stopped scientists and healthcare bodies from appreciating the importance of physical activity for overall health. Nobody is saying that we shouldn't exercise just because we haven't yet been able to fully dissect and isolate its mechanisms via traditional reductionist scientific methods.

Unlike some of the single-component problems that medicine and

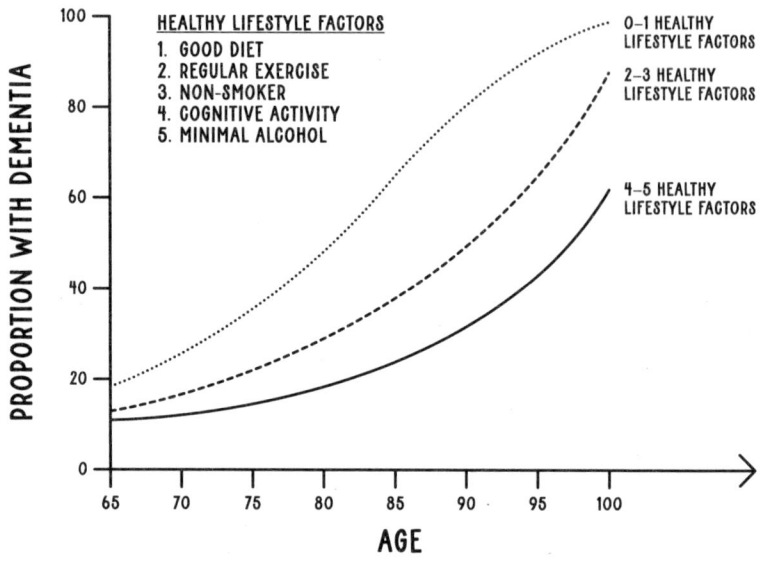

FIGURE 1. Adults 65 years or older grouped by the number of healthy lifestyle factors they have and percentage diagnosed with dementia between 65 and 100 years old. The 5 lifestyle factors are diet, exercise, cognitive activity, smoking, and alcohol. Those who had 4–5 healthy lifestyle factors (solid black line) had half the risk of being diagnosed dementia at all ages compared to those who had 0–1 healthy lifestyle factors (dotted line). Those with 2–3 factors were in the middle (dashed line). Modified from Dhana et al., *BMJ* 2022.

science have historically tackled, like infections and broken limbs, our cognitive function and health are determined by a lifetime of exposures—experiences and the conditions around us—as well as the way all those exposures interact. In our brains, these exposures have trained an algorithm so complex and so unique to each person that it is literally *impossible* to understand the function of the whole by isolating the individual components.

Luckily, we have a large body of science that suggests that we can take the Team One approach and "play the game" of brain health without having to understand the ins and outs of the source code. The Chicago Health and Ageing Project (figure 1) is a nice example of this. One analysis from this study looked at nearly 2,500 adults aged sixty-five or older and examined five main factors associated with dementia risk—diet, exercise, cognitive activity, smoking, and alcohol.[14] The researchers found that those who had four to five healthy lifestyle factors had *half* the risk of being diagnosed with dementia at any age compared to those who had zero to one healthy lifestyle factors. So the combination of challenging your brain with cognitive activity plus a good diet, regular exercise, not smoking, and not drinking too much seems to be associated with a 50 percent reduction in the risk of dementia!

One critical component missing from the Chicago study, though, is the effect of an intervention. This was another observational study where people were simply asked about how they lived, and then their risk of dementia was determined. That doesn't prove that these lifestyle factors were the reason why some individuals in the study had half the dementia risk of others. So, what about studies that apply the same principles in an attempt to directly improve the cognitive function of their participants?

Though there are many now, the first study to really test the idea of playing the game of brain health was FINGER (Finnish Geriatric Intervention Study to Prevent Cognitive Impairment and Disability).[15] More than 1,200 individuals aged sixty to seventy-seven who were at high risk of dementia were randomised to either a control group or an intervention group. The intervention group received two years of dietary change, an aerobic and resistance training exercise programme, a cognitive function training programme, and active monitoring and treatment of their heart disease risk factors. Compared to the control group, the intervention group saw significant gains in cognitive function over the two-year study, including improvements in overall cognitive function, processing speed, and decision-making.

If we were applying a proper reductionist approach here, we would demand to know which of the interventions, or which combinations, were most important. We would want to know all the mechanisms they acted through and how their effects could be measured. But in reality we have to be comfortable not knowing, because they *all* matter, and they will affect the brain in myriad ways that can never be measured. They all do their part, both individually and in synergistic alliance, to build headroom by bolstering brain function and resilience across innumerable pathways and networks.

The message is pretty clear now. In order to navigate toward an evidence-based and personalised approach to long-term cognitive function, we first have to step away from the source code of the brain—the amyloid and the microglia. Instead, we need to leverage the components of our lifestyle and our engagement with the world around us that drive and support brain health. In essence, we need to learn how to *play the game*.

Like the owls in the preface and the aliens playing *Angry Birds*, if you invest time and effort in adapting to a new challenge, your brain will direct the necessary resources to do that. Building headroom is, therefore, a matter of challenging your current capabilities and providing an environment that lets the brain respond accordingly, even if we don't understand how it all works at the biochemical level. That's great news, because it means, by playing the game, you have the power to future-proof your brain *right now*.

PART TWO

Winning the Brain Game

CHAPTER 6
THE RULES OF THE GAME

After reading the last couple of sentences and seeing the graph at the end of the previous chapter, you might be forgiven for thinking, "This next bit is where he's going to tell me to do all the things that I already know I should be doing." And, if I'm going to be completely honest, you'd be absolutely right. There's no getting around it, really, because most of the actions you can take to improve your cognitive function today—and your brain health long-term—will already be familiar to you in one way or another. Having some familiarity with the terrain is good news when we think about the long game of brain health because that can give you a head start or help you realise that you're already doing more for your brain than you might think.

As mentioned in part 1, the goal is to future-proof your brain from dementia, and the strategy to do that involves building a cognitive buffer we can rely on—in moments of stress but also as we age. The coming chapters will provide some of the tactics you can use to put that strategy into motion. But whether these tactics are new to you or not, I hope I can present them in a way that might help to make them stick. Because it's not exaggerating to say that your current and future brain depend on it.

THE PRIZE

Some play games for fame or fortune. Others for the fun of it all. The goal of this particular *brain* game, however, is building headroom. We do this by taking part in activities that help build a neurobiological buffer against the processes of ageing, allowing the brain to adapt and maintain optimal cognitive function for as long as possible. Though we are often told that this isn't the case, we can improve almost any function, including brain function, by challenging our current capabilities. The additional headroom this process gives us—the extra capacity and robustness we can use to take on the world and weather its storms—is the big prize in the brain game that we are all working toward.

We all need as much headroom as we can get because our lives are unpredictable, and the future is largely unknowable. Therefore, we want to head into that future with the confidence that our brains can handle whatever is thrown at us. For example, we know from scientific research as well as personal experience that our cognitive function declines when we're sick, stressed, or sleep-deprived. And the reality is that we will *all* face challenges like these.

The goal isn't to create a perfectly optimised and complex set of circumstances and habits and expect that we'll always be able to operate at 100 percent with no interruption. Though this will occasionally happen if we put the right structures in place and things go our way, the more common and realistic scenario is that we work to be able to function well even when the conditions and situations we face are less than ideal. Because the scenario that we really want to *avoid* is the opposite one, which seems to be increasingly common: a scenario where, as we get older, the effects of every illness, every injury, every sleepless night, and worsening physical health accumulate, diminishing our overall cognitive function and contributing to cognitive decline.

The thing about headroom is that you don't need it every day. But you want to make sure you have additional capacity in reserve when you need it most. And though it's difficult to quantify and feel our headroom sometimes, doing the activities that help to build headroom can also improve our cognitive function on a day-to-day basis while decreasing our risk of dementia in the long term. This is the essence of a future-proof brain, which is especially important now that we're lucky enough to routinely live far into our eighties and nineties.

For our brains to age well, we need to actively engage with and attend to the factors that are in our control and influence our cognitive function. As you'll see, this doesn't mean strictly controlling your entire life or striving to be perfect the entire time, but a consistent *resolve* to engage with the world around you and challenge yourself, while resisting the myth that your physical and cognitive function is destined to decline as you age. So the stakes are incredibly high, but the fact that small changes can have a big impact when done together gives me incredible hope for our collective cognitive future.

Before we dive into some details on how to play the game of brain health, however, let's think about the rules of the game. These rules aren't rigid, because there's nothing in biology that we can be 100 percent certain about. But the way we consider, approach, and act upon health information is often as important as the information itself.

STACK THE DECK IN YOUR FAVOUR

Whenever I talk about the fact that a large proportion—perhaps even the majority—of dementia cases may be preventable, the two most common reactions are disbelief and resistance. People are either amazed and surprised that this might be true or certain that it isn't. Both responses are completely reasonable.

When we think about our long-term health and cognitive function, it's quite easy to be filled with feelings of despair. We've already discussed how our brains focus on negative messages, and the general portrayal of our collective health by scientists and the media can be very stark. As a result, we might be forgiven for thinking that the increasing burden of dementia, as well as the unstoppable onslaught of technology, social media, and other environmental stressors truly does make us doomed.

Now, don't get me wrong, there is some truth in all of this. As a population, our overall physical health has been declining over recent decades, largely driven by the mismatch between our biology and the modern environment.[1] And, as discussed in part 1, there probably isn't going to be a miracle brain drug any time soon. But this story of brain doom is in fact only half of the story. We've already seen evidence that you can decrease dementia risk by focusing on individual risk factors, and the truth is that there's a huge amount that can be achieved simply by continuing to invest time in the activities that support our health and our brains.

If dementia prevention really is possible, this, understandably, leads to complicated feelings for many people. Maybe they've had a loved one or a close family member who experienced dementia and they wonder if they should have done something differently. This is where we have to remind ourselves that dementia is common, rarely the result of any single factor, and *definitely not* anybody's "fault." I truly believe that each of us is doing the best we can with the information we have at the time, and as a society we're still figuring out how a wide variety of factors come together to influence an individual's overall risk of dementia.

Though the big-picture constituents of brain health, like diet and physical activity, can dramatically impact our day-to-day cognitive function as well as our long-term risk of cognitive decline, we still have to remind ourselves that the brain is incredibly complex. It's not uncommon for me to talk about the benefits of something like physical activity for the brain, only to receive a comment along the lines of "My family member exercised every day and still got dementia." Comments like this are both understandable and expected because we already know that no single variable is going to guarantee a certain outcome. We also don't want to diminish the impact of a devastating disease or oversimplify its causes. On the other hand, there are several potential scenarios where the individual in question still had a better outcome than they would have done otherwise.

Maybe this person had better day-to-day cognitive function because of their exercise routine, improving their quality of life even though they eventually were diagnosed with dementia. Maybe their dementia symptoms were less severe because of their history of physical activity. Or maybe their active lifestyle meant that their rate of cognitive decline was slowed, and they were diagnosed with dementia years later than they would have been otherwise. All these scenarios are consistent with what we know about the relationship between physical activity, cognitive function, and cognitive decline.

Most of us struggle to think about how our habits and lifestyle affect our long-term health because we're dealing with probabilities rather than certainties. If we return to the graph from the Chicago Health and Ageing Project at the end of the previous chapter, at eighty years old, somewhere around 20 percent of individuals who had at least four protective lifestyle factors were diagnosed with dementia. So even though their health-promoting lifestyles weren't enough to eliminate all of their dementia risk, they still had about half the risk of those who only had one (or zero) healthy lifestyle factors. When it comes to the brain game, then, the most successful strategy is really about stacking the deck in our favour as much as possible.

Of course, there will always be people who do everything "wrong" and still live long lives without any health problems at all. This is part of the intrigue (for me at least) and frustration (for most other people) of biology, data, and statistics. But it shouldn't stop us from doing whatever we can to improve our odds of long-term brain health.

In many ways, the process of stacking the deck in our brain's favour is more like preparing for an athletic event than playing through levels on a computer game. As an athlete you want to play to your strengths but also identify and address areas of weakness or factors that might be limiting your performance. As a result, you will hopefully see measurable improvements in performance along the way and be happy with how you perform on the day of the event. However, you also have to acknowledge that whether you come in first place will depend at least partly on factors outside of your control. For example, in the 2012 Olympic men's 100-metre final, those who finished in second, third, and fourth places all ran personal-best times. Times that on another day might even have won them the gold medal. An additional four athletes set national records during the same competition. They just all happened to do it behind the unstoppable force of Usain Bolt.

This means that, even if we can't guarantee any specific long-term outcome, playing the game to build headroom can still give us meaningful progress, improvement, and daily wins to improve how our brains feel and perform, today and for years to come.

THE GAME IS A RACE

Thinking about the brain game as a lifelong preparation for an athletic event reminds me of a very different and much less glamorous race that I myself took part in during the summer of 2012—the world's first ever fully off-road ironman triathlon. The race took place across the south coast of the UK, starting with a twoish-mile sea swim followed by 112 miles of mountain biking overnight and then a marathon trail run, all within a twenty-four-hour time limit. Just describing the race reminds me that it probably didn't do my health any favours, and my knees have never been quite the same since. But on the upside, there are useful lessons I learned that can be helpful when thinking about the pursuit of our long-term brain goals.

Firstly, success for me may have been different than for the other competitors. We all have our own goals, and success looks different to each of us. At six foot two and 220 pounds, I'm not exactly built like a streamlined long-distance endurance athlete. A good friend of mine once told me that I run like a lion who has somehow figured out how to walk upright. If you're imagining something that looks like the *opposite* of speed of and grace, you're on the right track. So success for me in this particular race was simply making it to the finish line.

Secondly, I had to be very practical during my preparations for the race because 2012 was my first year working as a doctor. This meant that I had much less time to train for this race than for earlier ones I had done as a student. For most of us who have jobs, families, and other commitments and responsibilities, it's very unlikely that we'll ever have the time or ability to do everything perfectly. We have to focus our efforts on the areas where we're most likely to reap the most benefit.

In this case, I figured that if I could keep one foot moving in front of the other, I would probably get across the finish line. So I focused less on fitness and more on minimising the likelihood that I would either quit or get lost on the loosely marked course. I took multiple trips to the area to make sure I had biked or run the entire course by the time the race came around. I also started doing training sessions immediately after my night shifts in the hospital so that I knew I could keep going after missing a night of sleep. Any good coach will tell you that this is *not* the ideal way to train if you want to get the best out of your training or minimise your risk of injury. But I knew that if I had instead focused on the "perfect" training programme I would have failed to achieve it while also sacrificing my work and sleep for several months.

The race ended up taking place during the third-wettest summer the United Kingdom has experienced since records began in 1836. A torrential storm rolled in during the swim and lasted all night. The mountain bike part was especially arduous. Imagine a log flume made of mud where you have to bike yourself to the top of the ride and then hold on for dear life on the way down. For twelve hours. In complete darkness.

Aside from providing flashbacks to the muddiest I have ever been in my entire life, the storm ends up being an important part of this analogy, representing any one of many factors outside of our control that influence our long-term health. This could be, for instance, socioeconomic status, stress, genetics, or exposures from the environment, such as air and water quality. We all have our own storms to weather, but the key is to figure out the things that we have the capacity to influence, and to keep doing that until the race is over. Putting one foot in front of the other and doing what we can to make sure we don't quit.

In the race, a *lot* of people quit. Somewhere in the middle of the bike portion there was a rest station where you could go inside and get a snack and a hot drink. Most people arrived in the middle of the night, soaking wet and covered in bruises from falling off their bikes. Faced with heading back out into the rain and the uncertainty of what the next twelve hours would hold, many decided they'd much rather be dry and enjoy a nice cup of tea. Less than half of those who started the race finished it. Much like the overwhelming feelings we face when considering all the ways we should be living our lives differently in order to support our long-term health, the thought of going out into the dark, wet unknown was too much for many of the competitors, and they gave up.

There were several moments when I also thought about quitting. But in the end, I got back on my bike and finished the race. I don't tell you this because I expect you to be impressed by it. In fact, you might be forgiven for questioning the judgment of somebody who would sign up for an event like this. I also know for a fact that I wasn't a better athlete or better navigator than those who quit or got lost. But I do think I maximised my likelihood of success by focusing on what was most likely to hold me back—the high probability of getting lost or giving up—and the related factors that I could control with the time I had available.

This, essentially, is how I think we should play the game of brain health—think about the areas where we're most likely to see some benefit and match those areas to actions that we're able to consistently and reliably perform. Everything else ends up being a distraction. Therefore, the first rule of the brain game is that you should *Prepare for your own race*. What you choose to focus on can and should change over time, but only you will know how the factors involved in the game will apply to you.

PLAY THE LONG GAME

There are two more features of my race that I think map well onto the lifelong game of brain health. The first is that it is a *long* game. Hopefully decades long. Each stroke of the swim, turn of the pedals, and stride of the run is a small daily challenge or action that moves us closer to the goal of better brain health. And as the race wears on, each step gets harder, but our reward for continuing is that we get to stay in the race. Because stopping for too long results in elimination. Of course, this is where my carefully crafted analogy fails a bit, because if we're good at the game of brain health, then the race will last longer. In this case, that's part of success.

This brings us to rule two—*Never give up*. I will admit this is 100 percent stolen, because it also happens to be the tagline of the company that organised the wet and muddy ordeal that this whole story revolves around. But in this context, I don't mean "Never give up" as some kind of masochistic call to overcome our weaknesses and laziness in order to win at any cost. I mean it as a reminder that the most important thing is simply to keep your feet moving.

When the game is as long as the one you might embark upon to improve your brain health for a lifetime, your actions and the inputs you provide to your brain accumulate over decades. Though we might beat ourselves up about it, skipping a workout or two, having a few bad nights of sleep, or eating an entire cake in one sitting will make very little difference in the end as long as our steps in the race—workouts, sleep, nutritious meals—keep slowly accumulating.

The final piece of the race analogy revolves around something that I didn't know I needed beforehand, but which made all the difference on the day. Camaraderie. For me, this came in the form of a fellow competitor named Glenn whom I met on those dark muddy hillsides and have never seen again. For the first few hours of the bike portion of the race, we kept bumping into each other, and eventually we agreed to stick together. After a quick snack at the infamous indoor quitting point, we stepped back out into the rain together knowing that having to do it alone would have been that much harder. Ten hours later, as we neared the end of the marathon and I was mentally and physically exhausted, Glenn's words of encouragement were enough to help me get my head down and finish out the race.

This brings me to rule three of the brain game—*Don't go it alone*. This rule, like all of them, is open to a lot of interpretation. It means that sometimes it's OK to ask for a little help, whether that's for a few minutes, a few hours, or a few years. It also means that many of the actions we can take to improve our brain health and cognitive function are easier—or even enhanced—when doing them with others. For humans, as social animals, just the act of being connected to supportive and loving people improves how long and how well we live. This is a key tenet that will be reflected across many aspects of the brain game.

For most of us, other people will probably also provide the reason for even doing any of this in the first place. Nobody exists, thinks, or ages in a vacuum. Very few people worry about their long-term cognitive function or choose to change their lifestyle because they want to live an additional several years of solitude. For the vast majority of us, our *why* involves other people.

Maybe you want to spend more time doing the things you love with the people you love. Maybe you want to avoid being a burden to your family in your later years. Maybe you want to be able to roll around on the floor with your (great) grandkids or nephews and nieces, or attend (and remember) their graduations. Whatever it is, part of preparing for your own race is finding the *why* for your pursuit of headroom, because having a sense of purpose and enjoyment from the activities you engage in is critical to both well-being and long-term brain health.[2] This is what will provide the grounding and motivation you need to keep building on what you have and keep moving forward.

AIM FOR PROGRESS, NOT PERFECTION

Having thought about ways to approach and prepare for the game, we also need to think about how we process health information and use that information to make decisions about what we or others could do to improve our health. With the explosion of social media over the past twenty years, we have become increasingly exposed to the opinions and judgments of others, from faceless strangers and bots to (hopefully) well-meaning influencers who tell us that our perfect life and body would be achievable if only we had enough willpower and weren't so lazy. This wouldn't necessarily be a problem if we (a) didn't listen, and

(b) didn't internalise an expectation of judgment. But we're wired to listen to messages from others and use them to gauge where we fit into the world.[3]

In many ways, health information has been weaponised against us. Not on purpose, but simply because of how we react to the huge amount of information we're being exposed to. As a common example, you might see a list of "fifteen things to do to improve your brain health" on social media. In the best-case scenario, this list was generated and promoted by an expert in the field, with a good evidence base. You can even find lists like this in some of the top medical journals.[4] But what do we do with this information? Most of the time, we do nothing. Sometimes it's because decision-making becomes harder when we're exposed to large amounts of information, or because we're not in a position to act on the information at that exact moment in time. But more often than not, when faced with a laundry list of things to do that require us to change our behaviour, we rapidly realise how impossible it would be to do everything on the list, and we give up entirely. This is completely normal.

Even when we decide to focus on just *one* area of health, recommendations can still become overwhelming. For example, there are world experts in sleep and exercise—people whose opinions are absolutely worth listening to—who will say that you need to sleep eight hours every night or do four hours of aerobic exercise (biking, running, swimming, etc.) a week to see benefits to your health. But what if you currently only manage to sleep six hours a night? Or what if you have only an hour or two available for some kind of structured exercise each week? A perfectly understandable response would be to not bother trying to improve sleep or exercise at all because you know you're not going to hit those lofty targets. But when it comes to almost every aspect of our health and fitness, we lose out when we let perfect be the enemy of good. Actually, it doesn't even need to be good. Sometimes it just needs to be *something*. Especially when the more common alternative is worrying about the long list of ways that we need to change while simultaneously not changing anything because of the overwhelming feeling that comes from thinking we have to overhaul our entire lives in order to be healthy. This is the worst of all worlds.

Again and again, I've seen people either confused by contradictory health information or paralysed into inaction due to the insurmountable list of changes they think they need to make in their lives. Some of this problem can be solved by reframing the information to show that all those seemingly impossible health and lifestyle targets aren't as fixed as they might first seem. But more important than that is understanding that the tension between what we *think* we should be doing and what we're *actually* doing can negatively impact our health. For example, we know from work by people like psychologist Gloria Mark that having a mental list of tasks that we're not currently addressing is inherently stressful.[5] And when these tasks concern your health, seeing them on social media, and reading about them in the news *every day*, creates a lot of opportunity for stress.

When it comes to improving cognitive function and building headroom, there's a balance to be struck between action and rest. The brain and body *thrive* on stimulus and challenge but also need to be given the time to recover after experiencing them. Complementary opposites like this are so fundamental to our biology and the world in general that we see them everywhere in human mythology—yin and yang, shiva and shakti, fire and water. While I'm admittedly no expert in philosophy, the physiological implications of this relationship are clear. We *need* to be stimulated physically and mentally, and that stimulus also needs to be challenging because that's what drives adaptation. But rest and recovery are critical for that adaptation to occur. Work hard and then enjoy the fruits of your labours.

What most of us need, then, are relatively small but regular challenges, kind of like running a 5K race where we can push ourselves and then spend the rest of the day relaxing with friends or fellow competitors before recovering with a good night's sleep. But the constant psychological friction of cataloguing all the ways we think we need to change while not making those changes is more like my Ironman race—an endless self-inflicted beatdown with no opportunity for reprieve. In fact, though it's hard to test the effects in a controlled experiment, there is even some evidence to suggest that constantly telling ourselves that we're not doing enough may impact our long-term health.

One fascinating study looked at data from more than sixty thousand adult Americans, exploring the relationship between perceived physical activity levels and risk of death. Participants were asked whether they thought they exercised more, about the same, or less than other people like them. What the researchers found was that those who thought they were doing more exercise than their peers had the lowest risk of death, followed by those that thought they were doing about as much. Those who thought they were doing *less* exercise than other people like them had the highest risk of death. These results held even after accounting for age, sex, race and ethnicity, education, employment, income, marital status, multiple measures of health, smoking, and *actual* levels of physical activity.[6]

Put another way, all things being equal, those who felt they were doing less exercise than other people like them died sooner, regardless of how much exercise they actually did! Using similar data, another study found the same thing for cognitive function; it's almost as if by *thinking* they were doing plenty of exercise, participants enjoyed greater mental benefits.[7] Or maybe they were just unburdened by the expectations that many of us feel when we think we're not doing enough. As with any study like this where people are asked questions and their long-term health is assessed, it's possible that something else not measured or accounted for explains the results. But as Ellen Langer's work mentioned in part 1 shows, it is very clear that our perceptions change our physiology, which in turn affects our health.

Once you know that perceptions can have biological effects, it's easy to see how a discrepancy between what we're currently doing and what we think we need to be doing can sabotage our well-being. Frequently thinking that we're not doing enough can significantly increase stress and maybe even counteract the good work we *are* doing. As a result, we need to reframe what we think is "enough" exercise, sleep, or dietary change, as well as the ways we can achieve it. For instance, evidence suggests that people think they need to add a lot of vigourous exercise to feel like they have changed their physical activity.[8] This is despite the fact that lower levels of activity are also beneficial. In fact, setting lower exercise goals with a broader definition of what counts as exercise makes it more likely that you will actually stick with it, which also improves how you feel about your health.[9]

The importance of contextualising health information brings us some rules of the brain game that required a little introspection on my part. After spending most of my teenage years actively avoiding sports and generally being quite sedentary, it's fair to say that I then spent several years overcompensating. I devoured health-and-fitness magazines that served up unrealistic ideals of what being healthy looked like, as well as unrealistic expectations of the physical feats required. This contributed to me training twenty hours a week as a competitive rower at university and then taking part in increasingly punishing endurance races in my mid-twenties.

Looking back now, it's much easier to see (and admit) that my exercise escalation was largely driven by feelings of not doing (or being) enough. And while I do think there are many benefits to testing the limits of our capabilities, this shouldn't come at the expense of acknowledging what we're already doing. Because by discounting positive actions we're already taking, we may see less benefit from those actions, while at the same time increasing stress that reduces the impact of any other changes and habits we add. The last two rules of the brain game therefore provide the complementary opposites to the first three rules. While the first rules define our approach to *action,* the last two rules help to structure the necessary period of rest afterwards.

The fourth rule is that *Everything counts*. We absolutely need to do *something* and keep challenging ourselves to stimulate adaptation as part of the process of building headroom. And as you'll see in the coming chapters, even small changes can have a big impact. So we should let ourselves celebrate and acknowledge that. The kind of challenges that build headroom are also meant to build us up, not to tear us down. That's why the fifth rule of the brain game is *Be kind to yourself (and others)*. This might mean making sure we take the time to rest and recover, or being realistic about what we should be trying to do at any given time. And though there's certainly something (or many things) each of us could be doing to improve our brain health and decrease our personal dementia risk, value judgments shouldn't be made based on how we or others act on that information.

In the coming chapters, I'll cover frameworks for how to think about and tackle the areas where we can have the biggest impact on our brain health—and build the kind of headroom needed to improve cognitive function today and maintain it for decades to come. But for each of these, as well as when considering how they all might fit together, we have to remember the rules of the game:

1. Prepare for your own race
2. Never give up
3. Don't go it alone
4. Everything counts
5. Be kind to yourself (and others)

Remember that the brain game is a long one, and the goal is to slowly accumulate steps and actions to stack the deck in your favour. With that in mind, let the games begin!

CHAPTER 7
MOVE

As you have no doubt figured out by now, I've done a lot of exercise in my life. I've competed in rowing, running, triathlon, CrossFit, powerlifting, and strongman (that sport where people pick up rocks and pull trucks). I've coached athletes in most of those sports and several others. I've also done research looking at how exercise impacts brain function. As a result, you won't be surprised if I admit that I am a bit biased when it comes to advocating for the benefits of exercise—or any kind of movement, for that matter. But you might be surprised to hear that these personal experiences haven't always helped me spread the message of the importance of physical activity. More times than I can remember, people have told me they think I'm going to recommend some kind of gruelling exercise programme that requires hours of toil in the gym every day. To me, this really shows the complex relationship that many modernised societies have with physical activity and physical appearance.

In one way we idolise physical feats. The world's best are global superstars. Taking part in endurance events such as marathons and triathlons has also become baked into the common idea of what it means to be fit or healthy. Don't get me wrong: organised athletic events of all kinds are amazing, and I love it when people do any kind of physical activity that they enjoy and that also pushes them. But the downside is that for those of us not regularly engaged in physical activity, having certain kinds of events or activities held up as a benchmark of what counts as exercise can be daunting and off-putting because it encourages us to think being fit has to involve long and arduous sessions pounding the streets.

While endurance exercise is often promoted as a fitness ideal, lifting weights (also known as resistance training) can get a bad rap. Compared to the health and fitness benefits we associate with running, lifting weights is thought to be more about vanity. We might even imagine cult heroes like Arnold Schwarzenegger, Sylvester Stallone, or Dwayne "The Rock" Johnson, whose impressive physical stature has often (incorrectly) been assumed to be associated with lower cognitive capabilities. After all, isn't it true that we can have brains *or* brawn but not both?

Popular portrayals of resistance training can also be problematic in other ways related to how we think people should look. This includes creating a muscle-bound image of masculinity that is unrealistic while also implying that lifting weights is somehow not feminine. But lifting weights or building some muscle and strength isn't about looking like Arnie or Iris Kyle (the most successful bodybuilder—male or female—of all time). It's about building the kind of physical and cognitive headroom that allows us to remain independent and kicking ass for decades into the future. This is a message that often gets lost. And that's before we even consider having to navigate the endless raft of scantily clad influencers on social media trying to sell us their weight-loss and muscle-gain programmes.

All of this is then compounded by what paleoanthropologist Daniel Lieberman calls "the medicalization of exercise." Partly because of folklore but also due to the way exercise is studied—using rigorously regimented programmes based on a certain number of sessions of a certain set of exercises for a certain amount of time—we assume that physical activity can be prescribed like a pill, and that there is some strict amount or type of activity we have to do to get fit. For those of us just trying to be healthier, all these societal inputs make us assume that we don't have time to do the amount of exercise we would need to do to improve, and that any physical activity below that ideal level will be a waste of time. As a result, many people just don't see themselves as exercisers or athletes.

I'm happy to tell you that none of this has to be true.

Aside from my own personal interest in physical activity, one of the reasons I present movement first among the tactics we can use to win the game of brain health is that it's easy to see how each of the rules of the game applies to movement. My favourite example is that *everything*

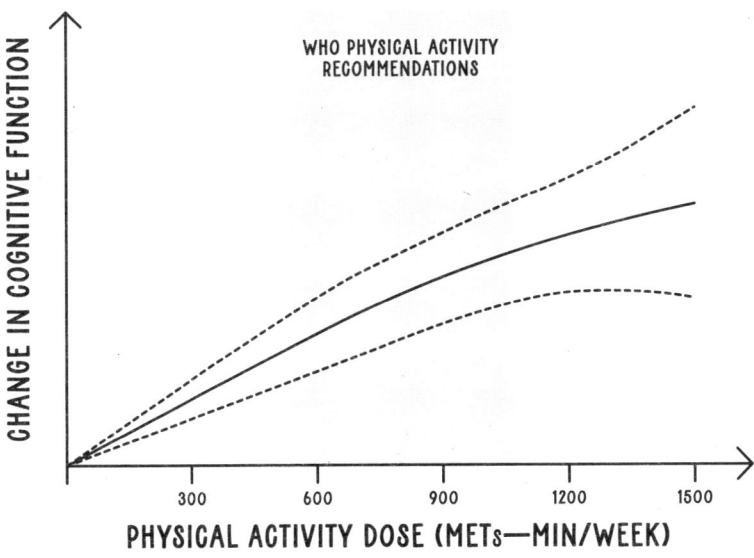

FIGURE 1. Results from a meta-analysis showing total physical activity dose along the bottom and associated improvements in cognitive function on the side. Physical activity dose is determined by multiplying how intense the activity is (metabolic equivalents, or METs) by the number of minutes you do it for. The box shows the standard World Health Organization (WHO) guidelines of 150–300 minutes of moderate-to-vigourous activity per week, which can be achieved with any combination of activities, including 45 minutes of housework, 30 minutes of brisk walking, 20 minutes of swimming/dancing/resistance training, or 5 minutes of sprinting per day. The key takeaway is that even small increases in physical activity can improve brain health and function, with almost all of the benefit seen just by doing a relatively short period of movement on most days. Adapted from Gallardo-Gómez et al., *Ageing Research Reviews* 2022.

counts when it comes to physical activity. For almost every health-related outcome you care to consider, *any* increase in physical activity above what you're doing now will, on average, reduce disease risk and be better for your brain (figure 1).[1]

Of course, whenever I say that, there are inevitably purists who feel the need to tell me that doing more exercise when you're already doing a lot may increase the risk of injury or overtraining. This is true and has affected me personally, as well as many of the athletes I've worked with. But I think we can agree that for most people the problem is too little movement rather than too much. If, on the other hand, you're currently training every day and have a training plan that balances multiple intensities of cardio training alongside resistance work (and you understand this sentence), you can skip ahead a couple of pages if you like.

Exercise really does have an impressive effect on brain health. A recent meta-meta-analysis (meta-analysis of meta-analyses) that included more than 250,000 participants from over 2,700 randomised controlled trials found that exercise significantly improved general cognition, memory, and executive function (planning and decision-making) regardless of age or whether individuals were healthy or already suffering from some degree of cognitive impairment.[2] Importantly, you can benefit from exercise no matter when you start. For example, a study of more than thirty thousand people in Norway followed for twenty years found that those who increased their fitness in their fifties and sixties decreased their subsequent risk of dementia.[3] Though not all studies find the same relationships, higher fitness and physical activity later in life may also be associated with lower Alzheimer's risk biomarkers related to amyloid and tau accumulation in the brain.[4] And even more importantly, movement and fitness have consistently been shown to reduce the risk of cognitive decline and dementia regardless of their effect on amyloid and tau.

As scientists have learned more and more about how physical activity benefits health, we have had to reframe some of our ideas about how movement affects our biology. Counterintuitively, in many ways it's not that *exercise* is itself beneficial. This is because exercise—structured and planned physical activity—is a modern concept that would be completely alien to most humans in history, even our very recent ancestors. After all, why would you waste valuable calories doing something strenuous that has no immediate purpose? Evolutionarily, we are hardwired to seek opportunities for inactivity whenever we can, because historically this was not something that was easy to come by. Put another way, the default human response is to avoid anything that looks like exercise unless it is absolutely necessary.

Unfortunately, though, our natural tendency toward being sedentary has some downsides in the modern environment. This is because our evolutionary history has inextricably linked physical activity to our biology. As a species that has spent tens of thousands of years moving—be that hunting, gathering, or farming for food, migrating for safety, or dancing for pleasure—movement regulates a whole host of pathways across the entire body that keep us healthy. One of my favourite quotes that encapsulates this comes from Iñigo San-Millán, who is an expert in both exercise physiology and human metabolism: "Physical activity is a canonical evolutionary characteristic of humans that remains embedded in our genes. The normalization of a lack of physical activity in our modern society has led to the perception that exercise is an 'intervention.'"[5]

What this means is that our physiology *requires* movement to function at its best. As a result, being sedentary negatively impacts our health. The nature of the modern environment, then, means that we've had to invent exercise to counteract the effects of not moving regularly. While different types of exercise do have different effects on the brain and body, a lot of the overall benefit comes from spending less time being sedentary. This is why *everything counts* when it comes to physical activity, and any increase in any kind of physical activity is expected to improve cognitive function.

As you'll see, a common theme in this book is that the function of the body is directly related to how we use it. Exercise affects the *entire* body, even if we're only working one part of it. Imagine you've gone for a bike ride. When we move the muscles in our legs, they start to take up glucose from the bloodstream for energy, which can help to regulate blood sugar. As our heart rate increases, increased blood flow from the heart to the muscles and the brain improves the health of those blood vessels, reducing blood pressure and risk of heart disease. That increase in blood flow to the brain, as well as the neurotransmitters like dopamine and noradrenaline released during exercise, then provide an immediate boost in well-being and cognitive function.[6]

When they contract, muscles also release a whole host of factors called myokines that go out into the body and support the function of organs such as the brain. Multiple other parts of the body also get involved. Myokines make up part of a bigger class of compounds called exerkines released by the liver, pancreas, and even bones during exercise.[7] Some of the best-studied examples of exerkines include brain-derived neurotrophic factor (BDNF)—a protein that supports nerve function and neuroplasticity—as well as the cytokine interleukin-6 (IL-6). IL-6 is a protein involved in inflammation that peaks during exercise, but this short spike in inflammation signaling actually *decreases* baseline levels of inflammation. In general, both higher BDNF levels—especially in the brain—and lower levels of markers related to inflammation are associated with better cognitive function and lower risk of dementia.[8]

Through the release of exerkines as well as the direct effects of exercise on the metabolism of all the organs involved in the response to movement, exercise activates anti-ageing pathways throughout the entire body, including in the liver and the brain.[9] One example of the critical anti-ageing pathways activated by exercise is autophagy—the process that cells use to clear out and recycle junky proteins and other components that accumulate with use and age. Though we're often told that fasting is the best way to kickstart autophagy and longevity in general, in humans, autophagy happens much faster and more consistently with exercise.[10] Amazingly, though we need to infer some of this from animal studies because it's hard to measure in humans, physical activity seems to be the only thing that helps to slow or reverse *all* the hallmarks of ageing—through autophagy and other means—in multiple organs including the brain.[11] This is why biochemist Bill Lagakos likes to say that "exercise is fasting in fast-forward." If you've ever gone searching for the fountain of youth, regular movement is as close as it gets!

A MOVEMENT FRAMEWORK FOR THE BRAIN

I like the idea of moving away from the concept of exercise as an intervention and instead thinking about movement as a core requirement of our physiology, because it allows us to be less rigid and prescriptive. It also allows us to have a lot more flexibility when we're building health- and brain-supporting movement into our schedules.

On the other hand, I know that simply saying "move some more" is spectacularly unhelpful. I've lost count of the number of times I've heard a doctor (including myself) hurriedly say this to one of their patients at the end of a consultation, everybody knowing, but not acknowledging, that this very vague advice will probably never be acted upon. So I do think it's helpful to have a framework to work from, allowing us to focus on physical activity in a way that can support our brain health and function but that also adapts to our interests, time, and capabilities.

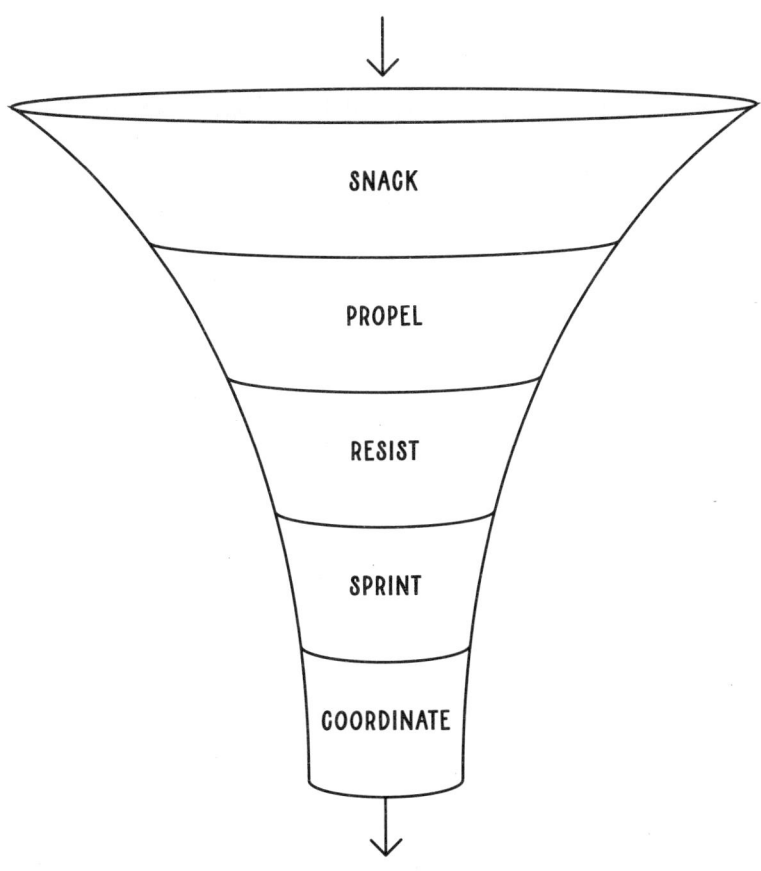

FIGURE 2. The movement funnel. Ideally we want to start at the top by focusing on the movement that represents the widest part of the funnel, before moving through and adding as we go. Many of the lower levels of the funnel have a similar importance, so they have a similar width.

Enter the movement funnel.

More than a decade ago, right as I was starting my PhD and spending my spare time writing blogs about health, I wrote a series on a movement framework for people who wanted to live longer and healthier lives without necessarily having to spend hours every day in the gym.[12] I've tinkered with it a little bit since then as we've learned more about how exercise supports health and brain function, and the shape has morphed from an upside-down pyramid to a funnel. But the core components remain the same, and unlike a traditional pyramid I remain convinced that it's better upside down (figure 2).

Aesthetically, a funnel makes sense to me because we want to start by focusing on the exercises that represent the widest parts, where we enter the funnel. A funnel is also something that we move *through*, adding and combining different exercise types and intensities as we go.

SNACK

By *snack* I unfortunately don't mean eating chips between sets of squats. I mean exercise snacks. These are our entry into the movement funnel. Thought to be first coined in a 2007 article by Howard Hartley in *Newsweek*, the term *exercise snack* made it into the published literature in 2014 when a paper showed that in people with prediabetes, doing six one-minute bouts of exercise before meals—either brisk hill walking or resistance training with bands—resulted in better blood sugar control than a thirty-minute jog.[13] Since then, multiple studies have found that breaking up movement into multiple small sessions across the day provides at least as much benefit, and sometimes even more benefit, than the same amount of exercise done as one long continuous session.[14]

It turns out there's a lot of magic that can come from very brief periods of movement. Practically speaking, these exercise snacks are simply a way to break up prolonged periods of being sedentary. In fact, the base of my original movement pyramid was called "sit less," which is fairly accurate but also a little too specific. Over the years, several studies have found that more time being sedentary is associated with lower cognitive function and a higher risk of both dementia and death. Though exercise does seem to offset most of the risk, spending very long periods being sedentary each day may be associated with increased dementia risk even in those who exercise.[15]

The reason "snack" is a better starting point than "sit less" is that sitting is a perfectly normal thing for humans to do. Even current hunter-gatherers and other less modernised societies spend a lot of time sitting or being sedentary—maybe even as much total time as we do when we're chained to a desk during the day.[16] The difference is that traditional forms of being sedentary don't involve several hours sitting in a chair or lying semicomatose on the sofa. Instead, they involve squatting or sitting on the ground, which requires our muscles to be much more active than they are when we're in a chair.[17] More traditional sitting positions result in more frequent movement because it's hard to hold one position for a long time if you haven't got some comfy cushions to hold you up.

So the problem is not necessarily the sitting; it's *how* we sit—fairly still and with minimal effort. A recent study of fifty thousand adults aged sixty years or older from the UK explored sedentary behaviour and later dementia risk, taking into account levels of physical activity.[18] What the study found was that only longer *unbroken* periods of being sedentary were associated with higher dementia risk. Put another way, if we accumulate a lot of time not moving during the day—which we often do for work or while we relax—it seems that we can offset that simply by breaking it up.

If this sounds too good (or easy) to be true, I get it. Over the years I've had several contraptions—rings, watches, and other wrist-worn devices—that measure sleep and movement. Many of them have a function that tells you to get up when you've been sitting still for a long period of time. I used to scoff at these notifications. After all, I do plenty of exercise. Just the act of getting out of my chair can't make *that* much of a difference, right? This idea was tested in a recent trial in sixty-to-seventy-year-old adults, half of whom received some coaching and a wearable to prompt them to sit less, based on personalised goals.[19] After six months, those who received the intervention spent around thirty minutes less per day sitting, and amazingly, their blood pressure reduced by an amount that would be enough to meaningfully reduce their risk of heart disease,[20] which is a major risk factor for dementia.

In addition to improving heart health, a wide range of studies suggest that just a few daily bouts of movement for less than a minute can significantly improve overall health and brain function.[21] For instance, a recent study found that three hours of sitting decreased blood flow to the brain, resulting in reduced executive function (rapid decision-making), decreased focus, and increased fatigue. All these effects of sitting were improved by doing some exercise snacking—fifteen squats every twenty minutes during the three-hour sitting period.[22] To do this squat snack you simply stand up, sit back into your chair without letting the chair take your full weight, stand up again, and repeat fifteen times.

A PANTRY FULL OF EXERCISE SNACKS

It's helpful to think of the snack level of the funnel in two parts. The first is simply taking a moment to break up periods of being sedentary, which might look like:

- Getting up to walk around or do some light stretching.
- Alternating between sitting and standing if your desk or work environment allows that.
- Sitting in different positions where your legs or body are doing more of the work to hold you up (Swiss ball optional).
- Sitting or squatting on the floor while watching TV (which can be surprisingly comfortable, and I do regularly despite sceptical looks from my wife).
- Literally anything that involves not being in the same position you've been in for the past two hours.

The second part of snacking is about adding more dynamic bursts. A large meta-analysis showed that several different types of movement can be used to break up prolonged periods of being sedentary and significantly improve cognitive function.[23] These included:

- Walking or climbing stairs
- Push-ups
- Squats, lunges, or calf raises
- Skipping
- Jogging or running (or dancing) in place
- Hopping
- Star jumps

In general, these snacks only need to last a minute or two, with interventions in most studies lasting no more than five minutes. As a starting point for your movement practice, think about breaking up your sitting at least every hour, with more dynamic movement a couple of times a day.

Many studies use the squat as an intervention because it requires minimal equipment and can be done by most people. However, for the purposes of these snacks, any movement that involves moving several muscles in the body would do the trick. It could be star jumps or push-ups. Or, if that sounds a bit too much like boot camp in the middle of the workday, try taking the stairs. In people new to exercise, bouts of as little as twenty seconds of climbing stairs have been shown to improve health and fitness without any additional exercise.[24] And, while I absolutely encourage people to purposefully head out to the stairwell for a few extra flights throughout the day, a great start is simply committing to take the stairs whenever you need to go to a different floor.

I know, I know, you've heard this many times before. But I promise it can make a big difference. For example, in nearly five hundred thousand adults who were part of the UK Biobank study, taking just five flights of stairs (fifty stairs total) a day was associated with a significant reduction in heart disease and strokes,[25] both of which are risk factors for later dementia.

Another study from the UK Biobank looked at intermittent vigourous movement measured with a wearable device, specifically in people who said they didn't exercise. Those who accumulated at least seven minutes of vigourous activity (like climbing stairs) per day offset the increased risk of worse health outcomes associated with being sedentary. Benefits were seen with as little as one to two minutes of activity per day.[26] Amazingly enough, these short daily bouts of movement were also associated with better health outcomes in people who regularly exercised. This is one reason I annoy my colleagues at work and make them take the stairs.

To recap, the top of the movement funnel, and the most important place we can all start to support our brain health through movement, is simply moving more frequently. Practically speaking, this is anything that breaks up long periods of being sedentary. More benefit will be seen with more intense exercise snacks such as climbing stairs or doing some squats, and more does seem to be better. But most importantly, these snacks don't require any equipment, getting changed, or heading to the gym. And they also benefit us regardless of how much time we spend doing exercises further down the funnel.

PROPEL

In 1949, at the age of twenty-eight, my grandfather Sidney Wood started a new job as a postman in London. This involved a lot of low-level physical activity—about two-thirds of his workday would have been spent walking, with some added stair climbing and cycling. Though he didn't know it at the time, the nature of this work meant my grandfather's postal colleagues were about to be included in what many consider to be the first systematic epidemiological study of physical activity and health.

In the late 1940s, epidemiologist Jeremy Morris began to explore the relationship between physical activity at work and heart disease. In their classic 1953 study, Morris and his colleagues looked at deaths due to heart disease in London transport workers. Specifically, they compared the outcomes of conductors, who walked up and down double-decker buses all day collecting fares, to the drivers of those same buses.[27] As the groups were demographically similar, this allowed Morris to examine the effect of spending most of the workday either sitting or walking. What he found was that conductors had around half the risk of heart attacks compared to drivers.

As any good scientist would hope to do, Morris sought to validate his findings in another group. This is where the postmen came in. Using 1949–50 data from the UK Treasury Medical Service, they compared postmen aged thirty-five to fifty-nine who pounded the pavements (as we call them back home) to telephone operators and clerks who did desk work. Heart disease rates were around 25 percent lower in postmen than in desk workers, and more senior postal workers who were less active than postmen but also spent a good amount of their day on their feet were somewhere in between.

Compared to being sedentary, walking has therefore been known to improve heart-health outcomes for over seventy years, though it took some time for scientists to fully appreciate how heart health also impacts the brain. Some of the first evidence came in 1978 from the Seattle Longitudinal Study, where following the same individuals over decades showed that cardiovascular disease was associated with more rapid cognitive decline.[28] And we now also know that, in addition to improving heart health, walking *directly* supports the health and function of our brains in both the short and long term.

As human beings, walking is our most fundamental form of physical activity. While nonhuman primates walk a lot more (and climb a lot less) than you might think—chimpanzees are estimated to take somewhere around five thousand steps per day—one of many differences between humans and other primates is how much we walk. For most of

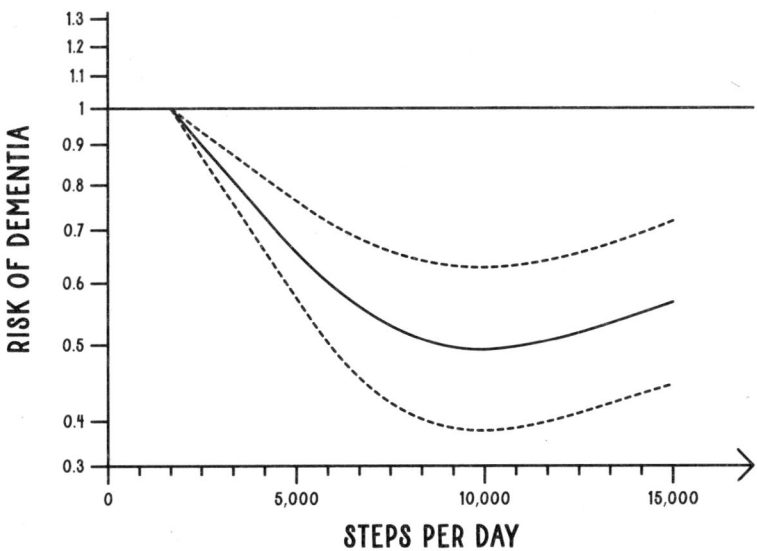

FIGURE 3. Steps per day and risk of dementia. Risk decreases linearly with more steps—the more the better but with no hard level of steps required per day—up to around 10,000 per day. After that, more steps can still be beneficial, but the risk of dementia doesn't seem to decrease any further. Adapted from del Pozo Cruz et al., *JAMA Neurology* 2022.

our history, humans are thought to have taken around fifteen to twenty thousand steps per day on average.[29] In modernised countries, the average is now around a quarter of that, with global and U.S. estimates suggesting that people take around five thousand steps per day. This large drop in time spent walking has resulted in hours per day of movement that we're not getting anymore, removing a critical signal to the body to maintain and improve function. And as we've already seen, even small amounts of physical activity can have a huge impact.

Since those first studies in the 1950s, the evidence has continued to accumulate that physical activity such as walking is directly associated with better brain health and lower risk of multiple chronic diseases, including dementia. And, as with exercise snacks, it doesn't take much to see a big benefit. For example, in a study of over seventy-five thousand adults who were mostly fifty to seventy years old, those who took four thousand steps per day had a 25 percent lower risk of dementia than those who took fifteen hundred steps per day. From there, more steps were better until around ten thousand steps (figure 3), and similar results have been found for many other chronic diseases as well as overall risk of death.[30]

As with exercise snacks, all of us could benefit from doing more walking. But up to that point somewhere around ten thousand steps per day the effect of walking is essentially linear. This means that the more steps you do compared to what you are doing now, the more benefit you see. For each additional thousand steps you do per day above fifteen hundred, the risk of dementia decreases by around 7–8 percent, and the overall risk of dying decreases by around 15 percent.[31] Walking, therefore, is a low-risk, free, and easy way to add brain-supporting movement to your day.

The linear relationship between walking and health also means that you don't need to hit a certain number of steps to see a benefit. In fact, the well-known target of ten thousand steps is still debated by two camps—those who are advocates and those who say the number ten thousand has more to do with marketing than science. This is because, as the story goes, that target came from Manpo-kei ("ten-thousand-step metre"), the name of a popular sixties-era Japanese step counter.[32] Decades later, it turns out that the overall benefits of walking do seem to increase up to somewhere around ten thousand steps per day, so maybe both camps are right. However, the scientist in me wants to say that a range of eight to twelve thousand would be more accurate, while also pointing out that anything is better than nothing regardless of the final number.

Though walking is a fundamental part of human movement and evolution, one reason it is so widely used in scientific studies is that steps are easier to measure than other physical activities. For my part, I'm a big fan of walking because it is a simple and accessible form of activity that provides a base level of fitness and movement that allows us to benefit even more from other activities in the rest of the funnel.[33] But that doesn't mean that other types of movement don't have similar benefits. And while not everybody can walk long distances in a day, they might be able to do other activities—cycling, rowing, swimming, propelling a wheelchair—that would have very similar benefits. This is the essence of the second level of the movement funnel—"propel."

Once you've started breaking up periods of sitting with some movement snacks, the next step is to add more extended periods of movement at intensities similar to a (brisk) walk or light run. This includes pretty much anything that might be considered "moderate" physical activity, such as dancing or gardening. Similar to "snack," "propel" also has two levels. The first is general movement, like walking, where anything counts, regardless of intensity. If you're not regularly taking several thousand steps per day, this is where you should start: simply by trying to build on what you're currently doing. For instance, you could aim to add a thousand steps or ten to fifteen minutes of your preferred type of movement in a day. If possible, you can build movement into your workday by having walking meetings, which may improve mood, creative thinking, and productivity at work in addition to adding some steps.[34]

PROPELLING YOUR BRAIN FORWARD

Nowadays it can be fairly easy to determine how much you're propelling yourself on a daily basis. If you have a smartphone with you when you're going about your day, all of them contain an app that estimates your number of steps. Though they're not necessary, pretty much any smartwatch or basic wrist-worn fitness tracker can also estimate steps with at least enough accuracy for you to track your activity trends over time.

After assessing your starting point, try increasing your activity by 5 to 10 percent per day—either adding steps or doing some more coordinated movement periods once or twice a week. The possibilities are almost endless, but include:

- Walking (obviously) or jogging
- Hiking
- Cycling or spinning
- Rowing
- Swimming
- Stair climbers or elliptical machines
- Dancing (in a class, in your living room, at a rave)
- Aerobics (classes, apps, or even that old Jane Fonda video)
- Golf

The next level of "propel" involves making things a bit brisker, up to the point where you get a little out of breath but could still hold a conversation if you had to. Once walking is "brisk" (at least 2.5 miles per hour or one hundred steps per minute), it counts as moderate physical activity. The amount of moderate-to-vigourous activity that people do in a day is one of the best predictors of their daily cognitive function.[35] And just like with steps, even small amounts of moderate physical activity can have a big effect. One analysis of data from the United States suggested that just ten minutes of moderate physical activity per day would be enough to reduce risk of death by 7 percent over a decade.[36] Adding thirty minutes of moderate physical activity per day might even be enough to overcome most of the health risks associated with being sedentary the rest of the time.[37]

Brisk walking and similar activities like cycling appear to directly reverse some of the impact of ageing on the brain.[38] As we age, several areas of the brain shrink over time, and this shrinking accelerates once we experience significant cognitive decline or dementia. One part of the brain that is particularly vulnerable to decreases in size with age is the hippocampus, which is critical to memory and is negatively affected in multiple forms of dementia, especially Alzheimer's disease. In one of the first studies to show that age-related brain changes in adults in their sixties and seventies could be slowed or even reversed, an exercise programme that involved forty minutes of brisk walking three times per week resulted in a 2 percent *increase* in size of the hippocampi over a year instead of the expected 1 to 2 percent decrease in size.[39]

The walking protocol in this study is both simple and effective and can be translated to any kind of activity that gets your heart rate up in a similar way. Participants started by walking for ten minutes three times per week, increasing by five minutes each week until they hit forty minutes. They then increased the intensity over time but remained walking. As with most exercise, intensity did seem to be important because those people who gained the most fitness on the programme saw the biggest increases in hippocampus size. This increase in hippocampal size was also related to increases in BDNF, which directly supports the health and growth of neurons. The release of neurotrophic factors like BDNF is thought to be one of the primary mechanisms by which exercise promotes neuroplasticity as well as improving the function of brain regions involved in memory (like the hippocampus) and decision-making (like the prefrontal cortex).[40] In this way, aerobic exercise increases headroom and the ability to learn, as well as future-proofing your brain by improving the function of brain networks that tend to decline with age.

The fact that just three walking sessions per week could reverse some of the aging-related changes in brain size still astounds me to this day. Multiple other studies have shown that brisk walking and similar activities can significantly improve cardiovascular fitness.[41] This increase in fitness is critically important for both dementia risk and brain health, with no minimum amount required to see a benefit.[42] Various aerobic exercises have also been shown to have clinically meaningful effects on mental health and well-being, for instance leading to decreased symptoms of depression.

Those who have higher fitness levels tend to perform better on cognitive function tests, have better white matter structure as they age, and have a lower risk of dementia long-term.[43] Aerobic exercise is particularly beneficial for improving memory as well as supporting overall cognitive function.[44] And most importantly, when it comes to our overall health, how fit we are is more important than our body weight or BMI.[45]

Summarising the two top levels of the pyramid at this point, the goal is to try to break up your day with small pieces of movement as much as you can ("snack"). After that, you can make those snack breaks longer or set aside some time to "propel" toward longer periods of activity. Once you've hit a good target (say thirty to forty minutes at least three times per week), you can try to get more bang for your buck by increasing the intensity of some of your movement so that you're regularly getting out of breath. And as you get fitter, this could look something like brisk walking, hill walking, light running, or any activity that feels similar—cycling (by foot or hand), rowing, swimming, propelling a wheelchair, skipping, etc.

And once you're doing that, it's time for the next level!

RESIST

At this point I hope that you're convinced that even small amounts of movement—including those that don't look very much like "exercise"—can have a big impact on our health and our brains. But if you're snacking regularly and doing some good moderate physical activity a few times a week and are ready for more, or if most of your current exercise focuses on cardio, it's time to lift some weights!

If the thought of pumping iron conjures images of sweaty, steroid-enhanced physiques in Speedos (you're welcome) or debilitating back injuries (scary but not a major concern), you're not alone. The most common comments I hear about lifting weights are from people who are worried about looking bulky or getting injured. But, interestingly, the type and amount of resistance training that most of us will benefit from tends to have exactly the opposite effects. And while it doesn't have to include a gym or lifting weights, moving our bodies against resistance is a critical component of maintaining the strength and function that we need for our brains to be at their best for as long as possible. For example, a study of female twins (comparing twins with different lifestyles helps to remove any effects of genetics) from Kings College London found that leg power was an important predictor of how slowly cognitive function declined over the next ten years, as well as later grey matter volume.[46] Building muscles builds headroom!

I've long been fascinated with the human capacity for strength. More than a decade before I ever set foot in a gym, I remember sitting close to the TV at Christmas every year watching the World's Strongest Man competition. This was the era of Jón Páll Sigmarsson and Magnús Ver Magnússon, two Icelandic four-time champions who dominated the competition for more than a decade. In nearly fifty years of competition, only the United States—which has a population more than a thousand times larger—has won or been on the World's Strongest Man podium more times than Iceland. Being half Icelandic myself, this was a huge source of personal pride when I was a kid. Iceland didn't become a hot (pun intended) tourist destination until several years later, so watching these compatriots of mine on TV was one of the few times I got to see Iceland represented on an international stage.

Something that has continued to fascinate me about strongman competitions is that if you scale them down, the fundamental principle of what the athletes are doing is critical to all of us. The muscles and movements needed for a mountain-sized human to pull jumbo jets, carry ship anchors, and lift enormous boulders are the same as those required to take out a bin, carry a load of shopping, and lift a heavy box onto a shelf. In many ways these abilities are also critical to survival, cognitive function, and mental health. But they are also increasingly being lost.

Just like the size of our brains, the size and strength of our muscles tends to decline with age. By the time we get into our fifties and beyond, we're losing about 1 percent of our muscle mass per year, and strength is lost two to three times faster.[47] Muscles also have their own version of dementia—the point at which the loss of function is enough to impair daily activities—called sarcopenia. Sarcopenia and cognitive decline are directly related, with increasing physical frailty frequently tied to increased risk of later dementia.[48] Part of this is due to the decreased activity and increased number of illnesses people experience as they get more frail, but muscles that are sarcopenic can also create an inflammatory state in the body that seems to directly impact the brain.[49]

Though some brain and muscle losses are an inevitable part of ageing and can be caused by chronic diseases that affect both the body and the brain, the loss of muscle and brain function are also intimately connected to what we do and don't do with our bodies as we get older. Recalling Ellen Langer's stereotype-embodiment theory from part 1, if we *think* we're supposed to get frail and weak as we get older, we stop engaging in activities that maintain muscle and strength, and our prophecy becomes self-fulfilling.

In chapter 4 ("Dominance of the Environment") I mentioned a study of mine that showed that leg strength in older individuals was strongly associated with how quickly they processed information.[50] More specifically, we found that of all the physical-activity variables we had access to, relative leg strength was the most important. The word *relative* is important here because the way we analysed the data accounted for differences in body size that can affect muscle mass. The real takeaway is that you only need your legs (or body in general) to be strong enough for *you*.

Keeping relative strength in mind is important because sometimes it can be easy to be left feeling a little lacking in the "gains" department. The first time I ever took part in a strongman competition, my wife turned to me as the other competitors filed in and said, "These guys make you look so *tiny*." Just what every man loves to hear. The differences were even more stark when I recently met with Hafþór Júlíus Björnsson—

former World's Strongest Man who played The Mountain on *Game of Thrones*—at his gym in Reykjavík. As we chatted about brain health, I had to work hard to keep my cool while he casually did sets of shoulder presses using dumbbells that each weighed nearly as much as I do.

The extremes of human jackedness aside, what does strong *enough* mean? This is a surprisingly tricky question to answer because every study uses different machines and techniques to measure strength. However, a consistent message seems to be that those whose strength and muscle mass is in the top third of the population tend to see most of the benefit in terms of both longevity and dementia risk.[51] Therefore, you could start by imagining a room full of people similar to you and thinking about how many you could beat in an arm-wrestling match. If it's not two-thirds, you have some bicep curls to do! Similarly, when it comes to having strong enough legs, being able to lift twice your body weight in an exercise like the leg press would be an excellent target. Luckily, as most people don't do any kind of regular resistance training, being in the top third of the population doesn't necessarily require a huge amount of time or herculean efforts in the gym, as you'll see.

Though I am a self-confessed lifting enthusiast with a clear bias toward resistance training, I have still been amazed by the amount of evidence that supports the importance of muscle mass, strength, and resistance training for enhancing and maintaining cognitive function and mental health. This is important no matter how old we are. For instance, in school-aged youth, resistance training can positively affect focus and academic performance.[52] Unfortunately, due to changes in physical activity patterns, young people are increasingly at risk of having inadequate muscle and strength to support their health. Strength in the general population of young people seems to be decreasing, and one recent analysis estimated that one in ten young people is already sarcopenic.[53]

Though there are a number of complex factors involved, decreasing muscle mass and strength may be contributing to the increasing burden of psychological distress in young people. For instance, lower grip strength is associated with a higher risk of future depression and anxiety.[54] Sarcopenia is also associated with a higher likelihood of having depression.[55] Some of this may again be due to a common disease process that causes both loss of strength and increased depression symptoms, such as a chronic inflammatory condition. It's also possible that those who are at risk of depression are less likely to engage in activities that build muscle and strength. However, regardless of the cause, there is evidence that resistance training can directly improve mental health.

In a trial of resistance training in young adults in their twenties, lifting weights twice a week for eight weeks resulted in large, clinically meaningful improvements in depression symptoms.[56] The effects were biggest in those who had worse anxiety or depression symptoms to start with but did not depend on how much strength an individual gained. That means that the simple act of taking part in a resistance training programme was enough to significantly improve mood.

A recent large meta-analysis of interventions for depression symptoms that compared multiple types of exercise found that in some studies, strength training had an effect on par with medications and therapy.[57] This doesn't mean exercise is a replacement for standard treatments, and I have to admit that more large trials need to be done, but these results are in line with the wide number of ways that we know that our muscles support our brains.

The connection between muscle mass, strength training, mood, and cognitive function is important for those struggling with their mental health but also as we think about building headroom and future-proofing our brains with the goal of supporting long-term cognitive function. For instance, depression and dementia are intimately linked and often occur together as we age, with one increasing the risk of the other.[58] And since our muscle mass tends to decrease with age, building a buffer of muscle and strength also makes it more likely that we'll have more strength, well-being, and cognitive function later in life.

Muscle mass and resistance training can positively impact our cognition in a number of ways, including lowering inflammation, improving blood pressure and cardiovascular health, regulating blood sugar, and protecting mitochondrial function, as well as raising the levels of growth factors that support the production of new cells and connections in the brain. (For the nerds, these include a veritable alphabet soup of BDNF, VEGF, and IGF-1 in addition to other signaling molecules like lactate, taurine, osteocalcin, irisin, MOTS-c, and Lac-Phe.)[59] Specific to resistance training seems to be an increase in the growth factor IGF-1, low levels of which are associated with both sarcopenia and dementia.[60] Because our muscles are our biggest users of blood sugar, doing resistance training to build more muscle may also be the best form of movement to improve blood sugar control—especially important for those with prediabetes or type 2 diabetes who are at higher risk of cognitive decline and dementia.[61] A recent meta-analysis found that regular resistance training also decreases at least one major marker of inflammation in the body (C-reactive protein, CRP).[62]

As scientists are continuously discovering new pathways activated by exercise, we don't necessarily know exactly how or why aerobic and resistance training are different when it comes to how they act on the brain. But we do know that different areas of the brain and different cognitive functions are preferentially supported by different types of exercise. This means it isn't necessarily a matter of cardio or weights being better—both muscle mass and fitness are important. But the reason that "resist" comes after "propel" in the funnel is that, for people who are sedentary, even brisk walking may be enough to start building muscle and improving muscle function.[63]

When comparing different types of exercise and their effects on the brain, resistance training seems to be particularly good at improving decision-making or executive function. Some colleagues and I recently summarised studies of resistance training and brain structure, and though the number of trials was low, they consistently showed that resistance training had a protective effect on the white matter, which is responsible for maintaining fast connections within the brain.[64] Also, those who were older or already experiencing some cognitive decline appeared to benefit more. As IGF-1 levels are related to white matter structure, this is probably one mechanism by which resistance training can improve and maintain the white matter of the brain as we age.[65]

Contrary to popular belief, then, lifting weights is not just a young person's game. In fact, it's a game that we should all play if we want to become as old as possible. And most importantly, it's never too late to start. There are dozens of studies that show resistance training improves health and cognitive function in older individuals, including those who are frail due to sarcopenia or osteoporosis, or who have limited mobility.[66]

Several decades ago, the prestigious *Journal of the American Medical Association* (*JAMA*) published a small study called "High-Intensity

Strength Training in Nonagenarians."[67] Ten frail individuals, the oldest of whom was ninety-six, took part in leg training three times per week for eight weeks, which resulted in significant increases in muscle, strength, and walking speed. More recent studies have found that resistance training initiated at retirement provides several additional years of improved muscle function, and individuals in their eighties respond just as well to resistance exercise as those in their sixties and seventies.[68] In general, studies show that resistance training has benefits for cognitive function across all age groups, for men and for women—the latter both before and after menopause.

Women gain muscle and strength relative to where they start just as quickly as men do,[69] and several studies also show that women can perform *more* repetitions of a strength exercise at a given intensity (a certain percentage of their maximum) than men can.[70] Lifting weights is important to help maintain muscle and strength before, during, and after menopause, and can help to maintain bone strength as women get older. Therefore, though muscle mass tends to decrease steadily over time for all of us, the best way to combat this is to focus on resistance exercise (and protein, see the next chapter). In fact, a famous study by evolutionary anthropologist Herman Pontzer found that metabolism doesn't necessarily slow down as we get older, as we're often told. Instead, it mainly slows down as we lose muscle mass.[71] With gyms and fitness trends increasingly focusing on the importance of muscle mass and strength for women and older people, I'm happy to see that people are catching up to these important findings.[72]

When it comes to what a resistance training programme should look like, there are some general guidelines but also a lot of flexibility. Just one session per week for a few weeks is enough for people to see improvements in muscle and strength.[73] Most study protocols use five to eight machines that any gym would have, making sure to train the whole body. This might include a leg press or leg extension, a hamstring curl, a horizontal pressing motion (like a chest press or push-up), a rowing or pulling motion, and a vertical pressing motion (like a shoulder press). These are done for one to three sets of five to fifteen repetitions, one to three times per week.

A nice example is the protocol from SMART (Study of Mental and Resistance Training), which had participants in their sixties and seventies do three sets of eight repetitions of chest press, leg press, seated row, hip abduction, and leg extension two times per week for six months.[74] This protocol resulted in improved global cognitive and executive function that was maintained for eighteen months after the end of the study.

Training in a typical gym does have some upsides—the machines are very similar, no matter where you are, and require minimal prior experience to get started. But a resistance training programme doesn't *have* to involve a gym. The legendary strength coach Dan John describes five basic human movements that would be an excellent way to build a resistance training programme anywhere, with any kind of equipment:

- Push (a movement pressing weight away from the body)
- Pull (a movement pulling weight toward the body)
- Hinge (bending over at the hips—usually picking something up off the floor)
- Squat (bending at the knees)
- Carry (walking with something heavy in your hands at your sides or in your arms in front of you)

You can pick pretty much anything in each category that allows you to work hard against some resistance—for instance, with resistance bands or objects you have at home. During the Covid-19 lockdowns I did a squat workout that started with some warm-up sets of squats with no weight, then some sets holding my seventy-pound dog, and finished with some sets holding my (weight not disclosed) wife.

As with all exercise, what matters with resistance training is that it challenges your muscles. Even the studies with participants nearing their eleventh decade call it "high-intensity" resistance training for a reason. But exactly how that challenge happens matters much less. All the research to date shows that you don't have to lift *heavy*; it just has to feel physically challenging.[75] If a squat with no weight, push-up on your knees, or rows with yoga bands is challenging, that's all you need to do initially. The minimum effective dose is also low. A group of top sports scientists recently estimated that four sets per week per body part, with six to fifteen repetitions per set, was enough to get improvements in strength and muscle mass.[76] It should be hard enough that the last few repetitions are a challenge to complete, but if that takes twenty or thirty repetitions with a lighter weight or your body weight, that's OK too. This can be done in a single session or split over multiple sessions. If you're tight on time, they suggest doing exercises as a circuit—completing sets of each exercise back-to-back rather than doing all your sets of one exercise before moving on to the next—and even avoiding long warm-ups and stretching.

A BEGINNER'S GUIDE TO RESISTANCE TRAINING

Though my hope is that eventually it won't be, I know that for those new to resistance training the gym can be an intimidating place. And while there are some relatively inexpensive gym options, I also know that not everybody has the ability to go to the gym or hire a trainer to give them a training programme. Starting out at home is a great option, especially if you get some adjustable dumbbells or resistance bands that have handles and a door anchor that secures the bands while you use them (these are available widely online). I like both these options because you won't have to keep buying more equipment as you get stronger. Here is an example home workout (done as a circuit of six to fifteen reps of each exercise back-to-back, three times through, resting as needed):

- Squats (weights held at your sides, to your chest, or in front of you for balance)
- Push-ups (hands on the wall, a chair, or done on your knees is easier, in that order)
- Rows (bands, weights, and milk jugs filled with water all work well)
- Shoulder press
- Thirty-second carry—pick something up (e.g., shopping bags with books in them) and walk with it
- Bonus: bicep curls

If you do hit the gym, ask a staff member if you're uncertain how to use something or where to find it. Another secret tip is to pick out the strongest-looking person in the room and ask them. While often physically intimidating, they're frequently the most supportive of others in the gym. Here's a great go-to gym workout (three sets of six to fifteen reps):

- Leg press
- Chest press
- Rows

- Shoulder press
- Thirty-second carry—pick up some dumbbells and walk with them
- Bonus: bicep curls

That last sentence might come as a surprise, but while long warm-ups and stretching absolutely have their place, they're not really needed for the average resistance training workout. It's usually enough to warm up with a couple sets of a few repetitions with lighter weights, or just your body weight, to practise the movement and get into the right positions. For people new to exercise, resistance training done in a controlled and progressive manner is also associated with very low risk of injury compared to other activities, such as running.[77] Increasing your muscle mass and strength with resistance training helps to stabilise joints, which has been shown to decrease back pain, as well as knee and hip pain from osteoarthritis.[78] While you should absolutely seek professional guidance if needed, in many cases, those with joint or back pain need *more* resistance, not less. Resistance training in athletes also decreases their overall risk of sport-related and overuse injuries. Adding some resistance will therefore help you build a solid foundation as you work your way down the funnel and start to think about moving more quickly and with more coordination.

SPRINT

The movement funnel was designed to help describe the way somebody can build a practice of physical activity from the ground up. When we're just getting started with adding exercise to our daily routines, any additional movement—even a small amount of it—makes a big difference, and that's the place to start. Exercise snacks and walking require no equipment or preparation and can be done pretty much anywhere. But as we start to build on that foundation, it's clear that intensity does matter. That was the case in "propel," where a lot of movement of any kind is amazing but adding some extended periods of brisker activity that gets the heart rate up and makes us out of breath will provide some additional benefit. Intensity is also important at the "resist" level. As you get stronger, you need to make sure you keep finding ways to add challenge, be that with heavier weights, boulders, or family members.

The importance of being challenged is grounded in one of the most basic aspects of biology and evolution: we adapt and improve in response to stimuli that push our current capabilities. In the case of physical activity, after you've built some fitness and strength and have seen some resulting brain benefits, it's time to sprint. If we're being technical, the scientific literature usually defines sprints as short bursts of very high intensity lasting less than thirty seconds. However, practically speaking, most of us can think about sprints as anything from a few seconds to a few minutes, with these slightly longer efforts often called high-intensity interval training (HIIT). Or, as I sometimes like to call it, moving really quickly with a rest between sets (#MRQWARBS).[79] Sadly, my version never really stuck.

When it comes to some of the brain benefits of exercise, and benefits of exercise in general, the pathways tend to be intensity dependent. This means that for a given total amount of time spent exercising, doing shorter periods of more intense work (with some rests built in) can result in more activation of adaptation pathways and greater fitness gains.[80] In some cases, a certain level of intensity might be required for a pathway to be fully activated. This brings us to a fascinating and important molecule that has had its ups and downs in the world of exercise: lactate.

Often feared and misrepresented as a metabolic waste product that is the source of muscle burn during intense exercise—neither of which are true—lactate is actually a critical regulator of many brain-supporting pathways. More intense exercise leads to more lactate production—often called *anaerobic* exercise due to a reliance on high-speed energy production that occurs without (*an*) oxygen (*aero,* meaning "air")—where the build-up of lactate is helping to offset acid accumulation that causes the "burn." Lactate supports multiple aspects of brain and physical function, and is even being researched as a therapy for many types of brain injury because of the way it activates pathways that support the growth and recovery of neurons.[81] In particular, lactate drives the production of BDNF—the critical growth factor that supports neuronal function and BDNF levels in an intensity-dependent manner (more intensity leads to more BDNF).[82] So at least part of the reason intensity matters for some of the benefits of movement is that more intense exercise results in the accumulation of lactate, which directly activates BDNF production.[83]

BDNF that is produced in the body during exercise doesn't necessarily get into the brain, because it isn't easily transported across the blood-brain barrier (BBB), the tight network of cells and junctions that regulates what can get into the brain from the blood. This is where lactate comes to the rescue. The brain is a big fan of lactate and has transporters that ensure that the more lactate we produce, the more lactate gets into the brain.[84] Once lactate is in the brain, it increases local BDNF production that directly supports brain function.[85] Remember that BDNF (as well as many of the other exerkines) is almost like a cognitive tonic—supporting neuroplasticity and the strength of new connections—which helps to build headroom.

The relationship between lactate and BDNF seems to explain some of the ways that sprinting is good for the brain. For instance, one study had volunteers cycle as hard as they could for thirty seconds, recover for four and a half minutes, and repeat that for six rounds (thirty minutes total time). Compared to a non-exercising group, the sprint group saw significant improvements in several measures of cognitive flexibility and working memory twenty minutes after the sprint session. The more lactate (and BDNF) produced, the bigger the improvement in cognitive function.[86] Even *very* brief bursts of activity can improve brain function. Rounds of six seconds (yes, you read that right) of maximum effort cycling with one minute of rest immediately improves some measures of focus and concentration.[87] Over several weeks, this type of training improves fitness, leg strength, and memory.[88]

Slightly longer intervals have also been shown to have significant long-term benefits for the brain. In one of the longest studies of exercise and brain function done to date, researchers in Australia took adults aged sixty-five to eighty-five and randomised them to three groups: (1) no exercise, (2) thirty minutes of moderate physical activity (similar to the brisk walking described in "propel"), (3) or a twenty-five-minute HIIT protocol. The HIIT protocol consisted of four minutes of running with three minutes rest, repeated four times. The exercise groups did their sessions three times a week for six months. The moderate-intensity group did see some benefits, but the HIIT group saw much larger improvements in memory function as well as maintenance of the size of the hippocampus when it would otherwise have been expected to decrease in size with age. This improvement was sustained for at least *four years* after the end of the study.[89]

The HIIT protocol used in this study is known as the Norwegian 4 x 4 protocol, which has consistently been shown to be a time-efficient way to improve fitness.[90] In a study of sedentary middle-aged adults in their fifties, a two-year training protocol that included doing the 4 x 4 workout one or two times per week resulted in such significant improvements in fitness and heart structure that the scientist who ran the study, Benjamin Levine, has been quoted as saying that the hearts of the participants looked almost twenty years younger.[91]

When it comes to the length of the sprints we do, we have a fair amount of flexibility, because a huge range of times and intensities has been found to have similar benefits. For instance, twenty minutes of alternating fifteen-second sprints with fifteen seconds of rest increases fitness almost as much as the 4 x 4 method.[92] One of my rowing coaches at Cambridge was a big fan of this fifteen seconds on/off protocol because it was a way to quickly improve fitness without causing huge amounts of fatigue.

To build your own sprint training programme, the exact protocol probably doesn't matter that much. The shorter the sprint and the longer the rest period, the harder you can work while you're moving. Any exercise that uses multiple muscles at once will work. As you gain confidence, you can work toward sessions that have longer one-to-four-minute bursts with the same amount of rest. The goal is to go as hard as you can at a pace that you can hold for all the rounds. But the great thing about hard-effort workouts is that, even including a warm-up and the rest periods, these sessions don't need to be more than twenty to thirty minutes.

This last part is important when it comes to intensity, because more is not necessarily better—especially when you don't have hours every day to train and recover like a professional athlete. Think about getting some good work done in a short period of time while enjoying a bit of the "burn" as lactate is increasing BDNF in your brain. But that's it. Even if *during* the workout you're nearing your limits, *after* it's done, you should leave feeling energised, not completely exhausted. Movement is supposed to be fun, after all . . . I promise.

> ### SPRINTING FORWARD
>
> If you're new to sprinting, try adding some short bursts toward the end of your propel-level workouts. Slowly build up the speed over time until you can push hard for a few rounds with the kind of structure outlined below. Another way to add some sprinting to your go-to workout is to do some short bursts of quick body-weight movements at the end. Work as fast as you can (safely) and look to get a bit of a burn in your chosen time window. Options include:
>
> - High knees / running on the spot
> - Mountain climbers
> - Burpees
> - Star jumps
> - Body-weight squats
> - Skipping jumps (rope optional)
>
> If you then want to add some specific sprint workouts into your weekly routine, one to three times per week, build in some sessions that look like this:
>
> - Warm up for five minutes on your chosen exercise
> - Sprint for ten to sixty seconds
> - Rest for two to four times as long as you sprinted for
> - Repeat for ten total minutes
> - Cool down and head home!

Any aerobic-type exercise can be used, including running, cycling, rowing, swimming, elliptical, skipping, etc. Running can be done on hills or stairs if you prefer. Cycling, the elliptical, and rowing are easier to do on a machine at the gym, with cycling perhaps the most user-friendly if you've never done it before.

For those wanting an extra level of sprinting nerdery, here are some protocols that have been used in scientific studies and that you can try out yourself:

INTERVAL LENGTH	REST TIME	NUMBER OF SETS
8 seconds	12 seconds	30 (10 total minutes)
10 seconds	4 minutes	6 (25 minutes)
15 seconds	15 seconds	40–50 (20–25 minutes)
20 seconds	3 minutes	2 (4 minutes)
20 seconds	10 seconds	8 (aka "Tabata," 4 minutes)
30 seconds	4 minutes	4–6 (20–25 minutes)
60 seconds	3 minutes	8 (30 minutes)
60 seconds	60 seconds	10 (20 minutes)
4 minutes	Single maximum effort	1 (4 minutes)
4 minutes	3–4 minutes	3–5 (20–40 minutes)

COORDINATE

All the levels of the movement funnel are good for—and support—your brain in different ways. But once you have some strength and fitness, there's a whole host of fun things you can do with them. In addition to simply going out and enjoying your newfound physical capacity by engaging with the outside world, carrying and running and jumping with abandon, there are a number of other movement types to consider that involve more complex movements and reactions. These activities also seem to have an outsized benefit on the brain because they work your brain and body *together* at the same time. They also often include a good dose of fun.

When I think about having fun while moving, I immediately think of Darryl Edwards. In a former life, Darryl ran computer systems for investment banking firms, a lucrative job that involved long hours and little time to think about anything other than work. As a result, he faced some significant personal health challenges that led to him completely changing his career. Starting with himself, Darryl has been on a mission to bring joy back into movement for, as he calls us all, "children aged four to ninety-four." In 2023, both Darryl and I were inducted together as honourary fellows of the British Society of Lifestyle Medicine, a recognition that only a small handful of people receive each year.

I first met Darryl a decade earlier in 2013 when I snagged a speaking spot at a small health conference he organised in London. It was only a month or so after I started my PhD—the first time I ever spoke about diet and health in public. In many ways, my journey into the world of communicating about health science started with the opportunity Darryl gave me.

In a TEDx Talk that has been watched more than a million times, Darryl talks about the problem with traditional approaches to exercise, including the "no pain, no gain" mentality that results in many people choosing (perhaps sensibly) to avoid the pain entirely and not bother with the exercise at all. As we've already seen, this mentality doesn't align with the science of movement, because *everything counts,* and pain is entirely optional (though some people do like that kind of thing). However, Darryl goes one step further and says that, when it comes to movement, we should instead seek pleasure, comfort, and joy. This aligns with the brain game rule *Be kind to yourself*—ideally we want factors like movement, diet, and sleep to be pleasurable and joyful.

When Darryl started training himself as his first client, he faced a conundrum. He knew he needed to move more but also knew that he *hated* exercise, at least in the way it had previously been packaged and sold to him. As a result, he came up with a method he calls Primal Play—re-creating the movement, games, and fun he had when running around with his friends as a kid. Darryl's social media is filled with him, as well as "children" aged four to ninety-four, crawling, chasing each other, and climbing trees.

My most vivid memory of Darryl is from *another* conference where he was in charge of movement sessions for all the attendees. Standing in front of a group of relative strangers in the morning Arizona sun, Darryl called me up to demo some moves. We played a game of static tag—standing in front of each other trying to tag the other person's thigh while they do the same. We did some slow-motion pushing and pulling against each other to create some resistance without weights. Then, at the end, he suddenly and casually threw me over his shoulder and started running around. This is one of Darryl's signature moves.

Despite having (almost) never set foot in a gym, Darryl is both fit and incredibly strong. He's overpowered me and dragged my face through the dirt more than once—each and every time with a huge grin on my face. But while I think we could all do with getting our hands (and faces) a little dirty from time to time, this is not a requirement of the method. Most of Primal Play is noncontact and low risk, with a particular focus on adding coordinated movement to exercises that can fit into any level of the movement funnel. Other examples might include slow crawling with your chest facing either the floor (like a bear) or the sky (like a crab). I've even seen Darryl lead a room full of a thousand people doing slow-motion noncontact play-fighting as if they were acting out old-school Batman comics (sound effects optional but encouraged).

"Coordinate" is the final step in the movement funnel, but it could be applied to any other level or be a way to enter into the other levels without necessarily needing to take a more traditional approach to exercise. Climbing a tree provides some pretty good resistance, and a game of tag can look a lot like some mini sprints. But there are a huge number of studies showing that, even within more structured activities, adding coordination can boost the brain benefits of pretty much any kind of movement.

In the sports science world, movements or sports that require a lot of coordination are often called *open-skill*, as opposed to *closed-skill*, movements that focus mainly on pure fitness or strength. For instance, cycling and running are closed skill, whereas any sport that requires you to move in less predictable patterns and respond to the environment are open skill. This includes ball sports (soccer, basketball, rugby, lacrosse), racket sports (pickleball, tennis, badminton, padel), and board sports (skateboarding, surfing, skiing). The open-skill activity you choose can be tailored to your level of comfort and abilities. In a study of healthy elderly men in their sixties, both brisk walking/cycling and table tennis improved some elements of reaction time, information processing, and working memory over a non-exercise group, but the benefits were greater in the table tennis group.[93]

A large analysis of studies where people were assigned to different exercise types also found that coordinative exercise was found to be the most beneficial for improving cognitive function.[94] In particular, when two interventions have very similar levels of intensity, the one that includes a coordination component often has a bigger effect on cognitive function. For example, one trial in nine- and ten-year-old children compared running to more complex coordination drills involving things like balls, rackets, and skipping ropes. Both groups improved working memory better than a group that didn't do any exercise, but the kids who did the coordinative movement improved the most.[95]

Though it is hard to measure in real time, open-skill movements are training your vision, reactions, planning, and coordination skills, all at the same time, in addition to working your heart and muscles. Coordinating these skills across multiple brain networks requires a greater effort for the brain, which is probably a big part of where the benefits come from. Coordinative exercise also seems to result in greater increases in myokines and factors like BDNF. For example, one study had people do a workout running around a track, either with or without obstacles (cones to weave through and bars to jump over or pass under). All the participants did both workouts in a random order, and blood tests were taken before and after each one. Both workouts resulted in increases in BDNF as well as VEGF (vascular endothelial growth factor), which is important for the health and growth of blood vessels, including in the brain. However, the increases in BDNF and VEGF were larger after the obstacle run than the regular run.[96] Another study randomised participants in their sixties and seventies to take either dance classes or traditional exercise classes, twice a week for six months. Both groups saw similar improvements in fitness and cognitive function, but only the dance group saw an increase in BDNF, as well as bigger improvements in multiple areas of their brains—including the hippocampus—on an MRI scan.[97]

Scientists aren't entirely sure why open-skill exercise often results in more BDNF production—it may be something about the nature of the exercise and how it engages the brain, or it might be that the types of movements involved (more starting, stopping, twisting, and bending) activate the muscles in a greater way to produce more BDNF. It's probably a bit of both.

The benefits of controlled complex movements also translate to other activities that might initially appear more sedate but can become incredibly challenging. For example, several studies have found that tai chi interventions significantly improve cognitive function in older adults.[98] Though the studies are all very different and use a variety of different practices, meta-analyses of yoga trials have found benefits for memory, executive function, attention, and processing speed; improvements in depression symptoms; and increased levels of BDNF.[99] Pilates improves cognitive function in both pre- and postmenopausal women, with one study finding similar improvements after four weeks of Pilates training compared to using gym equipment (treadmill, bike, elliptical) to do aerobic exercise.[100]

Not only do these activities help with strength, balance, and coordination but the nature of the movements may have some additional benefits. Both controlled and rhythmic breathing, which are very common in many Eastern-derived movement practices, as well as twisting and bending movements, may help to move fluid through the brain and spinal cord.[101] This fluid flow is critical to clearing waste from the brain but decreases with ageing in a way that is thought to contribute to cognitive decline and dementia.[102] Maintaining good fluid flow through the brain requires healthy blood vessels—for which exercise plays a special role—as well as changes in position that move the spine.[103] In this way, coordinative movements may have a special effect in terms of getting *all* of the brain and body moving, with cognitive benefits to match.

COORDINATE AND PLAY

In many ways, humans are especially well adapted to complex open-skill and coordinative movements; just think of children as they learn to move and play. The best part is that this kind of movement often doesn't require a gym or equipment. Darryl Edwards recommends animal moves—crab walks, bear walks, climbing, balancing on beams or low walls, and anything that involves a chance to move through the environment by running and jumping. If you have a workout partner, you can chase, push, or carry each other. All of this builds coordination, fitness, and strength.

Options for open-skill activities that can replace "propel" sessions include:

- Racket sports (tennis, table tennis, squash, pickleball, padel)
- Team sports (soccer, rugby, [tag] football, basketball)
- Board sports (surfing, skateboarding, skiing, snowboarding)
- Chasing your children/dogs/partner around the house
- Dancing (in a class, in your living room, at a rave)

Other coordinative activities you can try include:

- Yoga
- Pilates
- Tai chi
- Martial arts (karate, judo, jiu jitsu, aikido)
- Barre or any other activity involving balance and control

MOVING THROUGH THE FUNNEL

Adding more movement to our day is one of the best ways to slow the processes of aging, immediately improve cognitive function, and decrease the long-term risk of dementia. But assuming you're working out in order to add more life to your years rather than to spend as much time in the gym as possible, treat movement as a funnel that you add to over time. Snack to break up being sedentary, add longer lower-intensity propel sessions plus shorter sprint sessions to build plenty of cardiovascular fitness, and then resist to build muscle and strength and gain an extra cognitive boost. Ideally, find a way to move every day, alternating between these different activity types.

As the final element of the funnel, any of these layers can then be augmented or incorporated with movement that requires you to coordinate. Do some basic yoga poses as an exercise snack, replace a brisk walk or a sprint session with a soccer game, get some resistance with a Pilates class or by wrestling with your kids/dogs/spouse. All of these things provide benefits that can help you build physical and cognitive headroom and future-proof your brain. If you're ever uncertain about how to move, let your imagination and your environment inspire you. As Darryl Edwards says: "The world is your gym, [or] better yet, your playground."

CHAPTER 8
NOURISH

Of all the lifestyle factors that can influence our health, I think it's fair to say that nutrition has the potential to be the most confusing and the most polarising. Because, obviously, nothing brings people together like a calm, reasonable discussion about carbs.

Physical activity, by comparison, is a breeze to talk about. Pretty much everybody agrees that movement is good for you, and that most people would benefit from doing more of it. And while you can certainly get stuck on the details of what kind of exercise programme is optimal, we can be safe in the knowledge that pretty much any movement you do has a good chance of being beneficial for your brain.

Diet, on the other hand . . . not so much. Part of this stems from the endless stream of information and discussions related to what the best diet might be. This is also complicated by the fact that what constitutes "best" in these discussions often has more to do with weight loss than with helping to protect and maintain cognitive function.

We all need to eat in order to survive, and the foods we gravitate toward are shaped by myriad factors ranging from culture to accessibility and affordability. So perhaps it shouldn't be surprising that everyone has an opinion about what constitutes the "right" way to eat to support human flourishing—and those opinions often change with the release of new research that lionises (or demonises) a particular food or way of eating. Considering our constant exposure to many different opinions regarding nourishment, it's no wonder that many of us find it difficult to know which voices are worth listening to.

With that said, it's clear that what we eat directly affects our cognitive function, well-being, and long-term dementia risk. There is an ever-increasing amount of evidence showing that nutrient deficiencies contribute to a large number of health conditions, and that dietary interventions can help to slow or reverse disease. As a result, experts since Hippocrates have promoted the idea that food is medicine.[1] However, there has been a backlash against this idea, because medicalising an activity that we have to partake in multiple times a day takes away the joy, comfort, and social connection that food has traditionally been (and should continue to be) tied to. By overanalysing everything we put into our mouths we add stress to our meals, which brings its own sets of problems.[2]

You've likely experienced this phenomenon when eating with others in a social setting. Sometimes it's just a sideways glance from someone as you look at the menu. Other times it's an open declaration—"I'm going to be bad and order [insert delicious, usually less-than-nutritious food]." More than once, knowing they are sharing a meal with a doctor, my friends have commented outright, "I'm worried you're going to judge me for what I order."

That makes me sad, because I don't want anyone to feel judged. Which is why, before I discuss the ways food can support brain health and function, I first want to acknowledge that judging ourselves or others for what we eat is not helpful and can even be harmful. The manner in which we talk about how food can impact our health or appearance can negatively affect our relationship with it.[3] As the title of the chapter suggests, eating should be an opportunity for nourishment rather than a source of stress, especially since we know that chronic stress can itself have deleterious effects on the brain.

Our intimate relationship with food is one reason I'm not going to provide a specific, hard-to-follow diet to promote brain health. The other reason is that the research consistently shows that there isn't a specific diet I could even recommend. Looking at the research through the lens of future-proofing the brain, I can make a strong case that there is no one-size-fits-all way to eat. There are some basic brain-supporting dietary parametres we can consider, but a million different ways to implement them. The framework I use allows us to distill all the food-related research (not to mention the accompanying noise) down to two basic ideas that will help you maintain your brain health over the long term.

Maximise brain-boosting nutrients. Fuel for *your* needs.

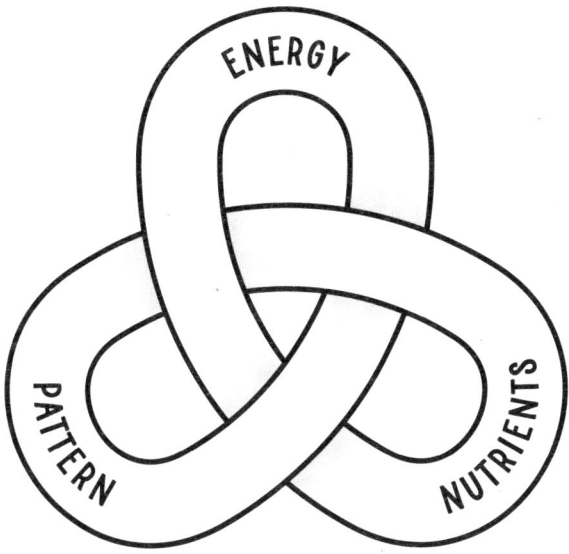

FIGURE 1. The three main components of nutrition that supports brain health.

A NOURISHING FRAMEWORK FOR THE BRAIN

One of the most amazing things about humans is our adaptability, which includes our ability to thrive in a wide variety of food environments. This is great news, because it gives us a huge amount of latitude in terms of the range of diets we can eat and still support our health and our brains. Having watched a wide variety of diets succeed and fail across a range of different scenarios, I see three components of a diet that are by far the greatest predictors of whether it is likely to support long-term brain health (figure 1):

1. Nutrients
2. Energy
3. Pattern

These three factors are tightly intertwined. Your brain, like any other part of the body, needs certain nutrients to function at its best. You (obviously) need to consume food to provide those nutrients as well as to meet the brain's incredible energy demands. But overeating and moving into a state of energy excess works against brain health. This means you need to fuel appropriately for your own requirements, which is why the most important brain-game rule for nourishment is *Prepare for your own race*. Choosing a dietary pattern that works best for you will allow you to take in those necessary nutrients and feel nourished and satiated while also ensuring you are taking in the right amount of calories. Let me explain in more detail.

NUTRIENTS

When I think about the brain and its many functions, my first thought always goes to the nutrients required to run all that complex squishy machinery inside the skull. As the primary source of the wide range of nutrients that are critical for brain function, our food plays a huge role in ensuring that we live as healthily as possible for as long as possible.

Some of the most important work on nutrients and health was done by Bruce Ames, a former professor of biochemistry at the University of California, Berkeley. The latter part of his career was focused on how nutrients status affects aging, which perhaps contributed to the fact that he was still writing scientific papers at ninety-two years old.[4]

Though there are some nutrients and vitamins that we can make ourselves (like vitamin D, which is made when our skin is exposed to sunlight), most come from our diet. These nutrients help form the structures of our cells, help produce the hormones and neurotransmitters that send and receive all the signals in our body, and generally make sure we can adapt and respond to our environment to survive and thrive. In the building that is your body—which is mainly made up of protein, water, and fat—all the other nutrients are the rivets, nails, glue, screws, appliances, fixtures, and everything else that makes the building function as a home.

One of Ames's main ideas was that nutrients are directed to different functions based on their availability—something he called *triage theory*.[5] When I worked in the ER department as a junior doctor, the first person patients saw was a triage nurse, who decided how urgently somebody needed to be seen. In our ER we had three different areas based on the seriousness of the problem, and patients were directed accordingly. For a patient, the process of triage can be very frustrating. Even with a broken arm, you might get bumped down the waiting list by somebody suffering from a cardiac arrest or a stroke. But when resources are limited, you need to make game-time decisions on where to allocate those resources.

Perhaps unsurprisingly, the brain and the body triage nutrients in a very similar way. For example, we can see the way the body prioritises different functions by looking at athletes who don't consume enough calories from food. When they don't have enough energy to support all the activity they're doing, athletes experience a state called *low energy availability*. They're fatigued and can't think clearly. They are also more easily distractible, tend to have a lot of gut symptoms, and see a decrease in the hormones that drive metabolism (like thyroid hormones) and reproduction (like testosterone and oestrogen).[6]

This all makes perfect sense—if you're working with limited resources, you start by cutting off energy investment in processes that you can survive without. In fact, our bodies are much smarter with their resources than we tend to be—the minute the budget gets tight, they cut up the credit cards and cancel all the TV subscriptions. Constantly replacing cells in the gut or investing in the process of building a new human (reproduction) both require a healthy budget, so these are paused until the next influx of steady caloric financing arrives.

Though it's harder to see and feel, Bruce Ames's triage theory shows that the same thing happens when we're low in certain nutrients—they get directed to the processes needed for survival at the expense of long-term investment in repair and longevity.[7] One example of this comes from the Illinois Brain Ageing Study. Participants had brain scans, cognitive function tests, and blood tests for multiple markers of nutrient status.[8] They were split into two groups: those whose brains were ageing quickly—their brains were smaller and had less white matter, and they performed worse on all cognitive function tests—and those whose brains were ageing more slowly. Those whose brains were ageing more slowly had higher levels of omega-3 fatty acids, choline, vitamin E, and the colourful antioxidants lutein and zeaxanthin that are found in fruits, vegetables, and egg yolks. In fact, across multiple studies, higher levels of B vitamins, omega-3 fats, antioxidants, and vitamin D have consistently been linked to healthier and younger-looking brains.[9]

Results like these are important to all of us because inadequate intake of critical nutrients is also incredibly common (though in some places, this has been helped by the fortification of foods—iodine in salt, vitamin D in dairy, iron and folic acid in flour).[10] Nutrient intakes differ by country, but in the United States and Europe around 15 to 25 percent of people have inadequate intakes of most B vitamins, with even higher deficits of the minerals iron, magnesium, and calcium, as well as the antioxidant vitamins C and E. Due to differences in both intake and requirements, the prevalence of nutrient deficits also differs by sex—women are more likely to get inadequate B12, iron, iodine, and calcium, while men are more likely to get too little magnesium, zinc, and some of the other B vitamins. In addition to other dietary components like omega-3 fatty acids, many of these missing nutrients are critical for brain health, and increasing their intake is associated with improved cognitive function and decreased dementia risk.[11]

In terms of the effect of diet on our health, nutrients are the great leveler. What matters is that you get enough of them, with the source being less important. For example, many dietary protocols aimed at improving health suggest limiting red meat, including the Mediterranean-DASH Intervention for Neurodegenerative Delay (MIND) diet, which has gotten a lot of press in recent years. However, some studies support the potential benefit of including unprocessed red meat in our diets for both mental health and cognitive function as it is associated with a lower risk of both depression and dementia.[12] This is probably because meat is a rich source of protein and many other nutrients the brain needs, including B12, iron, and zinc. Randomised trials show that red meat doesn't negatively impact important health markers such as blood sugar or inflammation, and lean unprocessed red meat has a minimal effect on markers of heart disease risk.[13] For other health outcomes like cancer, increased risk in those who eat red meat is probably due to a poor-quality overall dietary pattern that doesn't include enough fruits and vegetables, which are also critical for brain health.[14] Higher fruit and vegetable intake is consistently associated with lower risk of dementia, bigger brains, and slowed cognitive decline. So, if it fits with your preferences, health, and an overall brain-healthy dietary pattern, red meat can absolutely be included as a source of protein and other nutrients in your diet.

The fact that the nutrients themselves matter more than where they come from also gives us some latitude in terms of the way we source our food. Far too often we're told that for food to be as healthy as possible it has to be organic, wild, or grass-fed. But, while less intensive farming methods can absolutely have important benefits for animal welfare and the environment, the reality is that most people can't afford the cost of taking those things into consideration. Importantly, these stories about food also aren't usually true. Conventional farming results in food that is just as nutritious, and the effects of pesticides or other contaminants that might come along for the ride are usually overblown and pale in comparison to the benefit of eating the food itself.[15]

I'll make the same argument about fish. Species like salmon and tuna are incredible sources of omega-3 fatty acids, as well as other important nutrients, which have been shown, time and time again, to support brain health. However, due to concerns about microplastics and other contaminants, many people are reluctant to add fish to their plate. These concerns can be offset by eating smaller fish and shellfish, but regardless of the type, the brain benefits derived from eating fish far outweigh the potential detriments. For example, studies on both children and older adults have found that the benefits of eating fish more than offset any increase in mercury intake, the net result being better cognitive function and reduced dementia risk.[16] This is because fish includes a whole host of beneficial nutrients, including selenium, which counteracts the potentially negative effects of mercury. So, even though the picture can get complicated, the evidence consistently suggests that the benefits of nutrient-dense foods like seafood outweigh the potential downsides that people tend to focus on. Plus, these foods are delicious.

NUTRIENTS FOR BUILDING AND MAINTAINING A BRAIN

A lot of what we know about nutrition and the brain comes from looking at the nutrients required for a brain to develop in the first place (figure 2). Understanding how different nutrients affect cognition before and after birth gives us an idea of the brain functions they can influence. And, as you might expect by now, many of the requirements of the developing brain are also essential for keeping the brain healthy for the long term. For instance, iron is incredibly important for the develop-

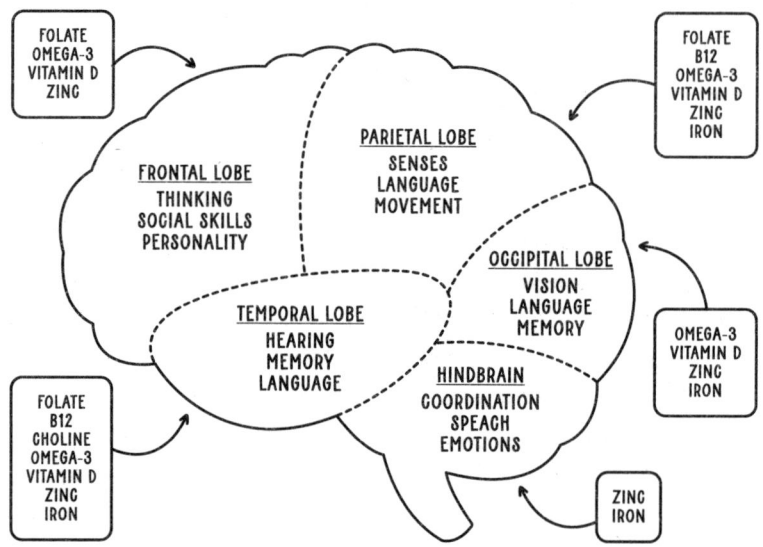

FIGURE 2. Brain regions, their functions, and nutrients known to be critical for their development and health. Adapted from Na et al., *Nutrients* 2024.

ment of the white matter during pregnancy and early infancy, but being anaemic or having low iron later in life is also associated with degeneration of the white matter and higher dementia risk.[17] One study of women at the menopausal transition found that cognitive function was higher in those with better iron status, even if they weren't anaemic.[18]

Similarly, long-chain omega-3 fatty acids like DHA (docosahexaenoic acid, often found alongside EPA, or eicosapentaenoic acid) that are typically found in seafood are so critical to brain development that the mother will sacrifice her own stores if needed, just to make sure the baby gets enough.[19] The importance of DHA for the developing brain is thought to be why women are better at converting other forms of omega-3s (like alpha-linolenic acid, ALA, commonly found in nuts and seeds) to DHA than men are.[20] Later in life, omega-3 status is associated with long-term dementia risk, and supplementing with omega-3s can slow the rate of cognitive decline and improve symptoms in those with depression.[21]

However, one big issue with research into specific nutrients is that we tend to apply the reductionist approach and treat them individually. If each nutrient is a different transistor or wire in your broken radio, by focusing on one nutrient at a time (for instance, saying that getting more omega-3s will prevent dementia), we are essentially assuming that everybody with a broken radio must have the same malfunctioning component. As a result, there is a long history of clinical trials where one specific nutrient was given as a supplement to treat or prevent a given disease, and no effect was found. People then assume that supplementing or increasing intake of that nutrient "doesn't work." Considering how different each of our diets are, it doesn't take much to imagine that there might be a group of people (or radios) where that one nutrient *would* help, but by mixing them in with a bigger group of radios that are broken for other reasons, that result gets lost.

One of the best examples of this is again omega-3s, which have been tested in multiple large clinical trials of dementia prevention, sometimes without success (and yes, I do recognise that I just recommended that you eat more fish and mentioned potential benefits of supplementing with omega-3s). While there are multiple potential reasons for the failures of these trials, I think the main failure is our application of the reductionist approach. For example, in many trials of omega-3s, participants weren't tested to see if they were deficient in omega-3s in the first place.[22] Focusing on omega-3s also ignores the many other beneficial nutrients that we also get from seafood, and the other nutrients needed for omega-3s to do their job in the brain. To better illustrate this idea, rather than send you away with a long list of nutrients to treat as individual transistors in your radio, I'm instead going to describe the journey of a signal being transmitted through the brain—and the nutrients that make it possible.

THE BRAIN'S NUTRIENT CASCADE

Sometimes, when you think about processes in the human brain, you can quickly become amazed that they happen at all. For me, at least, this is the case when I think about the complex balance of communication that is continuously happening across billions of cells in our brains. Even if we really simplify it, it's clear that there are multiple points in the process where one or more issues might arise in a way that can be tricky to fix with a reductionist approach.

If you want anything to happen in the brain, your neurons will need some energy. B vitamins, for example, are often touted as being important for energy because they support the function of the mitochondria—the "powerhouses" of the cell, where most of the calories from our food are turned into energy that the cell can use. There are eight main B vitamins: B1 (thiamine), B2 (riboflavin), B3 (niacin), B5 (pantothenic acid), B6 (pyridoxine), B7 (biotin), B9 (folate), and B12 (cobalamin). They come in many different forms, but in one way or another, all of them are essential to brain function and energy production. The process of generating energy always produces a bit of wear and tear in the form of oxidative stress (the body's equivalent of rust, where the components of our cells become damaged by free radicals). Therefore, antioxidant vitamins like vitamins C and E—and antioxidant molecules like polyphenols, which are found in fruits and vegetables—from the diet are needed to help keep that oxidative stress under control.

Once we've generated some energy, our neuron might want to generate a signal to communicate with another cell. The mitochondria and the energy they produce are critical for regulating the movement of minerals—sodium, potassium, and calcium—that transmit the signal along the cell. If that signal is travelling along an axon in the white matter, we already know that having enough iron is going to be important for making and maintaining the white matter structure so that the signal can travel quickly and efficiently. As the white matter is mainly made of fat, some of those fats need to come from the diet (like omega-3s), and many are made from scratch by the brain from glucose or ketones and then attached to other dietary precursors like choline.[23]

Once the signal gets to the synapse to be transmitted to the next cell, a whole host of things need to happen. Tiny little sacs (vesicles) filled with neurotransmitters sit at the synapse ready to be released. Though these neurotransmitters are often recycled after use, to make them in the first place you might need an amino acid (from protein), or a nutrient like choline, in addition to various other vitamins that regulate the process of manufacturing the neurotransmitter. For example, if you're a synapse that releases serotonin—involved in mood, sleep, and memory—you need vitamin D to stimulate the production of the enzyme that makes serotonin from the amino acid tryptophan.[24]

For the synapse to accurately and quickly release the neurotransmitter it needs DHA in its membrane, which is why DHA in the brain tends to be concentrated in the synapses. But the DHA you eat or make doesn't just magically arrive at the synapse. First it needs to get into the brain, which may be impeded by insulin resistance like you see in type 2 diabetes.[25] Then, because it's a fat and fats don't mix well with the water that surrounds all of our cells, the DHA needs to be attached to something (called a *headgroup*) that will let it sit in the membrane of the cell and do its job. That headgroup is usually choline or a related compound like ethanolamine, which you also need to get from the diet. Attaching DHA to these headgroups, or changing around the headgroups, relies on a process called *methylation*, which is dependent on at least four of the B vitamins—riboflavin, B6, folate, and B12.[26] DHA also becomes even more important in the setting of inflammation or injury, because it is used to make anti-inflammatory compounds (resolvins and protectins) that help to repair the brain.[27]

As the final step in this process, the neurotransmitter gets released into the synapse and binds to a receptor on the next cell to pass the signal along. At many of these synapses, the binding of the neurotransmitter to the receptor on the other side is modulated by minerals that are released with the neurotransmitter, such as magnesium or zinc.[28]

So just in the act of passing a single signal, every nutrient shown in figure 2 plays an important role. But the truth is, you don't need to remember all of that. The goal was just to illustrate that a whole host of nutrients need to act together in order to achieve a certain outcome in the brain. This means that looking at them one by one doesn't really make that much sense, even though each of them has been shown to play an important role in cognitive function, mental health, and dementia risk. You may also recognise many of these nutrients being important for heart health. There's a reason so many doctors will tell you that what's good for the heart is also good for the brain: they rely on similar building blocks, and anything that negatively affects the heart can also affect the brain.

One of the best examples of the ways that nutrients interact in the brain comes from several trials looking at the effect of B vitamins and omega-3s on cognitive decline. A lot of this work is based on the research of David Smith, former professor of pharmacology at the University of Oxford. In the late 2000s, Oxford ran the VITACOG study, which randomised participants with mild cognitive impairment to either a placebo or B vitamins (B6, folate, and B12). They found that B vitamins slowed the rate of brain shrinkage and cognitive decline.[29] As we might expect, the benefit of the B vitamins was greatest in those who had elevated homocysteine—a marker of methylation and B vitamin status in the blood that is increased in those who need more B vitamins (especially riboflavin, B6, folate, and B12).

There's a twist, though, because in follow-up studies the homocysteine-lowering B vitamins given in the VITACOG trial were found to only be beneficial in participants who had a good omega-3 status. Multiple trials of both omega-3 supplements and B vitamin supplements for cognitive function and dementia prevention have found that you need both to benefit.[30] This makes perfect sense when we think about how DHA depends on those B vitamins to get into the synapse and do its job.

As multiple nutrients interact to have a given effect in the body, it is often easier to study them when given together—for instance, as a multivitamin. And while the evidence for multivitamins is also mixed, because they each have different nutrient combinations in different doses and forms that may or may not be the best lineup for any given individual, there are an increasing number of studies that show the benefit of providing multiple nutrients at once. For instance, an analysis from the COSMOS (Cocoa Supplement and Multivitamin Outcomes Study), which included more than five thousand U.S. adults over sixty, showed that taking a daily multivitamin resulted in improvements in overall cognitive function and memory equivalent to being two years younger.[31]

It can be easy to get overwhelmed trying to keep track of all these nutrients and their interactions, which is why the most brain-healthy diets are ones that include a range of nutrient-rich foods. Rather than having to make sure you juggle every nutrient individually, focusing on nutrient-dense foods like those mentioned in the breakout box on page 128 will make it much more likely that you hit multiple important nutrients at the same time. And when you get them from food, a whole bunch of other potentially important nutrients come along for the ride, many of which we're only just starting to appreciate.

Some of these bonus nutrients are what Bruce Ames called *longevity vitamins*. We don't make them ourselves, and they're not essential for survival, but they do seem to support long-term health. These include a compound called ergothioneine, which is found in mushrooms and is gaining a lot of interest for its effects on cognitive function and heart disease risk.[32] However, the group of longevity vitamins with the most evidence is probably the carotenoids—lutein, zeaxanthin, beta-carotene, and lycopene—that make fruits and vegetables red, orange, or yellow, and astaxanthin, which makes shrimp and salmon red or pink.[33]

These carotenoids have a variety of antioxidant functions in the body and are associated with improvements in the health of both the brain and eyes (which have a lot of nerves and receptors and are directly connected to the brain). The brains of individuals with Alzheimer's disease also tend to have lower levels of carotenoids.[34] Similar benefits are linked to a related group of (usually) coloured antioxidant molecules called polyphenols. These include the flavonoids, which make berries red or purple, and a host of related compounds found in fruit, chocolate, tea, and coffee.

There are a huge number of studies showing that giving people the equivalent of one or two cups of berries a day (blueberries, cranberries, cherries, strawberries, etc.) can improve cognitive function in both the short and long term.[35] This may be because of direct actions in the brain, but polyphenols in berries and other colourful foods also affect the function of the gut and blood vessels,[36] as well as potentially impacting many of the hallmarks of aging. Berries are full of fibre and include nutrients that can improve blood sugar control.[37] Frozen berries—and all frozen fruits and vegetables, in fact—are an incredible food hack. They can reduce cooking preparation time, are often more affordable than the fresh version, and can retain a higher nutrient content over time.[38]

The polyphenols in tea and coffee are also thought to be why people who consume them regularly (two to four cups per day) might have a lower risk of dementia, especially as these are the major source of antioxidants in some people's diets.[39] Similarly, eating high-polyphenol dark chocolate (80 percent or darker) may help to improve blood flow to the brain and decrease cognitive fatigue.[40] In the COSMOS trial, some participants were given an extract of polyphenols from cocoa that seemed to be beneficial for those with lower-quality diets (and lower antioxidant intake).[41]

With the idea of bolstering overall nutrient status in mind, Bruce Ames developed a nutrition bar containing fruit polyphenols, DHA, and a multivitamin, which, in multiple studies, improved markers of health and risk of cognitive decline within two weeks—without having to otherwise change the diet.[42] But even if berries or chocolate don't give you superhuman cognition on their own, the worst-case scenario is that you enjoyed a tasty, nutrient-dense snack.

All these studies converge to provide the basis for the first rule of eating for brain health: *maximise nutrients*. By filling your plate with whole, nutrient-dense foods instead of just upping your intake of whatever so-called superfood is currently *en vogue*, you can harness the power of nutrient synergy to provide your brain what it needs.

NUTRIENT-DENSE FOODS LINKED TO LONG-TERM BRAIN HEALTH

I'm not one to throw around the term *superfood*. And if you did ask me for superfoods, I'm more likely to recommend blueberries and liver (though not necessarily together) than anything fancier or more elusive. Honestly, all whole, nutrient-dense foods are super in their own way. You should choose to eat the ones you want based on your background, each food's cost and availability, and your personal preferences. That said, here is a list of foods that pack a wallop in terms of nutrient density. I've bolded each food that appears in more than one nutrient category so that you can get maximum bang for your buck. There are quite a few, which increases the odds that there will be several you'll want to add to your meals.

Foods High in Iron
- **Liver**
- **Red meat**
- **Lentils**
- Chickpeas
- **Leafy greens (kale, spinach, chard)**
- **Eggs**
- **Poultry**
- **Seafood**

Foods High in Omega-3 Fatty Acids
- **Seafood**
- Walnuts
- **Eggs** (if the hen's feed is enriched)
- Chia seeds
- Flaxseed

Foods High in B Vitamins

Liver
Eggs
Salmon
Milk
Tuna
Quinoa
Oats
Brown rice
Lentils
Peas
Bananas
Avocados

Foods High in Vitamin D

Liver
Eggs
Salmon
Dairy (especially fortified varieties)
Tuna
Mushrooms

Foods High in Magnesium

Avocado
Beans
Spinach
Bananas
Whole grains

Foods High in Zinc

Oysters
Beef
Lamb
Poultry
Eggs

Foods High in Carotenoids (Like Lutein and Zeaxanthin)

Carrots
Sweet potatoes
Spinach
Bell peppers

Pumpkin
Broccoli
Dark leafy greens
Peas
Cantaloupe
Butternut squash
Tomatoes
Papaya

Foods High in Polyphenols

Olive oil
Blueberries (as well as raspberries, blackberries, and strawberries)
Apples
Spinach
Onions
Almonds
Walnuts
Dark chocolate

Foods High in Choline and/or Ethanolamine

Eggs (yolk)
Liver
Seafood
Beef
Dairy (milk, yoghurt, and cheese)
Soybeans
Kidney and mung beans
Potatoes
Quinoa
Oats
Cruciferous vegetables (brussels sprouts, cabbage, and broccoli)
Dark blue/purple berries

ENERGY

When it comes to energy, the brain is incredibly demanding. A well-worn fact is that the brain uses 20 percent of our energy but only takes up 2 percent of our body weight. If you want the brain to do *anything*, it's going to need a lot of energy. And the food we eat helps to provide it.

Throughout history, our ancestors often struggled to consistently ensure they had enough energy to support our large, hungry brains. Food was scarce, and the body will always sacrifice nonessential components in order to survive. We've already seen this in the example of athletes experiencing low energy availability. In fact, this can happen quite quickly; one recent study suggested that the brains of marathon runners eat the fat in their own myelin to provide energy![43] Luckily the effect was reversed in the recovery period after the race, and there's no evidence that these kinds of short-term changes in athletes are problematic. But it shows how energy hungry the brain is, and what it is willing to sacrifice when fuel is in short supply.

There's evidence that low energy availability over longer periods of time *does* decrease volume in critical areas of the brain, and that this is associated with higher dementia risk. If you're eating fewer calories than your body needs, it's forced to triage. You'll maintain enough brain function for day-to-day activities—probably for decades—but you likely won't have enough energy to invest in additional reserves. By comparison, having a well-nourished and energy-replete brain ensures that it has a savings account for the future. Eating *enough* food lets your brain build headroom—additional size and function that can provide a buffer later in life.

One reason having a brain buffer is important is that brain size tends to decrease with age, and several studies have demonstrated a strong link between the amount of brain volume lost over time and the risk of cognitive decline and dementia.[44] Therefore, when we consider diet, it's critical to think about whether the foods we're eating are providing our brains with the energy they need to maintain their volume. Because the bigger the brain you have, the more headroom you have to protect against aging-related neurodegeneration and cognitive decline.

Of course, as you might expect, it's not as simple as throwing back as many milkshakes and multivitamins as you can in order to maximise your brain gains. When it comes to energy and the brain, you can have too much of a good thing. Eating to energy *excess* over long periods of time can impair metabolism in the brain and increase inflammation and oxidative stress. This can also lead to brain volume loss as well as a higher risk of cognitive decline and dementia.

Therefore, in addition to supplying nutrients, food critically affects our brain health by making sure we are appropriately fuelled. Achieving health-promoting energy balance is exactly the same as fuelling a car in a Formula 1 race. At the start of the race, teams have to decide how much fuel to put in the car. (In previous decades they used to refuel rapidly during pit stops, but it turns out that filling up a car with a firehose is pretty dangerous.) In a sport that's often decided by hundredths of a second, and in which every ounce can make a difference, there's a fine balance that has to be struck—too much fuel makes the car sluggish and puts too much wear on the tyres. But too little fuel and the car risks not making it to the end.

Luckily, humans are much more adaptable and operate in a much wider window of energy balance than an F1 car does, but finding a balance is still important for our brains as we age. Consider, once again, the Bolivian Tsimané tribe, who we heard about in part 1. Comparing data from the Tsimané to their more globally integrated neighbours, the Mosetén, researchers have developed a model of how energy availability appears to affect the brain. Though both groups live lifestyles closer to our hunter-gatherer or subsistence farming past, and both have very low dementia rates—even when living into their eighties—the Mosetén lifestyle is closer to what you and I likely experience than that of the Tsimané.[45] As a result, the Mosetén are also more likely to have diseases associated with excess energy intake, such as obesity or type 2 diabetes, which can then have a knock-on effect on their brains.

A large research collaboration, including academics from four continents, looked at the relationship between energy status and brain size in the Tsimané, Mosetén, and U.S. and European adults. Across these groups, there is a continuum of energy availability—lower in the Tsimané and higher in the United States and Europe, with the Mosetén somewhere in between. Across this continuum there also seems to be a bell-shaped relationship between energy availability and brain volume (figure 3).

At the low end, higher energy availability (measured using BMI and cholesterol levels) is associated with higher brain volumes. This tells us that when food availability is scarce—as was more common during most of our evolutionary history—brain volume is sacrificed. In that setting, higher energy availability is better. When food becomes available, and energy budgets allow, more energy is invested in making

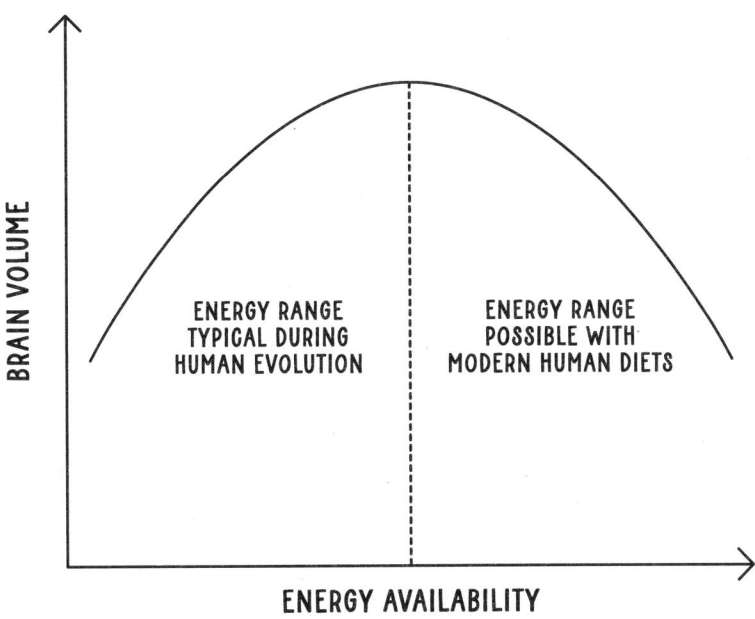

FIGURE 3. Proposed energy model showing how brain size (volume) relates to total energy availability. During the typical conditions our ancestors experienced, more energy meant more resources could be invested into the brain. However, modern humans are increasingly at risk of excess energy availability, shown on the right side of the graph. Here, being exposed to too much energy for long periods results in a smaller brain. Adapted from Kaplan et al., *PNAS* 2023.

brains bigger. However, there is another side to this equation. At very high energy intakes—as is more common in the modern food environment—we can enter a state of *excess* energy availability, which is associated with both more atherosclerosis (the damage to blood vessels that drives heart disease and strokes) and smaller brains. We know that the loss of healthy blood flow to the brain will impair its ability to maintain its size and function, but other aspects of excess energy availability, such as higher inflammation and blood sugar, also contribute to this effect.[46]

Based on the available data, it's also likely that changing energy availability is affecting dementia rates in the United States, which generally decreased during the twentieth century. One example of this is from the Framingham Heart Study, which has followed multiple generations of people from Framingham, Massachusetts, since 1948.

Nearly seventy years after they started the study, researchers reported that dementia rates had been steadily declining in their participants over time.[47] Over that same time frame, brain sizes in Framingham had also been *increasing*. As brains in Framingham got bigger over time, this seemed to provide physical brain headroom that then protected against age-related declines in brain size and function, decreasing the risk of dementia.

The trends in the Framingham cohort show that the biggest jump in brain size happened in those born in the 1940s, compared to the 1930s, with a slower increase afterwards. Though I can't prove this is the cause, these changes track with the big increase in food availability in the United States after the Great Depression and World War II ended. As food became more available, brains seemed to get bigger as a result.

The problem, however, is that now we're at the tipping point seen in figure 3. As our food system has become more modernised and industrialised, it has become easy to enter a state of excess energy availability that can negatively impact our brains. The Framingham cohort also shows this. Even though most risk factors for dementia decreased over time, both obesity and type 2 diabetes—diseases of excess energy availability—increased, just as they have done in the population overall.[48]

Several large studies show that obesity and type 2 diabetes are associated with smaller brain volumes, faster cognitive decline, and a higher risk of dementia.[49] For example, the English Longitudinal Study of Ageing showed that those who had prediabetes experienced faster cognitive decline than those who had normal blood sugar, and this decline was even faster in those who had type 2 diabetes. So, while our recent history shows the importance of getting enough energy for the brain, it's now more likely that we'll experience the opposite problem and get too much.

The effect of excess energy availability on the rate of brain decline with age is thought to be why the Tsimané have a slower decline in brain volume with age compared to adults in the United States and Europe, with the Mosetén again somewhere in between. When we have too much energy available, our brains decline more quickly with age. As a result, in addition to the ageing of the population, the health effects of excess energy availability are probably contributing to the fact that dementia rates are increasing again.[50]

Depending on your starting point, both sides of the brain energy model might be important. Hunger and malnutrition are still common in many high-income countries, though fixing this would require a lot of changes at the societal (rather than individual) level.[51] It's also clear that athletes who expend a lot of energy, or people who follow very restrictive diets, can put themselves at risk of not having enough energy for the brain to grow and function at its best. Warning signs might include low hormone levels; gut symptoms or changes in bowel movements; loss of muscle, strength, fitness, or ability to adequately recover from exercise; and fatigue and poor sleep.

At the other end, the modern food environment makes it very easy for us to have access to more energy than we need. This is another element of mismatch that has resulted in society having to think about diets—a fairly recent invention—in the first place. In a 2023 essay, longevity researcher Charles Brenner put it this way:

> Caloric restriction extends animal lifespan when compared to [having] constant access to food. However, it is more accurate to say that unrestricted access to food is a life-shortening condition that is unlike conditions in the wild to which animals are adapted.[52]

This idea mirrors what we've seen with movement in the previous chapter. Just as the absence of physical activity is the main issue rather than exercise being a health-promoting intervention we've suddenly discovered, the downsides of excess energy availability in the modern diet have resulted in us actively having to work against them by inventing diets.

As a result of the negative effects of excess energy availability in the modern environment, multiple possible strategies have been implemented, including caloric restriction (eating less of what you're currently eating), intermittent fasting (IF, having periods where you eat a lot less or nothing at all), and time-restricted eating (TRE, only eating during a specific time window each day).

Intermittent fasting in particular has been touted as being beneficial for longevity by boosting mitochondrial function and cell-cleaning processes like autophagy.[53] However, most of these benefits are based on mouse studies, and many of the effects of fasting in mice don't translate to humans. For example, my colleague Kristi Storoschuk recently compared the effects of fasting on muscle mitochondria in humans and rodents. Not only were the effects of fasting much more variable in rodents than we're usually told, but these same effects were not seen in humans at all.[54] This is probably because fasting is a much bigger stress in mice than it is in humans (mice can die after just twenty-four hours without food).

This doesn't mean that caloric restriction, IF, and TRE aren't useful—they have all been shown to reduce disease risk markers in multiple human studies.[55] However, their effect is primarily through decreasing energy intake and reversing the negative effects of excess energy availability. Any further restriction beyond that is unlikely to be beneficial for the body or brain, especially if it also results in the loss of muscle, strength, or hormonal health.

Several clinical trials have compared these energy reduction strategies with one another, with any differences usually tied to which strategy resulted in the most sustainable reduction in calorie intake.[56] And on the other side, one of the reasons that IF and TRE sometimes fail to show large benefits in human trials is that it's still possible to do those diets without reducing energy intake if your overall diet doesn't change otherwise.[57] If you do want to try one of these strategies, pick the one that feels most sustainable in your own lifestyle. Maybe that's skipping the occasional day of food (IF). Maybe it's TRE and not eating after 6 P.M. (which often improves diet quality by reducing intake of late-night snacks and desserts). My own personal approach is to change the energy density of the foods to match my needs without having to change when or how much food I eat, as I outline below. All of these can work to make sure you're fuelling appropriately.

One of the most striking examples of the critical importance of energy availability on health is the recent expansion of diabetes and obesity drugs like Ozempic and Mounjaro, with more advanced formulations on the way. These drugs affect the incretin system, which regulates food intake and metabolism, and often produce profound decreases in weight and blood sugar that result in lowered risk of chronic conditions like heart disease.[58] This happens primarily by decreasing hunger and food intake—so much so that changes in shopping habits have been seen at the national level since these therapies became available.[59] In addition, these drugs can have direct effects on metabolism in ways that decrease the negative effects of excess energy availability, improving blood sugar regulation and insulin resistance.

The success of these drugs at improving health in people with obesity and diabetes, and the link between those conditions and cognitive decline, have attracted a lot of interest in using these medications to lower the risk of dementia.[60] Another thing that makes these drugs interesting with respect to cognitive health is that many cells in the brain have receptors that they can bind to. For instance, semaglutide (the active ingredient in Ozempic) binds to GLP-1 receptors, which are found on neurons, microglia, and astrocytes. One of the earlier versions of these drugs, exenatide—a synthetic copy of a protein isolated from the venom of Gila monsters—is a promising neuroprotective therapy that we're testing in my lab right now. By binding to GLP-1 receptors, exenatide improves the survival of neurons and can decrease neuroinflammation.[61]

As a result of both the possible direct effects of these drugs on the brain, and indirect benefits via changes in energy availability, multiple trials of drugs like semaglutide are currently in progress to see if they are able to treat or prevent cognitive decline and dementia.[62] Though there is a huge amount of work to be done to decide who should and shouldn't use these medications, their impact clearly shows how energy availability drives our overall health, with important implications for the brain. Taken together, this evidence supports my second rule of eating to help reduce the risk of dementia: *fuel for your* own *needs*. You need enough energy to build brain buffers and maintain cognitive function with age, but taking too much fuel on board can impair long-term health and performance.

ARE YOU FUELLING FOR *YOUR* NEEDS?

Now that you understand the risks of both too little and too much energy for the brain, you are likely asking how to determine whether you are fuelling for your own particular needs. There are a number of ways to assess this, including some simple tools to start with.

Physical Symptoms

People who are experiencing energy excess often feel fatigued—either immediately after meals or overall. They may also feel "hangry," that uncomfortable mixture of hungry and angry, within only a couple hours of their last meal.[63] Energy excess can also impact your mood. For example, multiple conditions associated with excess energy availability, including prediabetes and metabolic syndrome, are associated with a higher risk of depressive symptoms.[64]

Body Mass Index (BMI)

Though BMI is an imperfect tool to assess health, the risk of cognitive decline and lower brain volumes does seem to increase in those with a BMI over 30, especially when in conjunction with specific body measurements described below. Those with obesity who continue to gain weight over time are at increased risk of cognitive decline associated with changes in brain structure that can be seen by MRI.[65] On the other side, an analysis of DIRECT PLUS (the Dietary Intervention Randomised Controlled Trial Polyphenols Unprocessed Study), which randomised individuals with obesity to Mediterranean-style diets plus exercise, found that weight loss as well as lower consumption of processed food, sweets, and sugar-sweetened beverages like soda were associated with slowed brain aging.[66]

Measurements

Use a tape measure to capture measurements of your hips (at the widest point of the buttocks), waist (about an inch above your belly button), and height (toes to top of the head). Once you've recorded those numbers, divide your waist measurement by your hip measurement and your height measurement to create two ratios (waist-to-hip and waist-to-height). Studies suggest that having a waist circumference above 90 centimetres or 35 inches indicates energy excess. Similarly, a waist-to-hip ratio of more than 0.85 in women or 0.90 in men, or a waist-to-height ratio of more than 0.55 suggests you may be overfuelling—and are at higher risk of cognitive decline and dementia as well as a higher overall risk of death.[67] Maintaining a lower waist-to-hip ratio through midlife is associated with better brain and cognitive health in older age.[68]

Laboratory Testing

Your doctor can order basic blood tests to understand whether you are in a state of excess energy availability. Evidence of prediabetes or diabetes—

based on either fasting blood sugar (above 100 mg/dL or 5.6 mmol/L) or the longer-term blood sugar marker HbA1c (above 5.6 percent or 40 mmol/mol) suggest you may need to examine your energy intake. Elevated fasting glucose is one of five components of metabolic syndrome, which is primarily a disorder of insulin resistance and excess energy availability. Other components include an elevated waist circumference (see above), high blood pressure, low HDL cholesterol (below 40 mg/dL in men or below 50 mg/dL in women), and high triglycerides (above 150 mg/dL). Metabolic syndrome—especially with high blood sugar and high blood pressure—is associated with increased risk of multiple forms of dementia, but this risk is reversible if health improves.[69]

PATTERN

Now that you understand the importance of consuming the right nutrients, as well as maintaining a state of energy balance to support your specific needs, it's time to talk logistics. And that means adopting a dietary pattern—notice I am intentionally not using the word *diet*—to help you achieve those goals.

There are some important reasons that I think we should talk about dietary patterns rather than specific diets. First, and most importantly, whether diets even "work" is a significant point of contention. Most of this debate occurs within the hallowed halls of social media (of course), and usually revolves around weight loss.

Of course, this is *not* a weight-loss book. You can (and should) do a million amazing things to support your brain, your health, and your well-being without ever needing to step on a scale. Your weight is also a very poor measure of health; if your weight goes up a bit because you've added some muscle and bone tissue from all the resisting and sprinting you're now doing after reading chapter 7 ("Move"), that is definitely a good thing!

With that said, we *can* learn quite a lot about the process of dietary change from studies focused on weight loss. The basic principle of any weight-loss diet is to decrease the amount of energy that is consumed from food. Those who argue against dieting will say that this approach doesn't work in the long term because many people who lose weight by dieting end up regaining that weight. This is absolutely true.[70] But it's not that changing your diet doesn't "work," it's just *hard*. You might need to completely change where or how you shop, what you cook and how you cook it, and find the time and resources to do all of that. You might even need to change how you look at food and your relationship with it more broadly.

Participants in a research study can often white-knuckle a new diet for a few weeks or months, especially with frequent contact, support, or food supplied by the people running the study. But remove that support, or just let those participants exist in the real world again for a period of time, and they'll tend to go back to their previous diet and previous weight. This is normal human nature: behaviour change is hard, especially when it's something as ingrained as what and how we eat.

STARTING A NEW HABIT

There are many schools of thought when it comes to building new habits, but they all include the need to make the process easy and actionable as well as thinking in advance about where you might struggle.

Implementation Intentions

One of the main problems with building new habits is that they are often overly ambitious and far too vague. Implementation intentions take some of the guesswork out of this process. Rather than saying, "I want to lose weight," commit to a more specific plan of action. An easy way to increase nutrient intake and decrease calorie intake without feeling restricted is to add more vegetables to a meal. Try something like "every night this week I will add an extra serving of veggies to my plate." Similarly, rather than just thinking about exercising more, you could commit to a five-minute workout as soon as you get home from work. Better yet, schedule these activities into your calendar so you don't forget. When setting health-related goals, having an implementation intention significantly increases the likelihood of success. It increases commitment and makes the goal seem easier. The catch? It works best if you set and commit to one goal at a time.[71]

WOOP

Gabriele Oettingen is a psychologist who specialises in cognition and behaviour. As part of her research, she developed the WOOP (wish, outcome, obstacle, and plan) framework to help people better achieve their goals.

WOOP has a specific focus on thinking about the *obstacles* that might hold you back. Her studies show that using this framework makes people more likely to increase their physical activity or improve their diet (eat more fruits and veggies).[72] When considering a change you want to make, think about (or write down) answers to the following questions. This will make it more likely that you stick to your plan if something gets in your way.

1. **Wish.** What is it that you would like to achieve? Pick a wish that feels challenging to you but that you can reasonably fulfill within the next few weeks.
2. **Outcome.** Think about the best possible outcome of fulfilling your wish. How would it make you feel?
3. **Obstacle.** What might hold you back or stop you from fulfilling your wish? It might be an emotion, a belief, the time you have available, or a bad habit. Think both practically and deeply to identify all the likely obstacles.
4. **Plan.** For every obstacle, identify an action you can take to overcome it.

Maybe your wish happens to be to include more vegetables with dinner every night. You hope the outcome will be that you feel healthier, more energised, and proud of your eating habits. One main obstacle you identify is that you might feel too tired to cook in the evening. In that scenario, you plan to use a frozen vegetable mix or prechopped veggies or salads to make it easy.

There are a few ways to get around the fact that dietary change can be hard to maintain, starting with considering how that change fits with your life, your goals, and you as a person. Yes, this is the point where we have to get a bit "meta" and do some self-reflection.[73]

One of the most widely accepted theories of motivation and psychological need is *self-determination theory*—first introduced by Richard Ryan and Edward Deci, psychologists at the University of Rochester, in the mid-1980s. Self-determination theory says that humans need three basic things: autonomy, competence, and relatedness. Autonomy is the freedom to make our own choices, control our own behaviours, and set our own goals. Competence is feeling like we are capable and have mastery over our lives. Relatedness is the feeling of belonging and connection to other people.

Any change you make is most likely to stick if you achieve those three core needs as part of it. So, to start, it needs to feel like you're actively making a choice that aligns with your goals (autonomy). In chapter 6 we talked about finding your *why*, and the same applies here. As an example, I'll go out on a limb and suggest that most people aren't going to eat more broccoli because of the pure, unbridled ecstasy they feel when consuming it. Instead, there is a broccoli-driven future scenario they *want* to achieve, like bolstering their brain health and overall longevity so that they can live long enough to make their great-grandchildren eat their broccoli too. If, instead, you're working toward a broccoli-studded future because you feel like you *have* to, the likelihood of success is much lower.[74]

In addition to autonomy, we also need competence: we need to feel capable of sustaining our planned change. Maybe we prepare by subscribing to a Broccoli of the Month delivery service and buying the bestselling *Joy of Broccoli* cookbook. Or maybe we start small by cooking broccoli once every couple of weeks and hiding it in the macaroni cheese. Or we could go full-bore broccoli most days but allow for some breaks in the weekly broccoli fest if it feels too restrictive or repetitive.[75] All of these are evidence-based strategies to increase competence and make a dietary change more likely to stick.

The final piece of the puzzle is relatedness; making sure that you have support from others in your broccoli-laden journey will also increase the likelihood of success.[76] Have your family commit to the same culinary journey and take turns finding fun ways to make delectable broccoli dishes. Put the broccoli out first as an starter (we eat what's in front of us, so a simple trick is to start a meal with foods you want to eat more of).[77] Have a potluck dinner and share the joys of broccoli with all your friends. Create a Broccoli Bros group on social media and share your broccoli hijinks with other like-minded enthusiasts. And because nutrition loves a good food feud, you could even start an online rivalry with the Cauliflower Crew. The options for having your way with cruciferous vegetables are truly endless. What matters is whether you feel supported by and connected to others on your brocco-journey.

Beyond being a way for me to write "broccoli" as many times as possible for my own entertainment, these three core psychological needs should be part of our plan anytime we try to change any aspect of our food or lifestyle. To me they also explain one of the most successful weight-loss trials done to date. The BROAD trial enrolled people with obesity and metabolic disease (heart disease, high blood pressure, or type 2 diabetes), assigning them to either a control group or an intervention that involved completely changing their diet to one based on unprocessed whole plant foods.

Though the intervention did eliminate a lot of foods, participants could eat as much as they wanted, which provided autonomy. They were taught how to source and cook this new food (competence) and had twice-weekly meetings for three months that included social events and potluck dinners, which provided social support and relatedness. Not only did the intervention group improve a whole host of health markers compared to the control group, but nine months after the end of the intervention, they had maintained all those changes—including their weight loss.[78] This tells us that diets *can* work, but making sure they align with our goals and what we're capable of and supported to do will be very important. And that's the problem. Because, regardless of our intentions, most diets don't do any of those things.

IS THERE A BEST DIET FOR BUILDING HEADROOM?

This is a question I'm often asked. And the simple answer is no.

As I mentioned in part 1, much of my perspective comes from the intersection of scientific evidence and a healthy dose of trial and error. It would take me a very long time to list all my failures as a coach and scientist over the years and the lessons I've learned from them, but there are some relatable examples that stand out. For example, I have to admit that there were multiple times when I was convinced that a very specific type of diet was going to be the solution to a wide variety of health conditions in something approaching a one-size-fits-all manner. In 2004, as an undergraduate, I was a steadfast proponent of the "paleo" diet—a diet that supposedly had the least mismatch to our evolutionary biology, eliminating dairy, grains, and legumes. Not too long after that I was sure that low-carb diets were the answer.

Don't get me wrong, there are several specific scenarios in which each of those diets can be very impactful, but I have also seen people thrive on diets that look nothing like either of those approaches. I also remember a slew of athletes I worked with during my PhD who were struggling with both their health and their performance after commencing restrictive diets that podcasts and social media had told them would be optimal for their health. But the reality for them was that overly focusing on removing certain food groups from their diet made it nearly impossible for them to consume enough calories to train and compete at a high level.

Similarly, I remember working with two Formula 1 drivers who, unbeknownst to each other, chose to try the same specific diet in the same offseason. These drivers didn't have any of the usual issues we might have when trying to change our diet. At any given time, there were several people available to source and prepare the necessary food and make sure that their caloric and nutrient requirements were being met. But even with the hard parts of a dietary change being taken care of and carefully monitored, one driver saw their performance improve while the other went in the other direction.

These examples reminded me how different each human can be, which is why I think we can say that almost any dietary pattern can work provided it helps the individual get the nutrients their brain needs and maintain energy balance over time. Whether you prefer a plant-based vegan diet, a Mediterranean diet, an "everything in moderation" diet, or a low-carbohydrate or ketogenic diet, there are huge numbers of people who have benefitted from that approach, as well as scientific evidence to support it. The success all comes back to those critical two rules: *Maximise nutrients* and *fuel appropriately*.

That's why, to combat the modern food environment, you need to look beyond branded diets and think about overall dietary pattern. Because, if you look closely at most diets that claim to support brain health, the main commonality between them is that they follow these rules. They tend to increase nutrient density (the number of nutrients and minerals in a bite of food) and decrease energy density (the amount of energy in an average bite of food).

As long as our energy and nutrient needs are met, it matters a lot less where that food comes from. Tamar Haspel, a journalist whose expertise lies at the intersection of food and science, summarises this by saying that humans "can thrive on basically any diet out there except the one we have." *The one we have* refers to the diet and foods that are most easily and readily available to all of us in our modern food landscape—high in energy and low in nutrients.

While it's easy to fall into the trap of assuming that traditional human diets are the *best* diets for health (also known as the *naturalistic fallacy*), looking across the types of diets that humans eat in their more ancestral habitats can give us a window into just how different the dietary patterns that support human health can be. For example, Daniel Lieberman, the evolutionary biologist we met in chapter 7, recently looked at calorie sources from eleven different hunter-gatherer groups across South America, Africa, Southeast Asia, and Australia. The sources of calories varied widely from group to group. Animal foods made up as little as 8 percent or as much as 88 percent of the diet. Similarly, plant foods ranged from 3 percent to 87 percent of calories. Any calories that weren't from plants or animals (up to 22 percent) came from honey.

The amount of energy that came from the major macronutrients—carbohydrates (5 to 67 percent), protein (14 to 48 percent), and fat (10 to 65 percent)—also varied a lot. Similar findings have been found elsewhere, with carbohydrate intake generally decreasing (and therefore fat intake increasing) the farther away people live from the equator.[79]

If we're looking for a source of mismatch between more traditional human diets and the modern diet, it's unlikely to be the exact macronutrient balance or whether the food comes from animals or plants, because humans all over the world are thriving on a huge variety of diets from across the spectrum.

Instead, the mismatch between traditional human diets and the modern human diet comes from the relative intakes of whole, nutrient-dense foods. This is also the factor that unites most successful dietary interventions, which then translates to better brain-related outcomes. For example, several research groups have found that people whose diets better adhere to dietary patterns such as the Mediterranean or DASH (Dietary Approaches to Stop Hypertension) diet have better mental and cognitive health outcomes.[80] The details differ slightly across these dietary patterns, but generally they include a greater intake of vegetables, fruits and berries, minimally processed whole grains (like oats and brown rice), legumes (beans and lentils), lean cuts of meat, and fish. At the same time, they recommend reducing heavily processed meats (bacon and hot dogs), heavily processed carbohydrates (especially cakes, biscuits, and other baked goods), and fried foods.

The most well-known brain-specific diet is probably MIND (Mediterranean-DASH Intervention for Neurodegenerative Delay), which was developed by Martha Clare Morris, a nutritional epidemiologist at Rush University Medical Centre in Chicago in 2015, as a hybrid of the Mediterranean and DASH diets.[81] Among nearly one thousand older adults from the Rush Memory and Ageing Project, as part of a study that Morris led, those who had the better MIND diet scores had a lower risk of later Alzheimer's disease.

The MIND diet was recently tested in a large trial, where six hundred people over sixty-five with a family history of dementia were randomised to either MIND or a group that focused on decreasing calorie intake without changing their overall dietary pattern. After three years on their respective diets, the groups saw similar improvements in cognitive function.[82] Both groups also lost similar amounts of weight. Though this could potentially be considered a failure for MIND over a more standard dieting approach of caloric restriction, I think it just underpins the importance of overall energy availability, which decreased in both groups. Though they weren't told to, the calorie reduction group also improved their diet quality slightly. And as with the BROAD study, participants were encouraged to socialise with other group members via cooking sessions, trivia games, competitions, and holiday celebrations. We know that all these factors increase success, regardless of the diet strategy being employed.

Results such as this also underpin why I think it's more important to talk about dietary patterns than exact diets, because it's the overall picture of a diet that matters rather than any one of its individual components. For example, a study using dietary data from more than sixty thousand people in the UK Biobank found that higher adherence to a Mediterranean diet pattern was associated with lower risk of later dementia, as well as having benefits to cardiovascular health.[83] However, when they looked at each component of the Mediterranean diet individually, there was no individual food or food group that explained the relationship between the Mediterranean diet and dementia. This means that there's no real magic to the Mediterranean diet—the benefit probably comes from the overall pattern of eating more whole foods that are higher in nutrients and lower in energy density.

Knowing that pattern is more important than individual foods means we can be more flexible and practical when trying to apply these principles to our own diets. It's not that everybody around the world suddenly needs to ship in a ton of olive oil in order to prevent dementia—you can build a headroom-boosting diet using whatever is available locally and that you can afford.

TO SUPPLEMENT OR NOT TO SUPPLEMENT

As you consider your own dietary pattern—and what foods to eat in order to maximise nutrient density—you may wonder what role supplements should play. While I hope that most people are able to find a nutrient-dense dietary pattern that means they don't need to supplement, there is certainly evidence that targeted supplementation can fill nutrient gaps and improve cognitive function as a result. For example, if you cannot access (or simply don't like) certain nutrient-dense foods, you can add key nutrients to your diet through a supplement.

Long-Chain Omega-3s

Omega-3 status is one of the best nutritional predictors of dementia risk, and supplementation with omega-3s can decrease depression symptoms and improve sleep.[84] While plant foods do contain a version of omega-3s (ALA), the conversion of ALA to longer-chain omega-3s like DHA (important for the brain) and EPA (important for heart health) is highly variable, and most people also need to consume EPA and DHA from food. Those who aren't eating at least two or three 4-ounce portions of fatty fish (e.g., salmon, tuna, mackerel, sardines) per week should consider taking around 2–3 grams per day of an omega-3 supplement that has both EPA and DHA. This can come from algae if you eat a plant-based diet.

B Vitamins Involved in Methylation

Several studies suggest that B vitamin supplementation is associated with slowed cognitive decline.[85] Low B12 levels are associated with worse cognitive function even when people aren't technically deficient.[86] And, as mentioned above, B vitamins and omega-3s interact to improve brain health. In studies of homocysteine lowering with B vitamins, the most benefit is seen when keeping homocysteine under <13 μmol/L, but a variety of other lines of evidence suggest that less than 10–11 m/L is probably better.[87] If homocysteine is elevated, the interventions in those studies included supplements with around 500 μg of B12 and 700 DFE (dietary folate equivalents) of folate per day.[88] Some studies lowering homocysteine with B vitamins have also included around 20 mg of B6 and 1–2 mg of riboflavin (B2) per day.[89]

Vitamin D

Vitamin D insufficiency is common around the world, and more likely in those with low sun exposure or darker skin tones. As many as one in four adults may need more vitamin D.[90] Vitamin D deficiency (levels below 20 ng/mL) is associated with an increased risk of dementia and smaller brain volumes, with higher target levels (40–50 ng/mL) generally recommended to support athletic performance.[91] In a study of more than twelve thousand people from the National Alzheimer's Coordinating Centre, those who supplemented with vitamin D experienced a lower incidence of future dementia.[92] Though testing and tracking vitamin D is recommended, a dose of 2,000 IU of vitamin D3 per day is safe and results in most people achieving adequate vitamin D levels.[93] Vitamin D supplementation in this range is also associated with a significant reduction in depression symptoms.[94] Trials of both vitamin D and omega-3 supplementation have even suggested that they may directly slow some of the processes of aging.[95]

Magnesium

Insufficient magnesium intake is also common, with some studies suggesting that almost half of the U.S. population is not consuming the recommended amount.[96] Magnesium is critical for vitamin D metabolism, so ensuring good magnesium intake may be important for vitamin D levels.[97] Magnesium status can be tricky to measure, but if you're looking to boost your magnesium intake, you could consider a supplement that includes 50–100 percent of the recommended daily intake (around 200–400 mg). Avoid magnesium oxide and high doses of magnesium citrate, as they have lower bioavailability and can cause stomach issues.

Creatine

Creatine is found in meat and fish and is critical for energy-demanding tissues like muscles and the brain. Though we make our own creatine, creatine supplementation is popular with athletes because it can help support gains in muscle size and strength.[98] However, creatine is increasingly being investigated for a range of potential brain benefits. It can offset some of the negative effects of sleep deprivation on cognitive function and support multiple aspects of cognitive function more generally (memory and processing speed), especially in older individuals.[99] Multiple studies also now suggest that creatine may help the treatment of depression.[100] The standard dose of creatine monohydrate is 5 g per day, and that's the best place to start, but some studies have found benefits at doses of 10–30 g in depression, with resistance training, or after acute sleep deprivation—with very few side effects.[101] If you do choose to supplement with creatine, look for creatine monohydrate manufactured by Creapure, which is the form that is used in the vast majority of studies. One caveat is that creatine is often overhyped, and when it does work it primarily helps you do a bit *more* of an energetically expensive activity, like performing a few more reps in the gym or a complex memory task.[102] So, for the full benefits, you still have to make sure you challenge yourself.

What About Other Supplements?

There is a whole host of supplements that could be included in a section like this, each with its own set of evidence and explanation of circumstances where it might be beneficial. However, I've chosen to focus on supplements where either there is a strong link between deficiency and brain health or there is *positive asymmetry*—a high likelihood of benefit in the right situation with a low likelihood of risk. Beyond these—for now, at least—there are very few supplements that I would routinely recommend to a wide range of people. Of course, we have to acknowledge that supplements can be expensive, and quality can be quite variable. The best companies will independently test their products using a third party to assess purity and make sure there are no contaminants. Any good company should be able to send you a certificate of analysis showing that they've done this.

In some cases, blood tests of nutrient status can be helpful in deciding if it's worth supplementing, but it's also fine to use a high-quality multivitamin to cover your bases. However, it's important to understand that you cannot supplement your way out of a bad diet. As much as possible, when trying to eat to promote brain health, the goal is to avoid needing supplements by getting as many nutrients as possible from whole foods.

A BROWNIE IS STILL A BROWNIE

Another reason I prefer that people approach eating in terms of dietary patterns as opposed to diets is that many diets can make us think something is healthy just because it's "vegan" or "keto," regardless of whether that food sticks to the general rules of brain health.

You already know that if you eat more vegetables, fruits and berries, and lean meat and fish, you're also eating *less* of something else. In most cases, what you're eating less of is foods with the problematic combination of being calorie dense, hyperpalatable (easy to eat a lot of), and low in protein and brain-supporting nutrients. Many people have pointed the finger particularly at ultraprocessed foods, which get that designation based on levels of processing or the additives they contain. But while there is some evidence that eating higher levels of ultraprocessed foods is associated with worse mental health and faster cognitive decline,[103] there are also plenty of ultra-processed foods that are not necessarily problematic because they're not calorie dense, hyperpalatable, or low in protein. For example, a good high-quality protein powder is technically an ultraprocessed food. But protein powders can be an excellent way for, say, a vegan, an athlete, or anybody else to easily incorporate more protein into their meals if they need.

The standard Western dietary pattern is full of calorie-dense, nutrient-poor, hyperpalatable, low-fibre, low-protein foods. It's these characteristics that are the problem rather than the fact that the food is ultraprocessed. And while these foods don't need to be demonised, making them a regular part of your diet may not be the best choice for your brain. For example, one study had participants consume one of their daily meals as a typical Western diet option (a choice of either waffles or a main meal and dessert from a fast-food chain) for one week, which resulted in lower performance on a hippocampal-dependent memory test than that of a control group.[104] As you may recall, the hippocampus is strongly associated with memory and cognitive function and is particularly at risk in those who suffer from Alzheimer's disease.

Other studies have shown that overeating a typical Western diet or adding a few chocolate bars to your daily diet can start to cause insulin resistance and oxidative stress within just a few days, along with disrupted insulin signaling in the brain.[105] By contrast, one reason the Mediterranean diet has been a focus of brain health in recent years is that the improved food quality and nutrients like polyphenols combine to benefit the brain by improving blood sugar control.[106]

While you might appreciate that only eating burgers, milkshakes, and waffles may not be the best strategy for long-term brain health, it's surprising how often foods that fit into supposedly healthy diets aren't much better from a nutritional standpoint. To illustrate this, let's think about a nice big plate of brownies. Now look, don't hate me. I had to pick something as an example, and I love brownies as much as the next person. (Except my wife, who for some inexplicable reason isn't a big brownie fan.)

Okay, back to the brownies. You could buy them prepackaged from the shop or make them yourself in a number of different ways. Out of a box, the old-fashioned way. Or from scratch with a full set of ingredients the *old* old-fashioned way. You could make them without eggs or butter, and they'd be vegan. You could replace the regular flour and sugar with almond flour and some kind of alternative sweetener to make them low carb. There's probably even a Mediterranean diet version where you make them with nut butter, whole wheat flour, and olive oil. All of these brownies would be delicious, especially if you add a sprinkle of salt on top to make them extra-craveable by hitting the maximum number of taste buds. And while only the premade brownie would count as ultra-processed, each of these delectable treats is energy dense, easy to overeat, and low in fibre, nutrients, and protein. At the end of the day, a brownie is a brownie.

This is why *pattern* matters the most. Enjoying brownies occasionally doesn't influence your dietary pattern on its own, and they can fit into any diet you choose to follow as long as you're getting the necessary nutrients and fuelling appropriately overall. But we also need to acknowledge that it's easy to regularly blow our energy budget on platefuls of brownies regardless of how we make them.

HOW OUR FOOD CHANGES HOW WE EAT

Kevin Hall is one of the world's foremost researchers on the topic of how our food affects how much we eat. Unlike most nutrition studies, in which people are just asked what they eat, or trials like the BROAD study, where people are given a new way of eating, Dr. Hall locks people up in a "metabolic ward," where their activity, food intake, and metabolism can be recorded in intimate detail. With their permission, of course.

The first research study I ever did, which was part of my undergraduate thesis project, involved something very similar. Of course, as it was my first research project, my main job was just to do what I was told and not mess anything up too much. The Human Nutrition Unit that I joined at the University of Cambridge had a facility where people stayed and were fed diets that contained different amounts of sugar. The goal of this particular study was to see if sugar intake could be measured in the urine.[107] The method the team developed was then used in large epidemiological studies as a more accurate way of measuring sugar intake than asking people how much sugar they eat. Because, let's be honest, it's hard to remember if you ate two brownies or seven.

The focus of Hall's work has been on how the composition and processing of food affects how much we eat. What his group has found generally aligns with the core principles of dietary pattern that seem to influence health. First, they found that people will eat more when given meals of ultraprocessed food compared to when they eat similar meals consisting of minimally processed food. One reason for this is that the processed foods tended to be lower in protein, and participants ate more total calories until they had consumed the same amount of protein as when they were eating the minimally processed diet.[108] Later studies have consistently found that people eat more if the food requires less chewing, and that people are more likely to overeat if food is low in fibre and protein and has a high energy density.[109] The main issue, therefore, is less about food processing and more about food composition and energy density.

Other studies have found something similar. For example, in the week-long waffle-and-fast-food study, participants saw changes in appetite control in addition to the changes in memory function. As it turns out, we're not very good at judging our food intake when that food is energy dense (think foods high in sugar, fat, and refined carbohydrates).[110] This is probably because the perfect, craveable combination of carbs and fat is something relatively new to the food environment, providing us with energy in the absence of other components that the brain expects at the same time, like fibre, water, protein, and nutrients. Therefore, filling our plates with whole foods that contain those missing ingredients—and that require real chewing—is the perfect antidote to the modern food environment.

Though there's ample evidence that humans can thrive on a wide variety of diets from a wide variety of sources, the focus on protein is an important one. In Daniel Lieberman's study of hunter-gatherers, the protein intake from traditional diets was relatively high—30 percent of calories on average compared to around 15 to 18 percent in the average American diet. The relatively dementia-proof Tsimané also eat a lot of protein—just over 0.9 grams per pound of body weight (2 grams per kilogram) on average per day.[111] This is 2.5 times the U.S. recommended daily intake. And increasing evidence suggests that the Tsimané are probably closer to getting it right than we are.

Higher protein intakes can help us feel full after meals as well as supporting muscle mass and brain health. For instance, older adults who eat more protein lose less muscle mass as they age, and population studies generally suggest that people who eat more protein have a lower risk of cognitive decline and dementia.[112] Most importantly, as we get older, we probably need more protein in order to get the same benefit, and most protein recommendations are based on the physiology of younger people as well as focusing on avoiding deficiencies rather than promoting health.[113] One study in adults over sixty found that protein consumption around 50 percent above the recommended daily intake maximised the production of glutathione, an antioxidant linked to the reduction of dementia risk.[114] Improvements in muscle mass appear to peak at around double the recommended daily intake.[115] As a result, the current consensus suggests that we should each try to eat at least 0.55 grams of protein per pound of body weight per day but ideally closer to 0.7–0.8 grams per pound, rather than the recommended daily amount of 0.4 grams per pound.[116] This higher level of protein intake, particularly when combined with some kind of resistance training, best supports improvement and maintenance of strength and muscle mass, as well as overall health. And if you ever hear high protein is bad for your long-term health, recent expert reviews of the literature find that there is very little evidence to support this (as well as lots of evidence for the benefit of protein).[117]

Those who struggle to eat enough calories and enough protein as they get older, or in general, can lean on some of the benefits of the modern environment and consume some protein-rich processed foods. This includes protein bars and protein powders. There are even some surprisingly good protein cereals that I myself will sometimes eat if I don't have the time or energy to make a bowl of yoghurt and berries or heat up leftovers for breakfast (which is what I usually do). Of course, these processed protein-focused foods don't necessarily have a ton of other nutrients, so they're more of a supplement than a focus.

Also, bear in mind that just because something *says* it has a lot of protein doesn't mean it does, or that it's something you should be eating a lot of. Think protein biscuits, protein chocolate bars, and protein brownies (insert eye roll here—a brownie is still a brownie). As a quick check, there's a trick I learned from Ted Naiman, an engineer and family physician who also just happens to be my doctor, and who has amalgamated huge amounts of information on how different foods affect our hunger in his book *Satiety per Calorie*.[118] When looking for processed snack foods with a high protein content, make sure that they have at least as many grams of protein as the number of calories divided by ten (e.g., twenty grams of protein in a two-hundred-calorie protein bar), and ideally more than that. It's a fairly arbitrary cutoff, but it's easy to remember, and I've found that it works pretty well for both professional athletes and everybody else.

CALCULATE YOUR PROTEIN NEEDS

Many people do not consume enough protein, and this can be especially challenging as we get older and our requirements increase—especially if we don't have the time to regularly cook and prepare our own meals, and for those who are have decreased their overall food intake (for instance, if taking GLP-1 medications) or who embrace more plant-based dietary patterns. To understand how much protein you should try to eat per day, whether it's in the form of lean meats or beans, fill out the following form.

Lower End of the Range
0.55 g of protein x body weight (in pounds) = _____

Upper End of the Range
0.8 g of protein x body weight (in pounds) = _____

For example, a person weighing 150 pounds should work toward incorporating 82.5–120 grams of protein per day, or 30–40 grams per meal. The average skinless chicken breast contains about 56 grams of protein. A 3-ounce serving of fish is somewhere in the 16–26-gram range. A half cup of beans offers 7–10 grams of protein, depending on the type.

Another way to do this is based on how much protein would fill the palm of your open hand. As your hand is scaled to your body size, you don't need to weigh anything. For meat or fish, aim for two palms' worth per meal. For yoghurt, beans, tofu, or eggs, aim for at least three palms. Getting your protein from whole foods in this way can also help you get a bunch of other nutrients you need and help keep you fuller longer while providing appropriate energy for your own needs.

Where does this leave us when we're trying to improve our diet pattern to improve our health? If we want to avoid feeling like our diet is restrictive, often the easiest thing is to focus on *adding* rather than subtracting. In particular, add more foods that are nutrient dense but not energy dense—fruits, berries, vegetables of all kinds, beans and lentils, potatoes (a surprising nutrient and satiety powerhouse), and minimally processed grains like brown rice and oats—as well as foods that are both nutrient dense and rich in protein like lean meat, fish, fermented dairy products like cheese and yoghurt, soy products like tofu and tempeh, and eggs. Nuts and seeds make an appearance here too, but if you turn them into peanut butter or honey-roasted macadamia nuts, they can quickly end up looking something a bit like our brownie scenario.

A nice place to start might be implementing the recommendations used in the SMILES (Supporting the Modification of lifestyle in Lowered Emotional States) trial, the first randomised trial that showed you can improve symptoms of depression using diet.[119] Their recommendations were to improve diet quality by focusing on vegetables (six servings per day), fruit (three servings per day), legumes (three or four servings per week), low-fat and unsweetened dairy foods (two or three servings per day), raw and unsalted nuts (one serving per day), fish (at least two servings per week), lean red meats (three or four servings per week), chicken (two or three servings per week), eggs (up to six per week), and olive oil (three tablespoons per day) while reducing sweets, refined cereals, fried food, fast food, processed meats, and sugary drinks (no more than three of these total per week). Importantly, though participants were given recommended servings for each food, they were told to eat as much as they wanted.

Admittedly, the list of SMILES trial guidelines is long. But if you start by focusing on one or two of the recommendations and building from there, this will slowly shift your dietary pattern as well as providing more nutrients that can support brain health.

To improve dietary pattern when working with clients who want something a little more specific than the SMILES trial, I recommend the following (I also typically use this approach when putting together my own meals). Divide a ten-inch dinner plate into thirds (figure 4). Fill the first third with your lean protein of choice. Chicken, fish, lean beef, lentils—whatever works for you. Then throw your favourite

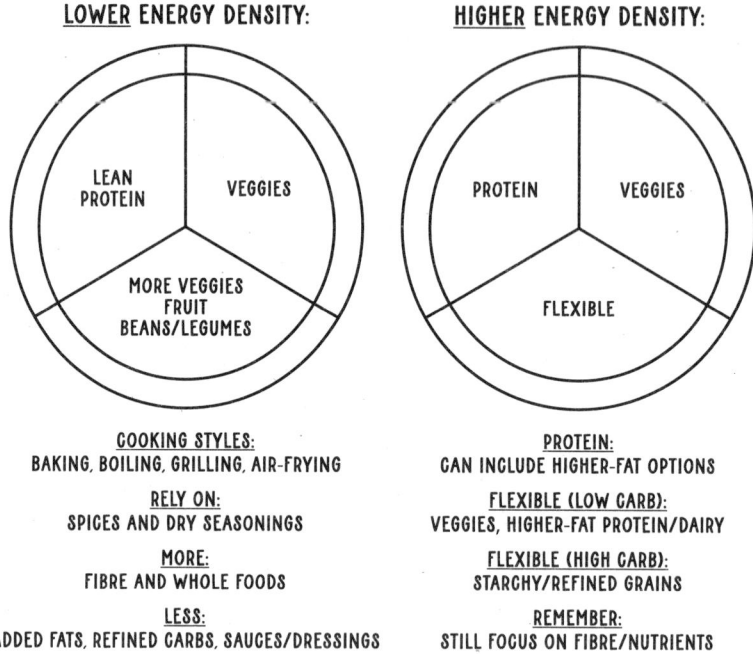

FIGURE 4. Options for plates based on energy requirements. Start with a protein choice—lean proteins for lower energy density or higher-fat protein sources if more energy is needed. Then load up with veggies and carbs based on preferences and goals.

nutrient-dense veggies and fruits into the second third of the plate. Again, eat the foods in this category that most appeal to you. The goal is to make it both nutrient dense and something you actually want to eat. In fact, studies have shown that just focusing on the fact that something is *healthy* often isn't enough to make people eat it consistently, and it's much better to focus on foods that hit your nutrient and energy goals but that you also find enticing and appealing.[120]

When it comes to the last third of your plate, you have some choices to make based on your body's (and brain's) current needs. If you are an athlete and need more calories to fuel your activity, putting a serving of brown rice, pasta, or other carbohydrate in the last section is probably your best bet (higher energy density). If, however, you are currently in a state of excess energy availability, consider filling the final third with more fruits and veggies. The protein choice can also be leveraged based on energy needs. If you're looking for a lower energy density, think about leaner cuts of meat and adding veggies to starches like pasta or rice to add nutrients and fibre. Also consider that some plant-based protein sources, like lentils and beans, provide both your protein and your carbs at the same time. If you need to increase energy density or are low carb, then fattier cuts of meat or types of fish, or more nuts and soy-based products, can come to the fore.

To be sustainable, a dietary shift should leave you feeling satisfied after meals, which is largely a matter of how full you are. One of the main downsides of Western diets is that they provide a lot of calories in not much space, so we feel like we need to eat more. Foods that are crunchy or require a lot of chewing can also help improve satiety (compare the work of eating a salad to the ease of throwing back a big milkshake). Randomised trials show that one of the reasons it's easier to overconsume foods that require less chewing is that the brain has less time to determine the number of calories being consumed.[121] The easiest way to navigate all this is to make sure your plate is mainly made up of foods that contain plenty of fibre or water and require chewing, which includes whole-food protein sources like unprocessed meats and beans as well as most fruits and veggies. The only caveat is that many salad dressings, sauces, and condiments quickly blow the energy budget, so they should be used judiciously.

The way you build your plate can change over time based on your needs. I always start by putting the protein on my plate, because that's the easiest thing to miss out on. Next comes the salad or veggies (or fruit like apples or berries, if you prefer), which might take up the entirety of the rest of the plate when my activity levels are lower due to work or travel. But when I'm training hard and need the energy, the last third of the plate might be rice, (sweet) potatoes, or pasta. Breakfast and lunch are often leftovers, so my plates usually look very similar throughout the day. (Actually, I usually just shove leftovers in a bowl and stick it in the microwave, because that's faster.)

Once you have a base like this that makes up the majority of your dietary pattern, it's OK to occasionally go outside of that. Sometimes I resort to higher-protein snack foods when I'm on the go. And though I usually cook all our meals at home, if we have takeaway, I tend to go for a grilled protein and veggie option (or two) and skip the fries. And though I don't usually eat desserts or sweets, that doesn't mean I never have them. Because brownies are delicious, no matter what my wife might think.

This is a very simple way to shape our dietary pattern to get maximum nutrients while simultaneously attending to our energy requirements. And it allows us to give the brain, an incredibly complex and energetically demanding organ, the range of vitamins and minerals needed to preserve cognitive function and mental health, ultimately decreasing the risk of cognitive decline as we age.

REMEMBER THE RULES

Instead of obsessing about one type of diet (or a specific superfood or nutrient), it's important to remember that supporting optimal brain health really comes down to enjoying more whole and minimally processed foods. These will automatically provide the wide range of nutrients that synergise to bolster cognitive function and protect your brain from decline. There's no need to eat foods that you hate. When it comes time to fill your plate, just remember the rules: *Maximise nutrients and fuel for your own needs.* That is the formula that will allow you to future-proof your brain today—and for decades to come.

HYDRATION

A major part of what we put in our mouths that gets less attention than it should when it comes to cognitive function is hydration. Even a small amount of dehydration can change our memory and focus, with greater effects once we lose around 2 percent of our body weight.[122] In my experience, many people spend a lot of time being mildly dehydrated without even realising it—reaching for caffeine or a snack instead of a glass of water when they feel fatigued or are having difficulty focusing.

In general, there are no strict guidelines for how much water people need to drink each day. For most of us, just making sure to drink when we're thirsty should be enough. At the other end, well-hydrated urine is clear and only very slightly yellow, so anything more concentrated or potent than that is a good indication that you should drink some more. It also doesn't need to be water—almost all beverages have a similar effect on hydration. Even caffeinated beverages usually contain enough fluid to balance the very mild dehydrating effect of caffeine, which is usually only seen at high doses.[123]

If you're very active or sweat a lot or feel that you're still thirsty despite drinking a lot of fluids, having a beverage that includes some electrolytes like sodium, potassium, and magnesium can help to retain the fluid you drink. However, you usually don't need a carbohydrate-based hydration drink unless you're doing very long (an hour or longer) or hard training sessions.

CHAPTER 9
STIMULATE

In most games, the final showdown—the final boss or the ultimate throw of the dice—isn't where the game is won. The game is won by leveraging strategies implemented many turns earlier and cashing in on the experience and assets they provided. This might be the resources collected in a board game or accumulated armour, skills, and weapons in a video game. The game of brain health is the same. As we draw toward our final years—as will happen to all of us eventually—we want to have as much armour and as many skills and reserves at our disposal as possible.

If there's one component of the game that best defines how we accumulate our lifelong brain resources, it's the way that we stimulate our brains. Considering that this book is called *The Stimulated Mind*, you probably could have guessed I was going to say that.

In many ways our brains are both overstimulated and understimulated at the same time, and it's probably a combination of the two that's contributing to the core fears many of us have about our brains now and in the future. But if we think about the trajectory of how we use our brains across the lifespan, ensuring that our minds remain *appropriately* stimulated no matter how old we are is going to be a critical component of winning the brain game.

This is because a crucial property of biological systems, including the brain, is that their function is driven by the challenges and stimuli they are exposed to. Not only that, but cognitive challenge is *required* for optimal brain function, just like the body requires physical activity.

WHAT DO BICEPS AND BRAINS HAVE IN COMMON?

Our individual biology is continuously shaped by the environment around us. In the brain, this adaptation allows us to learn and automate processes that we need to "survive" our daily lives—such as a doctor honing their skills in a specific surgery, my wife's ability to parallel park into spots that defy the laws of physics, or my *equally important* ability to identify that actor from the one cameo he did in that sitcom twenty years ago. (We both bring a lot to the marriage; it's not a contest, okay?)

Each of us can appreciate the amazing and unique abilities that we can develop, but we often underestimate how much this process is driving the overall health and function of our brains. I do think we have an inkling, though. For instance, most of us have spoken the cliché "use it or lose it" at least once when talking about the brain. Deep down, we know that our brains need ongoing stimulation to function at their best. Unfortunately, however, our definition of *using* it might not quite hit the mark. For example, we've all heard that as we age—or when we retire—we should make sure to add crosswords and other puzzles to our daily routine. But, while these kinds of activities can provide a nice mental break by requiring focus without a huge cognitive burden,[1] sometimes we're going to need to dig a little deeper to achieve the stimulus that really drives brain function.

To understand the importance of stimulating the brain, we have to bring together a few ideas from previous chapters. The first is that the brain is more than the sum of its parts. We can't just take a list of cells, proteins, and genes and automatically know how the brain will function, because each component is finely tuned and interacts with other components. Practically speaking, this means that we can't just tick off a list of things that are important for the brain—we need to have some idea of how they fit together.

The second idea is that the function of many organs or parts of the body is determined by the demands placed on them. This is true, for instance, in the immune system after exposure to infections, vaccines, or allergens.[2] Similarly, the liver can adapt to become better at metabolising compounds that it is frequently exposed to, such as alcohol or medications.[3] And, of course, our muscles, bones, and heart (and brain) get stronger when we exercise. But despite having studied these principles as an undergraduate and in medical school, as well as applying them to athletes trying to get fitter and stronger, I didn't begin to really appreciate the true importance of how they relate to the brain until several years later.

During my PhD, around the time I was learning how well neuroscientists were able to develop new therapies for strokes in rats while struggling to do the same in humans, I was invited to present at a small conference in Scottsdale, Arizona. The goal of the conference and the group that organised it was to explore ways environmental mismatch might be driving increasingly common chronic diseases such as type 2 diabetes and Alzheimer's disease. It was at this conference that Darryl Edwards first threw me over his shoulder to teach me some of the benefits of coordinative movement. This was also where I met Josh Turknett, whose *Angry Birds* parable in part 1 highlighted the problems with trying to win a video game by manipulating the underlying computer code.

Josh is a neurologist whose dedication to all things brain-related comes second only to his love of the banjo. Josh loves the banjo like I love bicep curls. And it was Josh who first made me realise that our respective hobbies have more in common than you might initially think. In his book *Anyone Can Play Music,* Josh wrote:

> You've probably seen the difference between the body of a seventy-five-year-old who's been working out in the gym all their life and one who hasn't exercised since their teens. The body of an older person who has continued to challenge it regularly not only looks healthier, but it is also much more *capable*. While harder to appreciate because they're hidden from view, our brains are the same. The more we challenge them, the healthier they look and the more capable they become.

If you look at the underlying biochemistry, the process of a brain adapting to a stimulus is very similar to how muscles respond to exercise.[4] And in the long list of factors that we know can influence the function of the brain, multiple lines of evidence suggest that stimulus is probably the most important; it's the key component of brain health that ties all the others together.

Imagine that you're a bicep who wants to get as big and strong as possible. In this scenario where you're suddenly a sentient muscle (or, technically, *several* muscles, if the anatomy nerds are paying attention), you know that decisions about nutrition, such as getting enough protein, will be important to support your gains. A healthy blood supply is also critical for bringing that nutrition to you. If you're a particularly astute bicep, you'll also know that rest and recovery are important for growth. But none of those things matter in the absence of a stimulus. Though I am sad to say it, chugging lots of protein shakes and taking a lot of naps won't make a bicep any bigger, because the primary cause of bicep growth is bicep curls. It's that stimulus that acts as the catalyst—it starts the growth process and brings in the extra blood flow and nutrients needed for growth to happen.

As your brain interacts with and responds to stimulus from the environment, it is doing exactly the same thing as my imaginary sentient bicep: directing blood flow and nutrients to active brain networks and stimulating growth and maintenance processes in those regions. This builds strength and capacity, improving function in the short term but also building headroom as a buffer that helps to keep those regions in good shape in the long term. Knowing this, and knowing that the brain is more than a sum of its parts, it becomes clear that cognitive function is a *stimulus-driven process*. As important as all the other factors that support brain health are, the effects of those factors are directed by *how* we use our brains in the first place. Therefore, in order to preserve cognitive function as we age, we need to take a long, hard look at whether our brains are getting enough stimulation.

In a recent paper, Josh and I proposed the idea of demand-driven cognitive decline.[5] In its simplest form, the idea suggests that one of the main reasons we experience decline in cognitive function as we age is that we stop challenging those functions in ways that strengthen them. When we're younger and our brains are initially developing, most of our time is spent learning new skills and building brain function. But once we're adults, we stop doing the brain's equivalent of exercise, and our brains lose function as a result. Thinking back to the rules of the brain game, perhaps the most important is this one: *Never give up*. After all, it is much easier to maintain what you have than to build it from scratch, which only grows more true as we age. But if you haven't yet begun, or don't know where to start, don't fret! We'll get to that as well.

STIMULUS KEEPS THE BRAIN SHARP FOR LONGER

Though we all have some idea that it's important to keep using and stimulating our brains for as long as possible, until very recently it was quite controversial to suggest that we could use this idea to enhance or maintain cognitive function, especially in older adults.

A shift began in the 1980s, led by psychologists such as Warner Schaie, who was a professor of psychiatry and behavioural sciences at the University of Washington, where I now work. Dr. Schaie is perhaps best known for founding the Seattle Longitudinal Study (SLS).[6] Starting in 1956, the SLS tested the cognitive function of individuals every seven years, continually adding new participants until 2012. In total, more than six thousand adults aged twenty-two to over one hundred years old took part in the study.

The design of the SLS allowed questions about age and cognitive function to be asked in a new way. Prior to this point, a study might just take a big group of people of different ages and measure how they perform in a variety of cognitive tests. What they would find is that as the ages of the participants increase, performance in functions like processing speed or memory steadily decreases. Therefore, we assume that each individual person will experience a similar decline in cognitive function with age.

But knowing the cognitive function of an average person twenty years older than you is not the same as knowing how your own cognitive function might look in twenty years. After all, you are not a statistic; you are a specific human in a specific context. What we *really* care about isn't group averages—it's individual changes in cognitive function that come with age.

By seeing the same participants every seven years, the SLS was one of the first large studies to look at changes in cognitive function *within an individual* over long periods of time. What they found was that cognitive function remains relatively stable until people are in their sixties. Most people also maintained similar levels of cognitive function into their seventies and early eighties.[7] While average cognitive function does decrease as people get older, that doesn't mean *everybody's* function is decreasing, or that we will all experience significant decline as we age. The takeaway here is that almost nothing is written in stone when it comes to how we age.

Even now, this idea is still pretty mind-blowing. By showing that significant cognitive decline is not an inevitability, Schaie and his colleague and wife Sherry Willis provided some of the first scientific evidence that pushed back against William Osler's ageist idea of forcing people to retire once they became "useless" in their sixties. In fact, data from the SLS was later used as evidence to support raising the retirement age in the United States.[8] In addition to busting myths about age, as we saw in chapter 7, the SLS was also one of the first large studies to link certain health conditions, such as heart disease, to changes in cognition over time.[9]

Where the SLS really excelled, though, was in exploring the influence of the environment, and how we interact with it, on cognitive function.[10] In particular, the SLS focused on what they called *complex environments*—ones that present a wide range of cognitive inputs and require complex decision-making. They found that individuals who experienced greater environmental complexity—a measure of the stimulus their brains received on a daily basis from their work and home environment—exhibited better maintenance of cognitive function.[11] The components of environmental complexity studied at the time—level of education, occupation, time spent reading, and relationship status—were relatively simplistic in light of the complexities of the modern world; however, they still form the bedrock of a framework for understanding how environment influences cognition.

Fresh from your tour into the mind of a bicep, I'd now like you to come back into your own body and imagine your cognitive function as a blade made of steel. The ideal blade is one that is aligned with its environment, shaped and honed according to what it's being used for. Over time it may accumulate some wear and tear, but this can be offset with some regular maintenance and care. And while it's perfectly reasonable to keep using that blade for its original use, the fact that it's made of metal means that it can be strengthened and reshaped over time if we put enough energy (heat) and effort into it.

I make this last point because effort is critical to the process. Just like with exercise, *intensity* matters. As a result, the process of the brain changing in response to experience may involve some cognitive discomfort. And when we really think about it, this makes perfect sense. Your adult brain has spent decades honing itself to become responsive to the needs of you and your environment. While it might not feel like it, we *want* our brains to be stable and only change if they really need to. If it were too easy to change your brain, chaos would ensue on a daily basis as your brain learned, unlearned, and relearned facts on a whim. Or maybe it would even be impossible to learn anything at *all*. Imagine having to remodel your house every time the weather changed—you'd spend all your time at home building walls and plumbing bathrooms and would never be able to do anything else.

For this reason, the adult brain is more like the lightbulb in this classic joke:

"How many psychologists does it take to change a lightbulb?"
"Just one, but the lightbulb has to really want to change."

What makes the brain *want* to change? A feeling that something is important but that the capacity to do it is missing. After all, if the brain can already complete a certain task, there is no reason for it to improve or adapt. Therefore, the real magic of neuroplasticity happens when we fail at doing something we want to do. This creates a feeling of agitation or stress that tells our brain that some new processes and wiring need to be developed.

If we want future-proof brains, learning and cognitive challenge are the equivalent of squats and sprints—the stimuli that make our brains bigger and stronger. But just as with training our bodies, sometimes training our minds can feel difficult. This discomfort, and our desire to avoid it, may be a major contributor to cognitive decline as we get older. As we've seen, our brains and bodies seem to age faster when we stop engaging in activities like learning and physical activity that were critical to our initial development as children and teenagers. And one reason we stop engaging in those stimulating activities as adults is because we *hate* being bad at things. We would rather avoid the gym and language classes entirely than risk the discomfort of failure. This is the exact *opposite* of what we should be doing. As psychiatrist Thomas Szasz put it:

Every act of conscious learning requires the willingness to suffer an injury to one's self-esteem. That is why young children, before they are aware of their own self-importance, learn so easily; and why older persons, especially if vain or important, cannot learn at all.[12]

Though his words are absolutely true, I'm a bit more of an optimist than Szasz. If we can overcome the friction and discomfort that comes from learning and failing, we can keep driving neuroplasticity and brain health no matter how old we are. Most importantly, this process will provide headroom that we can rely on as we age or when our brains come under pressure. Just as with physical strength, we improve almost any function, including brain function, by challenging our current capabilities. Like the owls in the preface, if you invest time and effort in engaging with a new challenge, your brain will direct the necessary resources to adapt to that challenge in a stimulus-driven process.

YOUR BRAIN IS WHAT YOU MAKE OF IT

The best part about the wide range of skills we can learn is that we ourselves can ultimately decide what we want our brains to be good at. We can choose if we want to dedicate our time, effort, and brain to be exceptionally well specialised to one specific area of performance or pick a broader range of stimuli and build more of a multipurpose kind of brain. No one approach is better than any other. But knowing that our brain adapts to what we expose it to allows us to craft our own goals and training programme and think about how one skill we learn might be helpful in other areas.

Any time your brain receives a new stimulus such as learning (or failing at) a new skill, a network of brain areas related to performing that skill becomes activated, instigating a biochemical cascade that improves the function of that network.[13] While different stimuli and skills activate different areas of the brain in different ways, the same basic processes are involved any time the brain is challenged. This includes making new connections or removing connections that are not needed or don't support the skill being developed, as well as activating maintenance processes like autophagy to make sure the neurons in that network remain in tip-top shape.[14] In this way, the brain is constantly shaping itself according to the inputs it is receiving, increasing function as well as acting as its own mechanic by staving off aging-related processes in the areas being stimulated.

One of the first examples of the way stimulus actively shapes the adult brain was a study where individuals in their twenties were taught how to juggle. Over the course of three months, participants in the juggling group had to learn a three-ball cascade—the classic manoeuvre you would see from somebody juggling three balls. Brain scans taken before and after the three-month training period showed that learning to juggle resulted in the brain getting bigger in areas related to coordinating vision and movement. And the bigger the changes seen in their brains, the better the jugglers performed. After the initial learning period, they stopped juggling entirely for three months, and a third scan showed that the juggling-induced changes in the brain had started to be lost.[15]

Though the juggling study is now more than twenty years old, it tells us almost everything we need to know about stimulus-driven changes in the brain. When we encounter a new challenge and learn a new skill, the areas of the brain where extra function is needed become activated. Over time, resources are invested in those areas, the effects of which can be measured in terms of their size or structure. And the more time that's invested in developing that skill, the bigger the changes. However, just as your muscles get smaller if you stop lifting weights, if you remove a stimulus, the brain will respond by reducing function in the area associated with that stimulus, because that function is no longer needed.

BRAIN BENEFITS OF THE DAILY GRIND

In addition to my predilection for bicep curls, you may also have noticed that the process of learning is a running theme of my career. I was a student or trainee of one kind or another until my mid-thirties—either in the classroom or in the hands-on world of coaching and doctoring. There's even a running joke in my house that I've collected more than enough degrees and I'm not allowed to get any more, even though that idea is occasionally tempting. However, considering that very little about the medical or academic training process teaches you how to run a research programme or teach and mentor students (or write books, for that matter), I still spend a large part of my job actively learning—

even though I'm supposedly in charge. Last year, when introducing myself to a neuroscience class, I joked (kind of) that I was in year 38 and still didn't really know what I wanted to be when I grew up.

In the most watched (and, in my opinion, still the best) TED Talk of all time, Sir Ken Robinson quips that the main purpose of the education system is to produce university professors. Therefore, as a university professor, I have to admit that I'm probably going to be a little biased about learning. But the reason I'm telling you all this is because some of the best evidence that learning is a critical stimulus for driving cognitive function comes from what we know about the effect of formal education. Of course, I know how it looks when somebody who has essentially been a professional student for most of their life tries to tell you how great education is for your brain. But luckily, you'll see that the benefits of learning don't *have* to come from formal education at all.

As mentioned in part 1, the *Lancet*'s Livingston report on dementia prevention included education as one of the factors that is known to significantly decrease dementia risk.[16] For example, in areas where education has improved and become more accessible over time, dementia rates have decreased in parallel. Those who complete a university degree also have a lower risk of dementia compared to those who left formal education after graduating secondary school. Of course, those who attend university or get graduate degrees might also get different jobs, live in different places, and have more time and resources to engage in other activities that also decrease dementia risk. This is important to consider, but the benefit of more education seems to hold even after taking that into account.[17]

It turns out that the level of education achieved is a better predictor of dementia risk than the number of years spent in school, which is consistent with the idea that it's the *stimulus* provided by education that explains its relationship with cognitive function.[18] Why might those two aspects of education—attainment and time in school—differ when it comes to their effect on the brain? The process of achieving a degree or a qualification requires you to not only take in new knowledge but also employ critical thinking and problem-solving skills. It's a dynamic challenge of continued brain engagement and adaptation that wouldn't be achieved simply by sitting in the classroom for the same period of time without making progress toward a specific goal. Active engagement in the process and challenge of learning is clearly important.

There has been a lot of debate about *how* education might decrease dementia risk. One of the most consistent findings is that those with higher educational attainment perform better (on average) on cognitive function tests. For example, one study by researchers at the University of California at Berkeley looked at data from nearly two hundred thousand people using an online cognitive-training platform. They found that the higher somebody's level of education, the higher their average peak of cognitive function was, and the later that peak occurred. On average, cognitive function tends to peak around the time we finish education—the time when we finish dedicating most of our time to the process of stimulating our brains.[19]

Part of the reason those with higher levels of education perform better on cognitive assessments is probably that people who spend more time in school simply get better at taking tests. But the broad range of skills and thinking we're (hopefully) exposed to in school also directly translates to improvement in focus, memory, and decision-making because those functions are being stimulated and trained.

The greater peak in cognitive function and brain health driven by more learning stimulus early in life creates cognitive reserve and resilience—upgrades to the brain's software and hardware that allow it to resist changes that happen with age—which make up two-thirds of my definition of headroom.[20] In part 1, we talked about the importance of developing greater capacity in our cognitive systems so that we have more buffer as we get older. As a result, we're less likely to ever experience dementia, and if we do, we might experience it later.

One difference between headroom and some common definitions of cognitive reserve and resilience is that the process of building headroom is a lifelong and active one. Sometimes we have to rely on our headroom when we're busy, sleep-deprived, or stressed. But when conditions and time allow, we should be actively building and maintaining headroom, because we never know when we're going to need it. This active process is typified by a lifelong quest to learn and engage with new things, which is why the third "R" of headroom is *resolve*.

Take, for example, the neuroscientist Rita Levi-Montalcini, who won a Nobel Prize for the discovery of nerve growth factor. Even in her nine-

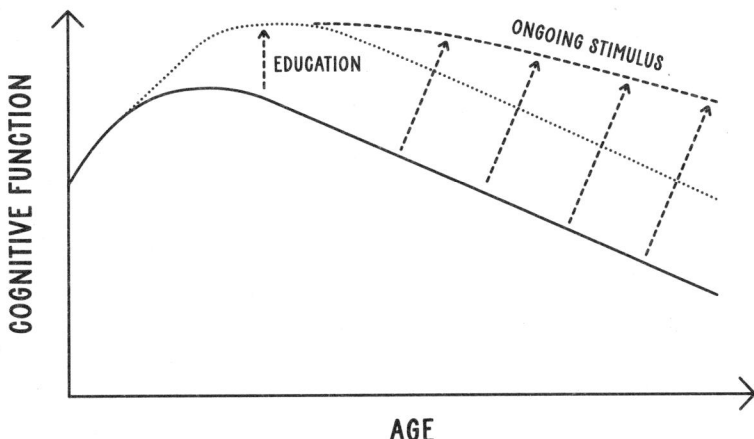

FIGURE 1. Stimulation-driven trajectories of cognitive function. Early life education increases function, providing higher function at a given age on average. However, without ongoing stimulation the rate of decline doesn't change compared to somebody with lower levels of education attainment. In order to slow the rate of decline with age, ongoing stimulus is required.

ties she continued to seek out new insights into neuroscience, discovering critical ways that the immune system influences the brain,[21] while at the same time starting a career in politics—serving in the Italian senate until her death at the age of 103. Now compare Dr. Levi-Montalcini's life of continued academic and civic engagement to the all-too-typical caricature of a dusty old professor (you know who I mean), wandering around the university halls becoming increasingly decrepit as they ride out their tenure without seeming to really engage with anything (or anyone) at all. Of course, I can't *prove* these differences are because of stimulus and engagement, but I think it's fair to say that all of us have met people who fit these different approaches to lifelong intellectual exploration, and whose cognitive functions have reflected this.

Beyond stellar scientists and academic clichés, there is research on education and rate of cognitive decline to suggest that stimulating our brains to maintain and develop headroom should be a lifelong pursuit. While higher educational attainment early in life does appear to increase overall cognitive function and therefore help you maintain a higher average level of cognitive function at a given age in later life, it doesn't necessarily *slow* the rate of cognitive decline as you get older (figure 1).[22] Slowing the rate of decline requires ongoing stimulus to maintain headroom. In the face of aging-related processes, you need to keep building that buffer. Unsurprisingly, the "stimulated mind" requires continued stimulation.

Remember that many of the areas of the brain that are most susceptible to ageing are those that are responsible for some of our most complex cognitive functions. These are also the brain areas that have the most environment-driven development after birth and throughout adult life. If we want to maintain the function of those areas of the brain with age, we need to keep providing stimulus, telling the brain that it's worth maintaining and keeping those parts of the brain around. But that's not what many of us typically do. As we saw with the pianist study in part 1, as we get older, we often let our learning and complex skills drop off because life and *adulting* get in the way.

Luckily, it doesn't have to be this way, and ongoing daily cognitive stimulus can come from both likely and unlikely places. After leaving formal education, most of us enter the workforce. Since work is the place we most consistently spend time using our brains, you won't be surprised to hear that the nature of our work influences our cognitive function later in life. In a large study of more than one hundred thousand people from the United States and Europe, cognitive stimulation through both education and work were found to separately decrease the risk of later dementia. Those who had both a high level of education (a university degree or higher) and a cognitively stimulating job had the lowest risk of dementia. Those who had a high level of education *or* a cognitively stimulating job were also protected against dementia compared to those who had neither.[23]

This last fact is critical because it means you can still get significant benefits from cognitive stimulation later in life, regardless of the educational opportunities you had when you were younger. Definitions of a cognitively stimulating job differ, but in this study, people were considered to have a stimulating job if they felt their job was demanding but that they had a lot of control over their work. A similar study performed in Finland looked at work-related monotony and risk of cognitive impairment and dementia.[24] What the researchers found was that jobs with less routine and monotony and more creative thinking, data analysis, decision-making, and need for interpersonal skills were associated with a lower risk of later cognitive decline and dementia.

At this point it's important to step back and think about what these studies are telling us. Clearly, longer and more intensive engagement with learning earlier in life helps to support and increase a range of cognitive functions. Cognitively stimulating work—be that due to the complexity and novelty of the tasks, the need for complex decision-making, or an active social environment—also supports cognitive function and prevents decline as we get older. However, there's nothing that says these stimuli *must* come from education or work. One main reason researchers study education and work is because most people do at least some of both. It's much easier to look at educational attainment than it is to estimate the cognitive stimulation somebody might be getting elsewhere in their life. Work also tends to provide a more consistent input over decades—even when we move jobs, the type of work is usually similar—compared to hobbies or other activities that might change, so the effect of cognitive stimulation over time is easier to assess when it comes from our jobs.

But we can't all get multiple degrees (and many of us have neither the means nor the interest), and not everybody gets to work in a job that they consider highly stimulating or complex. Luckily, there's evidence that similar function-boosting effects can come from a wide range of activities that we can all benefit from, regardless of our schooling or profession. For example, multiple studies in older adults show lower rates of cognitive decline and dementia in those who engage daily in hobbies (including reading, crafting, playing games, and even singing karaoke).[25] This suggests it's the ongoing engagement and stimulus that matter more than where that stimulus comes from.

CAN WE *REALLY* ENHANCE COGNITIVE FUNCTION?

There's a saying in coaching, medicine, and business: "You can't improve what you don't measure." As a doctor, you often rely on a specific marker of risk—for instance, blood sugar in somebody with diabetes—to track whether an intervention or medication is working. You might also have to track the intervention itself—for instance, the dose of the medication, and maybe even how frequently the patient remembers to take it.

When I was a rowing coach, a huge amount of the work revolved around measuring and tracking different variables. Often, there were dozens of rowers, each with slightly different training plans based on their current level of fitness as well as the goals of their crew for that part of the rowing season. For some crews, the goal was to show up at a race, row the boat in something approximating a straight line, avoid falling into the river, and have a lot of fun doing it. For others, the goal was to compete (and win) against some of the best rowers in the country. My job was to structure the necessary training programmes and track whether what we were doing was helping the crew get closer to their goal. Not all of this was an exact science, and experience plays a large role as well, but I had some numbers to help figure things out.

In exercise science and athletic coaching, decades of research have gotten us to a place where we have a pretty good idea of how a specific stimulus is going to affect performance. There's always some variability, and a good coach will work to tailor a programme to a specific athlete. But as we saw in chapter 7, we have some pretty good general parametres for what it takes to see progress in fitness or strength. By comparison, it's *really* hard to do this kind of measurement and tracking for the brain and cognitive function.

One reason the idea of enhancing cognitive function has been so controversial over the years is that it's really tricky to measure. Everybody knows that practicing a new skill or hobby will make you better at that specific activity. And even if older adults tend to get better more slowly than young people do on average, they still improve with practice.[26] But there's a difference between skill-specific training and a larger idea that challenging your brain could improve cognitive function overall. And though I strongly believe this is possible, and our ability to measure and track cognitive improvements over time will improve as research continues, for now, I admittedly have to rely on bigger overarching concepts about stimulus and function in the brain than I did as a coach counting reps in the gym.

When thinking about how a stimulus affects brain function, neuroscientists have a concept called *transfer*. There can be multiple levels of transfer, but the idea is to think about how getting better at one task improves or supports function in another task. *Near* transfer, where learning one task makes you better at a similar task, is more common. For instance, learning to drive one particular car will transfer over to driving any car. *Intermediate* transfer would be if learning how to drive a car made you better at operating an 18-wheeler—the skills are related but not quite the same. *Far* transfer is when learning one skill improves abilities in a completely unrelated skill—for instance, if your newfound driving skills made you better at speaking French.

As ridiculous as it might sound, there is actually some evidence that far transfer can happen, though it does depend a bit on both the stimulus and the unrelated skill.[27] One of the reasons education might enhance cognitive function broadly is that engaging in education requires you to practise your focus and attention while engaging your memory and critical-thinking skills. Of course, this will depend on how interesting and compelling you find the subject and the teacher, but success in a given class will usually require some engagement with the material and periods of sustained focus and attention. This process of *learning how to learn* often appears to transfer to other unrelated tasks where you need to stay focused, because being able to focus and direct your attention are skills in themselves.

Two of my very good friends and colleagues at the University of Washington, Chantel Prat and Andrea Stocco, are cognitive psychologists who (amongst other things) study how speaking two languages affects the brain. Multiple studies have found that being raised bilingual is associated with a lower overall risk of dementia, suggesting that learning and speaking multiple languages increases headroom.[28] People who are bilingual also tend to perform better on tests of very short term (working) memory and tasks that require attention and rapid decision-making (executive function).[29] In an attempt to explain this, Chantel and Andrea suggest that the constant need to select and control two different languages that you're fluent in improves your broader ability to control attention and deal with competing information.[30] Chantel has measured patterns of electrical activity in the brain associated with the ability to control attention, finding that they are often stronger in people who are bilingual.[31]

As with most things, though, this doesn't mean that those of us who grew up speaking only one language are forever at a disadvantage to those who speak more than one. For instance, monolingual people have a greater capacity for expertise in their native language because they're not having to contend with thinking about multiple languages at once.

And though bilingual people tend to be better at handling multiple tasks—like driving and speaking French at the same time—Chantel and Andrea's work shows that the brain networks that support their internal processing of information may also make them less reactive to sudden changes in the outside world—such as a pedestrian suddenly stepping in front of their car.

Though I trust their expertise as exceptional neuroscientists, I can't help but feel that maybe the last point is a little tinged by personal experience, because Chantel (monolingual) just happens to be married to Andrea (fluently bilingual) and frequently laments his lack of situational awareness. Come to think of it, my wife, Elizabeth (monolingual), often says the same thing about me (on a good day, I can stumble through several languages). I'm sure it's just a coincidence . . .

Luckily, you don't have to grow up bilingual to get some of the benefits of language learning. Even a few months of learning a foreign language can improve various measures of cognitive function in older adults, with related changes also seen on brain scans before and after learning.[32] Benefits have been seen both with in-person classes and language apps, and they may be most beneficial for people already experiencing some level of cognitive decline.[33] That's right, your Duolingo habit (assuming you made it a habit rather than giving up after three days) could actually be helping you to protect your brain from later dementia.

Beyond language, there are a host of other skills and activities that might serve to increase headroom and cognitive function. For example, physical activity also seems to improve the structure and function of those same regions of the brain responsible for the cognitive flexibility that comes from learning multiple languages.[34] In our paper on stimulus-driven cognitive function, Josh Turknett and I hypothesised that the activities most likely to benefit overall brain health and function are those that are linked to our unique human brains. These include language, music, social connection, and complex, coordinative movement-related skills like team sports and dancing. One of the main reasons for this is that these activities are rooted in the way that humans evolved to learn and interact with the environment, so they're most likely to align with the way that the human brain functions best. The nature of these activities also tends to require using multiple brain networks at once—

integrating activity across different skills related to memory, moving, hearing, seeing, and decision-making all at the same time.

Learning to perform these complex but very human skills and activities might be particularly good for increasing cognitive *efficiency*, which is another way that far transfer is thought to occur. By learning how to process multiple different types of information at the same time, the brain becomes more efficient.[35] When your brain adapts to processing complex stimuli, less mental energy is required to perform a given task. As a result, you have more available capacity when you need it, making it more likely that you can perform well when your brain is overextended or stressed. Cognitive efficiency is therefore another critical aspect of headroom.

Continuing to (or beginning to) stimulate the brain using complex stimuli may be increasingly important as we get older because one of the main changes we see with ageing is that networks in the brain become less stable and less efficient, which is associated with worsening cognitive function.[36] Challenging and stimulating those networks can help them to maintain efficiency and function as we get older. This brings us to one particularly interesting human-specific activity that may actively make the brain younger: music.

MUSICAL INTERLUDES

Throughout my entire childhood and adolescence, I was involved in making music in one way or another. One of my earliest memories is sitting in a group cello lesson, a child-sized instrument that was not much bigger than a violin sitting between my knees. I was probably four years old. The cello didn't last long, but over the next fourteen years I picked up (and put down) a number of instruments—piano, flute, trumpet, saxophone, bassoon. In secondary school I dabbled with electronic music, composing and recording pieces using computers and synthesisers.

I can't say I really enjoyed my early forays into playing musical instruments. It was something that I *had* to do because it was "good for me." Undoubtedly that was true, but what kid enjoys eating their broccoli or stumbling through a piano piece because of some unknown benefit they might get in the future? It was the stumbling that was my real downfall, because I was frequently consumed by the terror of having to practise—or, more specifically, having other people *hear* me practise.

Most of us can quickly conjure up a memory of listening to a kid learn how to play an instrument. Even though I never played one, when I think about this situation, I always imagine a violin. It's screechingly out of tune, painfully out of time, and sounds nothing like any kind of music you'd ever listen to outside of a torture chamber. And this racket continues endlessly as the young maestro in question perseveres for *hours*. That perseverance is admirable, though, and the imaginary kid has my utmost respect for doing what I couldn't.

The house I grew up in was right next door to what the Brits lovingly call a corner shop (though this one wasn't on a corner). It was a small Shop where everybody in the neighbourhood shopped when they didn't have time (or the need) to go to the supermarket. The shop was owned by the Johnson family, whom I saw every day of my life for fifteen years. Each time I opened the lid on the piano or extracted my saxophone from its case, I imagined my neighbours and the Johnsons standing in the shop listening to me fail to make music, over and over and over again. As a result of the imagined onslaught I was about to expose people to, I didn't practise. More than one teacher fired me for showing up week after week having made no progress.

The concept that I didn't appreciate back then, but which is critical to the idea of brain function being demand driven, is that you're *supposed* to be bad at stuff. It's in the sucking—and the slowly learning to suck a bit less—that the magic starts to happen. So, when I've alluded to the benefits of learning, and that neuroplasticity requires discomfort, this is what I mean. You have to spend time doing stuff you suck at.

As part of its job of adapting to your personal environment, the brain is constantly predicting what it expects to happen next. At the same time, it's also monitoring the world for differences between what it expects and what is actually happening. When we do a basic function like tying our shoelaces, or when a professional musician plays some Vivaldi, actions are performed as expected. Everything continues on as before.

But when we make a mistake, the brain detects an error between expectation and reality, and this is what opens up the door to the magical world of neuroplasticity. When the error detection mechanisms are triggered, the brain knows that new or stronger connections and patterns need to be generated to fix the error. This error detection can be measured based on electrical activity in the brain, and bigger error signals tend to be associated with better learning afterwards.[37] Activation of these signals also comes with—and is stimulated by—the release of stress-related neurotransmitters like adrenaline and norepinephrine, which is partly why mistakes feel uncomfortable.[38]

There's a whole body of research focused on the fact that failure is one of the best drivers of learning.[39] This is slightly ironic because formal education is generally geared around *avoiding* failure. There are even studies showing that students think making mistakes is bad while at the same time benefitting from mistakes by learning more quickly. But the fact that failure drives learning makes perfect sense because, as discussed above, the brain needs a *reason* to stimulate all the processes involved in improving its own connectivity and function. There are even parts of the brain that function better specifically when we expose ourselves to challenges that involve failure or discomfort, which may make us better at dealing with other challenging situations and exerting cognitive control—that is, doing things we don't feel motivated to do.[40] Just as we can learn to learn, we can (and should) learn to embrace scenarios where we might make mistakes and be uncomfortable.

Musicians provide one of the most interesting examples of the ways in which being less good at something might be good for your brain. As we know, age is the main risk factor for cognitive decline and dementia. However, people of the same age can have brains that function very differently and have very different risks of later decline. One way this has been studied is by looking at *brain age*. Using a machine-learning model based on thousands of brains, researchers can upload a scan of somebody's brain and ask how old that brain "looks." People whose brains look older than they should for their *actual* age tend to perform worse on cognitive function tests, and those with cognitive decline and dementia have brains that age more rapidly than they accumulate candles on their birthday cakes.[41] Factors we've previously discussed, such as physical inactivity, poor nutrient status, diabetes, as well as smoking and poor physical and cardiovascular health, appear to directly increase somebody's brain age, which then impacts their cognitive function.[42]

As part of some of the early work exploring how the environment can affect brain age, researchers compared brain scans of nonmusicians, amateur musicians, and professional musicians in their thirties. They found that musicians had younger-looking brains than nonmusicians, but that this effect was stronger in *amateur* musicians. Their theory was that playing an instrument was harder for amateurs. As a result, their brains were getting more stimulus and, accordingly, looked younger.[43] This aligns with multiple studies suggesting that active practice of music is associated with better cognitive function.[44]

Just as with language, the benefits of music extend to complete beginners. In one study, children taught a musical instrument of their choice for eight months saw improvements in multiple aspects of executive function, including attention and working memory.[45] Across more than a hundred other studies, musical training in children was also associated with improved measures of intelligence and memory.[46] In older adults receiving piano lessons for the first time, improvements in brain structure as well as working memory were seen, with bigger benefits in those who did more "homework" (more practice) between learning sessions.[47]

The multiple complex sensory and motor stimuli associated with music seem to be particularly good at driving neuroplasticity in the brain, even in adulthood. These stimuli include interpreting and learning complex visual and motor patterns (musical notation and precise body movements) while receiving continuous multisensory feedback. Learning to play music is associated with stronger connections between auditory and motor regions of the brain as well as the regions involved in integrating and transmitting multiple forms of information and making decisions.[48] Even very short periods of musical training appear to have this effect on neuroplasticity.[49]

While I'm not sure that my teenage self would have been more likely to practise his saxophone after hearing an impassioned and evidence-based case for how music might improve brain function, my own experiences with music ended up being overwhelmingly positive. In particular, this was because I switched from physical instruments to using my own body as an instrument. For singing. Just in case you were thinking about something else.

From the ages of eleven to eighteen, I took part in many choirs, both inside and outside of school, and did some musical theatre. Later on, I was also a singer in a band as part of my disgruntled-youth phase. Then, after a two-decade break—and leaning into the significant discomfort of practicing an old skill—I heeded the call of my adoring public and dusted off my vocal cords to sing and record the first dance song as a wedding day gift for my wife. Josh Turknett recorded the instrumental backing track, and more than a hundred people heard it without any obvious signs of distress or suffering.

I think one reason I enjoyed singing more than playing an instrument was the social nature of all these activities. I was particularly comfortable in a choir because the initial failures and mistakes were generally shared across the group, and we got to learn together with a common goal. Band practice was the same, with the added benefit of providing a reason to (occasionally) skip school and have an outlet for our teenage angst and shared desire for embarrassing hairstyles.

My experiences show how part of the benefit of playing music is social: Not only does it provide a way to connect with others, but the challenge of integrating into a group of musicians increases the cognitive complexity. This is a common theme across language too, as well as many of the other ways we can stimulate our brains for both fun and health. At its core, the idea is pretty simple: find something that you're new to and can actively learn and fail at. Importantly, it should also be something that you *want* to get better at, or else you're not going to keep doing it. And if it involves interacting with other people, that might provide some additional benefits and challenges. With that in mind, if languages and musical instruments aren't your thing, how about dancing?

"DANCE FIRST AND THINK AFTERWARDS"

While I'm not sure that Samuel Beckett was thinking about the cognitive benefits of dancing when he wrote these words, there's a lot we can take from them. Overthinking the potential downsides of failure or making mistakes is often what holds us back from engaging in activities that are fantastic for the brain. And this tends to get worse as we age. We marvel at the fact that kids will throw themselves into an activity, fail, get up, and do it again, yet we are rarely—if ever—willing to do that ourselves. If you take anything away from this chapter, having a bit more of a "try (and fail) first, think afterwards" approach to life is probably the best thing you could ever do for your brain.

As somebody who is much more acquainted with the modern and exercise-centric view of movement, I have to admit that I overlooked the benefits of dancing for a long time. But humans have been dancing for a lot longer than they've been going to the gym. As we saw in the "coordinate" level of the movement funnel, there's also something extra special about exercise that goes beyond the pure physical effects on our heart and muscles and also challenges our balance and complex motor skills. So perhaps it's not surprising that dancing is the form of movement that has some of the most impressive benefits when it comes to the brain.

In 2003, a seminal paper in the prestigious *New England Journal of Medicine* explored leisure-time activities and later dementia diagnoses in adults over the age of seventy-five. The single activity most associated with decreased dementia risk was dancing.[50] Since then, multiple studies have compared dance classes to other kinds of physical activity that have the same level of *physical* difficulty, such as brisk walking. While benefits are consistently seen in the physical activity groups, the results in the dance groups tend to be better—resulting in greater increases in hippocampus size on a brain scan and larger improvements in measures of cognitive function such as processing speed.[51] Across the many studies that have been done in adults in their fifties or older, dancing—especially ballroom and square dancing, which have a significant social component—results in consistent improvements in memory, attention, executive function, and mental health.[52] Dancing can also significantly improve mood; in one of the biggest analyses to date examining the effect of physical activity on symptoms in those with depression, dancing was the activity that seemed to have the biggest impact.[53]

If we wanted to apply some reductionist neuroscience to dancing, I think we'd struggle to figure out *why* it has the effect that it does. It's probably the combination of multiple factors—listening to music, learning new motor skills, physical activity, and the benefits of connecting with others in a social environment. Plus the even-more-difficult-to-quantify element of *fun*. As with the brain itself, dancing is probably more than the sum of its parts. The fact that dancing includes so many inputs means that it activates and requires coordination across multiple brain networks.[54] For this reason, dancing is being used as an intervention for a range of neurological disorders, including multiple sclerosis,

Parkinson's disease, and dementia.[55] This doesn't mean traditional medical approaches to those conditions aren't important, but dancing increasingly seems to be a powerful tool to support many aspects of brain health and function.

From what we've covered about the importance of *stimulus* for the brain up to this point, I hope it's clear that for many aspects of cognition, the function of the brain is stimulus-driven. Even the father of modern neuroscience understood the importance of stimulus. In 1894, Cajal is quoted as saying that "the ability of neurons to grow in an adult and their power to create new connections can explain learning."[56] So in reality, Cajal was talking about "stimulated minds" more than a hundred years ago!

Increasing brain function through stimulus can involve very specific skills (learning to juggle) or broader skills like those associated with education. Some of the most impressive benefits seem to come from learning skills that are uniquely human and require the coordination of multiple brain networks, such as languages, music, and dancing. And you don't necessarily need to do all of them; just pick one you think you'll enjoy and lean into that feeling of discomfort that comes from learning something new—that's your brain changing itself. However, we also saw from the studies of jugglers and pianists that *maintaining* a stimulus is important for maintaining the necessary adaptations in the brain. And this applies to more day-to-day activities in addition to your ability to tear up the dance floor.

As a result of the need for ongoing stimulus, the *Never give up* rule of the brain game underscores the importance of how we use our brains in many ways. You could take this rule as additional encouragement to go to that language or cooking class you always wanted to take, or as a reminder that we need to keep providing inputs to maintain what we've already got. For example, a study of more than two thousand adults in the United States ages thirty-three to eighty-three looked at the relationship between change in cognitive function over time and activities like reading, doing word games, attending educational lectures or courses, and writing. They found that people who engaged in more of those activities, especially if that engagement increased over time, had slower rates of cognitive decline. This effect was *greater* for those without a university degree, suggesting again that we can make up for differences in education by doing more cognitively stimulating activities later in life.[57]

Perhaps the first major example of how these day-to-day activities might be related to the risk of dementia was the same 2003 study that revealed the potential benefits of dancing in adults over seventy-five.[58] They created a cognitive-activity score where participants got one point for each day per week that they did one of the following activities: reading books or newspapers, writing for pleasure, doing crossword puzzles, playing board games or cards, participating in organised group discussions, and playing musical instruments. The researchers assessed the participants every twelve to eighteen months for up to twenty-one years and found that those who performed at least one or two cognitive activities per day had the lowest risk of later being diagnosed with dementia, even after taking into account initial levels of cognitive function. As all the participants were retired, it's studies like this that helped create the "use it or lose it" idea that drives retirees to the crossword section of the newspaper (even though they should maybe pick up a clarinet instead).

It's worth bearing in mind, though, that this study of retirees began in 1980. While I think the take-home messages will remain important long into the future, as we start to think about how to apply this information nearly fifty years later, it begs the question of whether we all need to focus on stimulating our brains like our grandparents did, or if there's a possibility of doing something a little more . . . modern.

SOME SURPRISING POSSIBLE BENEFITS OF MODERN STIMULI

At this point of the book, I've talked a lot about mismatch—how aspects of the modern environment such as retirement and how we eat and move (or not) are often poorly matched to the inputs our bodies and brains need in order to maintain a long life of health and function. As a result, when it comes to talking about *stimulus,* you might be forgiven for imagining that, like some cantankerous old-timer shaking his cane and complaining that things just aren't the same as they were back in *my* day, I would recommend eschewing the perils of modern technology.

The truth is that things *aren't* the same, and while there are several potential pitfalls related to technology use that we'll cover, I think some of the doom and gloom that exists around the use of technology is unwarranted, or at least should be reframed. Though exact estimates are hard to find—and if I found one it would probably already be out of date by the time you read this—it's clear that our brains are now being exposed to vast amounts of information that would have been unfathomable even to our recent relatives. It's also clear that how we use our brains is changing as a result.

One example of this is the *Google effect*—sometimes called digital amnesia—first coined by Betsy Sparrow and colleagues in a paper describing several studies exploring how our use of information is changing. For example, they showed that when participants learned facts before typing them into a computer, they were less likely to remember those facts if they thought that information had been saved (and therefore that they could access it later). Similarly, they found that people were more likely to remember *where* the information was stored rather than the information itself.[59]

It's important to point out that it wasn't that the study participants weren't capable of remembering facts. If they thought that the computer had erased rather than saved the information, they were more likely to remember it themselves. So our collective memories still work in the age of Google; it's just that we've shifted the way we use them. This makes a lot of sense when we consider the ever-increasing volume of information we're exposed to every day.

Of course, we can't rely on Google for taking exams or if we want to win at the local pub trivia night, so we do need to flex our memory muscles occasionally. But rather than try to remember every fact or detail we're exposed to, which would probably be impossible at this point, sometimes we can instead remember where to find those details if we need them again. If the goal is to have a future-proof brain, adapting to the world around us is critical. This is a nice example that isn't good or bad; it just shows how we can—and probably should—expect our brains to change as the world changes around us.

The same thing can be said for ways that we can beneficially stimulate our brains and build headroom using modern technology. This could be through formal brain-training programmes, but even regular video games, and technology use in general, have been found to be potentially beneficial. Recent work by Chantel Prat found that learning to write computer code has similarities to learning a language and requires similar cognitive skills, suggesting that coding could also provide a novel way to stimulate the brain while learning a skill that is often important in the modern world.[60]

All of this goes against the hypothesis that we're all on the path to *digital dementia*, a term coined by neuroscientist Manfred Spitzer in 2012. His idea was that more passive screen time, offloading of cognitive abilities onto devices, and increased distractions would negatively impact cognitive function. The idea really stems from a worry that technology will essentially result in the *opposite* of stimulus—removing the cognitive inputs that our brains thrive on. While this is of course possible, depending on how we choose to interact with technology, luckily, there seem to be several possible benefits from embracing more modern cognitive stimuli.

Perhaps the most obvious place to start is with technologies that are *designed* to stimulate cognitive function through online or app-based brain training. These apps have been met with a lot of skepticism—and rightly so—by the scientific community. Many programmes designed to train different cognitive functions like reasoning or memory have been shown to improve those specific functions, but usually only when tested in a format that resembles that of the training itself. In a sense, people were mainly training for the test rather than gaining broader cognitive skills to take out into the real world.[61] This is probably because most brain-training programmes are relatively rudimentary—a far cry from the kind of multisensory real-world stimulation that the brain is used to.

But while an app on your phone that you tap with your thumbs probably isn't going to replace learning a musical instrument, exploring a foreign country while practicing a new language, or throwing shapes on the dance floor, there is some evidence that even fairly simple brain training might impact cognitive function in unexpected and beneficial ways. Perhaps the first large study of brain training, and still one of the best examples of how brain training might result in beneficial transfer to other areas of life, is the Advanced Cognitive Training for Independent and Vital Elderly (ACTIVE) study.

Sherry Willis, who was a core part of the Seattle Longitudinal Study team, was one of the principal investigators of ACTIVE, which began in 1996 and took place in six major cities across the United States.

ACTIVE randomised 2,800 participants aged sixty-five or older to a control group or one of three brain-training groups: processing speed, reasoning, or memory. Memory training involved learning tools like mnemonics to memorise lists of words. Reasoning training involved searching for patterns in sequences of numbers or letters. Processing-speed training involved identifying an object on a computer screen that was flashed up at increasingly brief intervals, as well as having to divide attention between two search tasks. Participants did ten training sessions of around sixty minutes over five to six weeks, followed by brief booster sessions at one year and three years.

All three training groups improved at the task they were trained in, and this benefit was retained for at least five years after training. There was no evidence of transfer—those who trained in one area did not get better in the others—but five years after training, all three training groups had experienced less decline in quality of life and level of independence compared to the control group.[62] Those who were trained in processing speed were more likely to still be driving several years after the intervention, and both reasoning and processing-speed training were associated with a significant reduction in involvement in car accidents where the driver was at fault.[63] In general, the best results were found with the processing-speed training, probably because learning to divide attention and process information quickly provides additional cognitive efficiency—increasing headroom and reducing cognitive load when doing complex tasks like driving.

One of the most important scientists in the field of brain training is Michael Merzenich—former professor at the University of California, San Francisco—whose work in the lab was critical to our understanding of neuroplasticity in the adult brain. A lot of this work was summarised in his book *Soft-Wired*, which showed that the adult brain is capable of surprising amounts of neuroplasticity if we provide the right types of inputs. As part of this work, Merzenich built an online cognitive training platform called BrainHQ, which includes cognitive training tasks such as an updated version of the processing-speed training task used in ACTIVE.[64] Though I have no personal connection to BrainHQ, it is probably the brain-training platform that has the best evidence behind it, having now been used in hundreds of research studies.[65]

With that said, the availability and quality of cognitive-training technologies is only going to improve, with the most exciting development being the increasing promise of (relatively) inexpensive and accessible virtual reality (VR) training through headsets that people can buy and use at home. Unlike training your brain on a computer screen, VR can provide multisensory cognitive inputs that involve both vision and hearing as well as information processing and physical activity, which map more closely onto the ways that the brain is used to receiving complex stimuli.

One of the best-studied uses of VR does exactly this by implementing something called *dual-task training,* which includes physical activity plus elements of motor coordination or brain training. This type of training can re-create the benefits of coordinative or open-skill exercise that better align with how our brains evolved to learn and process information but in a virtual environment, and has been found to significantly improve cognitive function, even in those already experiencing some cognitive decline.[66] On a personal note, I must admit that I love VR boxing, which requires reacting to targets coming from multiple directions, allowing me to get a quick coordinative "propel"- or "sprint"-style workout while listening to my favourite music and looking ridiculous in my living room.

Though the evidence for VR is still accumulating, the immersive nature of it makes it very promising as a form of cognitive stimulus as well as being a tool for rehabilitation after traumatic brain injury or strokes.[67] It is also being used as a tool for training in specialties like medicine and surgery, where complex skills or emergency situations can be practised in a safe environment before being deployed in the real world. Compared to current approaches, VR might even end up being a better and more sensitive way to *test* cognitive function and track it over time, because it requires the integration of multiple senses. Some VR headsets can accurately track the movement of both your body and your eyes, so subtle changes like those seen after concussions or with Parkinson's disease could be picked up earlier, allowing for better intervention. VR is also being increasingly used in athletes, and though it isn't published yet, I have seen promising data showing that complex VR training involving both processing speed and executive function might decrease sport-related injury. This is thought to be due to increased headroom: by training to be better at dealing with multiple complex inputs, the athletes experience less cognitive load on the field and are therefore less likely to get themselves into positions where they get injured.

While the best ways to use and apply VR are still being figured out, we can (if we choose to) rely on a more conventional technological stimulus—video games. This idea often raises some eyebrows, but, again, I think with some reframing and practical application, video games can be a great addition to our toolbox of cognitive stimuli (as well as being fun).

Because of the immersive environments of many modern video games, several studies have shown that regular video game players have different patterns of brain connectivity than non-gamers. For example, regions involved in visuomotor coordination—that is, the process of initiating movements in response to visual inputs, needed during tasks like driving—often show greater activation in gamers than in non-gamers.[68] Video games can require navigating a large and complex world as well as solving problems, quickly reacting to the environment, and careful strategic planning. As a result, there is evidence that playing video games—especially if it is a novel stimulus—can promote certain aspects of cognitive function.

If I were to recommend the one video game that has the most evidence behind it, it is probably *Super Mario,* the recent 3D incarnations of which involve all the skills and activities mentioned above. In one classic study, researchers had sixty-to-eighty-year-old adults play solitaire, *Angry Birds,* or *Super Mario* for thirty minutes every day for four weeks.[69] At the end of the intervention, adults in the *Super Mario* group showed better improvements in a test of hippocampal function, which was similar to results they had previously seen in a group of undergraduate students.[70] Other groups have shown that playing *Super Mario* increases the grey matter in the hippocampus of older adults, and can improve feelings of well-being and working memory in individuals with depression.[71] Importantly, *Super Mario* doesn't have a monopoly on cognitive training, and it's probably the complex immersive nature of the game that is most important—other games, like *Minecraft* and various action video games, have been found to be beneficial in a similar way.[72]

When it comes to video games, and technology use in general, I think the bigger picture is going to be critical. In a recent review paper on digital dementia, most of the concerns about screen time and modern technology were actually related to how they might impact *other* aspects of lifestyle, including disrupted sleep, decreased physical activity, social isolation, and decreased academic and occupational engagement.[73] As a result, it's likely that digital dementia risk factors mirror more traditional dementia risk factors.

If technology use forms part of a broader lifestyle that involves attending to movement, eating well, sleeping, and being socially active with real people in real life, it can almost certainly be a net benefit to our cognitive function by providing complex novel stimuli that also help us to navigate the modern world. In fact, a very recent meta-analysis of more than four hundred thousand older adults found that greater technology use was associated with a slower rate of cognitive decline and a lower risk of dementia.[74]

It's also interesting to note that some of the most promising modern treatments for neurological diseases include some element of more direct stimulation that uses technology. This includes magnetic fields and electrical currents transmitted through the skull, such as transcranial magnetic stimulation (TMS), transcranial direct current stimulation (tDCS), transcranial alternating current stimulation (tACS), and transcranial random noise stimulation (tRNS), as well as stimulating the brain and nerves with specific frequencies of sound and light. These technologies that directly stimulate certain parts of the brain—triggering activity and adaptation—are particularly promising for symptom relief and treatment in scenarios like Alzheimer's disease and depression as well as directly supporting important brain functions like restorative sleep. Though they're still being developed, there are many clinical trials currently underway.[75] So, while we absolutely want to keep stimulating our brains by staying engaged with cognitive challenges and skills as we get older, it's also important to have as many options as possible available to help us avoid the loss of stimulus and function with age and treat neurological issues when they occur. Some of that may come from new and surprising uses of technology.

HOW WILL AI AFFECT OUR BRAINS?

With the ever-accelerating pace of technological advancement, it's worth taking some time to reflect on what that future might look like—and the influence that could have on our brains. As with most of these developments, the devil is in the details of how we use them.

Take, for example, large-language models (LLMs) like ChatGPT. One aspect of LLMs and AI that will eventually become relevant to all of us—if it isn't already—is their integration into our day-to-day work. This is where I think a simple litmus test can be applied. When you're using these tools, are they helping to support cognitive stimulus and the skills we want to foster and maintain, or are they doing the hard work for us and therefore causing our skills to atrophy?

I have colleagues who successfully employ LLMs as *cognitive orthotics*—tools to boost brainstorming and planning in a way that still requires them to be engaged in complex cognitive activities. And, like any diligent user of AI, they still have to chase down and confirm what the models say, because they're prone to making up their own facts and scientific references (often known as *hallucinations*).[76] If AI truly allows you to do complex work more efficiently so you can harness your own brain power for higher-level tasks, these tools have a lot of promise that will only increase over time.

However, it has also become increasingly common to completely offload tasks onto AI, with minimal forethought or cognitive input from the user. Every day I receive emails from colleagues that were clearly written by a chatbot, and more and more scientists are using AI to design experiments, analyse data, and write research papers. When this happens, it's almost like you can see the individual's skills (and cognitive function?) decreasing in real time. Or maybe those skills will never get built in the first place. If a student (or professor, for that matter) uses AI to design their experiment, analyse their data, and write it up for publication, how much science did that individual do? What skills did they learn, and how did it benefit their brain? Perhaps unsurprisingly, studies suggest that using AI tools for complex tasks can decrease activity in regions of the brain associated with that task because the brain is no longer engaged in the same way. As a result, less is learned and retained. This is fine if it saves you time that you can spend stimulating your brain in other ways but becomes a risk if you stop learning or maintaining critical skills.

The cognitive stimuli we get from our education and work, which we know are some of the most important ways to build and maintain cognitive function, can quickly be lost if we delegate the act of learning and critical thinking to AI. In an extreme version of this scenario, we might just become skilled at writing prompts for algorithms and not much else. I don't know about you, but that's not really the skill set I was hoping to take with me into the future.

While I do use LLMs myself, I primarily use them to help me write statistical code to analyse data. Just like with other aspects of technology, the algorithms available to help us understand complex data continue to advance and expand all the time. Though I often have to correct errors in the code to make it work the way I want, AI models can help me write code much faster. This means that I can spend more time asking questions of my data and thinking about what the results really mean, fostering the scientific skills that are important to me. By comparison, I wrote this book the old-fashioned way. I wanted to build the skill of communicating ideas in the written form myself, including all the procrastination, false starts, self-doubt, and trial and error that the process includes. In this way, I try to use AI to augment the stimuli and skills I want to build rather than offloading complex tasks that I should be really doing myself.

As the world continues to change, I think this same thought process can be applied to any new technology. Though it won't always be clear, start by asking whether a tool will bring you closer to or further away from the skills you want to learn and the core components of stimulus that the brain thrives on.

FIGHTING BACK AGAINST THE FORCES OF DECLINE

In part 1, we saw that retirement can be one of the periods when cognitive function is most at risk. Several studies in multiple countries have found that cognitive decline accelerates around the time of retirement, and those who retire *early* are at particularly increased risk of dementia—even after taking into account medical conditions that might force somebody to retire earlier than they would have otherwise.

While the mechanisms are complex, it certainly makes sense that part of what's driving the risk of decline after retirement is the cognitive, social, and physical slowing down that comes from no longer having a regular place of work. In line with this, at least one study showed that going *back* to work after initially retiring resulted in some benefits in cognitive function.[77]

I'm not suggesting the goal in life is to toil away for a corporation until your final days. However, it's clear that what we really want to avoid, either during our careers or after our transition away from standard working life, is a loss of the daily cognitive inputs that we get from work and related leisure activities. For example, a study of nearly six thousand people in multiple cities in France found that more time spent doing crosswords, playing cards, attending organizations, going to the cinema or theatre, and practicing artistic activities was associated with reduced risk of dementia in those over sixty-five.[78] So, as long as work is replaced by activities that can have similar cognitive benefits, such as taking up new hobbies and skills, attending group events or classes, travelling, or volunteering, there's no reason retirement should be a period of increased risk. And, yes, retirement can absolutely include some more time for rest and relaxation.

In addition to the day-to-day ways we can help to maintain our brains through regular stimulation, there are other inputs that are critical to ongoing brain health and function that we need to attend to, and these can be lost either slowly over time, or very suddenly.

In early 2019, barely a month after I started my job on the faculty at the University of Washington, I was bitten by a pit viper in the Costa Rican jungle. I was there on an otherwise perfectly pleasant work trip and had gone for a walk with some colleagues around dusk (which was silly because that's peak snake time) on what was supposed to be my last night in the country. I was crossing a stream and felt a sharp sting above my ankle, then looked down and saw the offending serpent slithering away.

Not knowing anything about snakes, my friend Ben and I decided it was probably best to head to the local ER, so we jumped into his truck and started the forty-five-minute drive down a mountain dirt road to get to the hospital. On the way, I called my wife back home in Seattle. To this day, she still points out that I started the call with every spouse's *favourite* words: "I don't want you to worry, but . . ."

About halfway to the hospital Ben received a text message, and as he read it, I immediately felt the truck pick up speed. The manager of the centre we were staying at had gone to find the snake and promptly dispatched it with a machete. He relayed that I had been bitten by a fer-de-lance, known locally as a *terciopelo*. The fer-de-lance has been dubbed "the ultimate pit viper" due to its aggression and general tendency to bite anything it comes across (it's a real "bite first, think afterwards" kind of reptile). Terciopelo bites require antivenom to prevent the main side effect of the bite—massive internal haemorrhage—and antibiotics to treat the bacterial infection that always comes along for the ride.

If you're ever going to be bitten by a terciopelo, I have a few general recommendations. Firstly, don't immediately google "terciopelo"; go to the Wikipedia page and look at the pictures of necrotic limbs requiring amputation. Secondly, try to make sure it happens in Costa Rica. With their huge expertise in treating these kinds of snakebites, and world-leading research and development in antivenom, even a relatively small rural hospital had everything they needed to treat me.

What followed was eleven days of general agony and slipping in and out of consciousness. As is typical of *tourists,* my doctor told me, I got (almost) every possible side effect of a terciopelo bite. This was particularly hard on my wife, Elizabeth, who not only had to worry about my health and well-being from thousands of miles away but found herself the sole operator of a 24/7 international information network responsible for regularly updating our family members (not to mention managing all the house- and dog-care duties required when your spouse finds himself indefinitely convalescing in a Costa Rican hospital).

Luckily, the antivenom did its job, and I managed to avoid one of the more unpleasant possibilities after a snakebite—compartment syndrome. This is where the swelling gets so bad that the leg starts to cut off its own blood supply. The treatment for compartment syndrome is surgically slashing open the lower leg from knee to ankle to release the pressure (a guy who got bitten a couple of days after me wasn't so lucky). My infection was a weird one, and it took several days and several different antibiotics to get it under control, by which time it had spread from my ankle up to the top of my leg. I also needed to have a large abscess drained, and I can still vividly remember being drenched in sweat, clinging to the bed for dear life as pus was forcibly squeezed out of my calf. Then, as a final treat to top off the whole ordeal, I got serum sickness—a delayed allergic reaction to antivenom that resulted in me being covered in whole-body hives for several days while they pumped me full of steroids and antihistamines. In telling the story now, this cascade of compounding misfortune is almost funny (to everyone but Elizabeth, who, quite literally, had requested that I *not* get bitten by a snake before I left for Costa Rica).

Even though my experience was a touch unusual, its utility here is to illustrate that unexpected events that completely wipe us out can occur to anyone at any time, which is why we want to build up as much of that valuable headroom as possible. As I hope will be the case for you if you ever become really unwell, I made it through unscathed (though not unscarred) because of the people and resources around me. Through friends and family, I had access to everything from local snake experts to doctors with decades of experience doing emergency medical evacuations.

On the ground, Ben drove to the hospital every day to bring me supplies and check in on me. As Spanish isn't one of the languages I can stumble through, he made sure to be there to figure out what was going on and translate what the doctors and nurses were saying. Elizabeth then flew down to implement my final rescue mission before spending weeks looking after me at home while I recuperated on the sofa. She somehow also managed to pick up my slack on a grant proposal with a tight deadline that we'd been working on together.

Throughout all this, Ben commented more than once that he was surprised by how calm and unflappable I seemed about the whole ordeal. And while I could probably try to make a strong case that my focus on cognitive stimulus, sleep, nutrition, and exercise had given me lots of headroom to deal with this unexpected scenario, I wouldn't want to take that much credit; all of this was possible because I had others to do the worrying for me.

Why am I telling you all this? In addition to being a good story, this tale does have some relevance to the brain. Despite being in good health beforehand, I was, obviously, incapacitated for quite some time. Even after I was home—after the infection was gone and my leg was healed—it took *weeks* for me to feel like my brain was working properly again. This is not unusual. The combination of being stuck in a hospital bed and the infection and inflammation left me about twenty pounds lighter. Overcoming the effect of just a few weeks being sick took a lot of work over several months.

As was the case with my own unavoidable downtime, periods of significant illness as we get older are associated with sudden decreases in both physical and cognitive function. An analysis from the Adult Changes in Thought study—where adults over sixty-five had their cognitive function assessed at regular intervals for several years—found that cognitive decline rapidly accelerated when a participant was hospitalised between assessments. And the more severe the illness, the more severe the decline.[79] There are studies that show that even just two weeks of forced bed rest in otherwise healthy people can significantly impair cognitive function due to the loss of critical inputs from physical activity and other cognitive stimuli.[80] And within a few weeks of an extended layoff, the speed at which we process information—one of the most basic functions of the brain—also starts to decline.[81]

If we think about all the accumulated illness we might experience over decades, each time losing a little fitness *and* a little muscle mass *and* a little cognitive function, it's going to add up. If we don't actively work to regain what we've lost afterwards, these losses are going to eat into our headroom and eventually decrease our overall capacity. As a result, we may end up thinking that we're just succumbing to the inevitable process of ageing when in fact it's the accumulated total effect of periods when our bodies weren't able to receive (and respond to) environmental inputs that has resulted in the system no longer running at the same level. So not only do we want headroom we can rely on during periods of illness, we also need to actively work to regain headroom afterwards so that it's still there whenever we might need it again.

KEEPING WHAT YOU'VE GOT

In addition to sudden losses of input caused by something like illness, a steady loss of normal inputs also puts us at a greater risk of dementia. This is particularly the case when it comes to our senses. Multiple studies have found that people who lose their hearing or eyesight with age tend to be at an increased risk of dementia—especially those who are at higher risk due to other reasons, such as age or medical conditions.[82] This increased risk seems to be directly related to the brain losing an important sensory input, because the risk is reversible—for instance, if somebody gets hearing aids for hearing loss or surgery if they're losing their sight due to cataracts. One study even found that having cataract surgery was as protective against dementia as an additional four years of education.[83]

There are a few reasons why losing a sense might increase the risk of dementia. The first is the direct effect of a loss of stimulus, with the brain adapting to the fact that certain regions or networks are no longer being used. But people who lose a sense are also less likely to engage with the world in ways that they used to, because they no longer feel able to navigate the environment as they could before. If people start to lose their sight or hearing, they also have to work harder to see or hear, which uses up more cognitive resources and decreases the headroom or cognitive reserve available to do other tasks. As a result, they may be more likely to stay at home and perform fewer activities, decreasing stimulus indirectly.

An important note, though, is that the loss of a sense is only important with respect to brain function if it was a sense that you previously had. Never having had sight or hearing doesn't seem to increase your risk of dementia, because the brain never experienced, adapted to, or expected those inputs. Instead, the brain puts extra resources into making the most of the networks and brain regions responsible for using the senses that it *does* have.[84]

The ongoing stimulation our senses provide to the brain is important for everybody, regardless of their age. Though the evidence is certainly not definitive, some physicians are concerned that constant use of noise-cancelling headphones may be associated with mental health issues in young adults because their ears and brains spend less time learning to filter out noise.[85] Loss of smell due to Covid-19 is thought to potentially be one of the reasons people experience brain fog after an infection: as the brain loses an input, function decreases in response (though a more direct effect of infection on both the brain and the nose is certainly part of the picture too).[86] Even the food we eat may play a role; slowly making food soggier and mushier as we get old might decrease the normal sensory input that our brain expects from our mouth, accelerating some aspects of cognitive decline.[87]

Luckily, none of this has to be bad news. We just need to know that the risks exist and work to minimise their effects as much as possible. In reality, though many of the types of decline people experience as they get older are simply tolerated and accepted (and expected) as an "inevitable" part of the ageing process, we have many options available to us to potentially avoid such a fate. As long as you find ways to ensure a wide range of both consistent and new stimuli through all the senses, and work to overcome any losses that might have happened through illness or long periods of rest, the brain will keep responding and functioning for decades to come.

In short, *never give up*.

STIMULATE YOURSELF

As you can hopefully tell, there are a huge number of stimulating and brain-boosting activities that help us support our headroom and cognitive function. Many of them are backed up by observational studies in which people are asked about their activities and then followed for some period of time to determine their risk of cognitive decline and dementia. These types of studies can't really prove the relationship between a given activity and cognitive function. However, a whole host of studies do show improvements in cognitive function when people learn a new skill or activity, so I've summarised some examples and protocols from studies mentioned in the chapter for you to try. Pick something that sounds fun, new, or that you can easily do for a period of time. Make sure to take opportunities to fail (and therefore drive neuroplasticity). Once you get really good at one thing, it's time to pick another!

Juggling
Learn a three-ball cascade, practicing ten to thirty minutes per day for six to twelve weeks. This is associated with improvements in white matter structure and spatial orientation skills.[88]

Languages
Most studies involve two to five hours per week (including homework) for a few weeks to a few months as part of a course or classes, with improvements seen in attention, working memory, and executive function.[89] Thirty minutes per day of an app (e.g., Duolingo) has also been found to be beneficial.[90]

Musical Instruments
Studies often use weekly music lessons (around sixty minutes long) plus at least thirty minutes of practice a few times per week for several months, finding associated improvements in some aspects of executive function and processing speed.[91]

Dancing
Ninety minutes twice per week for at least three or four months as part of a class has been linked to improvements in mobility, balance, cognitive function, and mood,[92] with longer interventions also showing improvements in hippocampus structure on an MRI scan.[93]

Brain Training

Performing exercises for at least one to two hours per week for around three or four months can bring improvements related to the function being trained, such as working memory or executive function, but additional benefits may be seen from tasks that train processing speed (like Double Decision in BrainHQ).[94] Computer-based brain training also seems to be beneficial in those already experiencing cognitive decline and can improve function in brain areas susceptible to aging.[95]

Video Games

Paradigms vary a lot, but around thirty minutes per day several times a week is what was used in the *Super Mario* studies. Meta-analyses suggest that a wide range of video games (including action/war games as well as driving and role-playing games) may be beneficial for overall cognitive function and attention. More complex games with interactive environments seem to have a greater effect.[96]

Addressing Sensory Loss

Most studies suggesting that hearing aids or cataract surgery decrease the risk of cognitive decline associated with sensory loss are observational, but in one clinical trial, hearing aids were found to be especially beneficial for those at high risk of dementia (for instance, due to lower education or higher cardiovascular disease risk).[97]

Novel Smells

Not all stimuli have to be actively engaged with. One interesting recent study had participants who were sixty years or older diffuse an essential oil into their bedroom air for two hours per night every night, rotating through seven different scents (one for each night of the week). After six months, the olfactory enrichment group improved on a memory task compared to a control group, with related changes visible on an MRI brain scan.[98]

We can apply these examples from the research more broadly. You could probably replace juggling and dancing with other complex coordinative motor skills, as discussed in chapter 7. If you prefer, you could learn to code or play chess instead of (or in addition to) learning a language or playing video games.[99] Think about it more in terms of the time and type of skills and stimuli that your brain is getting through these activities.

WHAT HAPPENS WHEN I RETIRE?

Even if we don't fully retire, we will probably divert a lot of our attention away from the daily grind of work life at some point later in life. Arthur C. Brooks is a professor at the Harvard Business School who teaches and writes about leadership and happiness. In his book *From Strength to Strength*, he describes what he calls *the striver's curse*. This is where individuals who are used to the success and accolades of a complex and competitive work environment struggle the most when they transition to retirement. Thinking back to self-determination theory as one of the core human needs for well-being, which was mentioned in chapter 8, losing the chance to express our expertise at work can translate into losing feelings of competence.

While this certainly makes sense from a psychological perspective, there are also elements of this phenomenon mirrored in some of the data looking at cognitive function after retirement. Though results differ across studies, some suggest that the rate of decline may differ based on the level of stimulus your brain became accustomed to earlier in life.[100] In particular, those with higher levels of education may experience more rapid loss of certain cognitive functions after retirement. For example, among more than two thousand adults from the Reasons for Geographic and Racial Differences in Stroke (REGARDS) study, those who attended university had higher levels of cognitive function before retirement but experienced a more rapid decline in cognitive function afterwards.[101]

Some of this may be due to the striver's curse. In the absence of the meaning and purpose achieved at work or through education, it's harder for people to engage in the unfamiliar environment of retirement without some kind of goal. But I would argue that a large part of this is due to the drop in stimulus. A brain that has spent decades being challenged on a daily basis is likely to need greater ongoing stimulus to maintain the same level of cognitive function. It's like an athlete who quits their sport and stops exercising altogether. They have a lot more strength and fitness to lose compared to somebody who never trained at that level.

The solutions to this problem are relatively simple, though not necessarily easy. Brooks recommends switching gears and leveraging new strengths as we transition to midlife and retirement. In particular, while the processing speed of the brain might decline a bit with age, this can be counterbalanced by an increase in crystallised intelligence—the components of cognitive function that make up wisdom, which we discussed in part 1. So, rather than being the person *doing* the thing, we could benefit by becoming the person *teaching* the thing—applying and leveraging our accumulated experience and finding ways to give back to the younger generations and our community.

This, I think, typifies what we see in preindustrial cultures where the active grandparent hypothesis originated. This hypothesis suggests that there was evolutionary pressure for humans to be able to live for decades after they reproduce by continuing to play an important role late into life, supporting the survival of their family and the community as a whole. As individuals get older, they become repositories for institutional knowledge. It allows them to take more of a role teaching and looking after the tribe. As we transition to new phases of work or leave work entirely, the key is finding a place in the world where we still feel useful and have purpose.[102] In a recent meta-analysis of more than thirty thousand people, a greater sense of purpose was associated with a lower risk of later dementia regardless of age, medical conditions, sex, or education level.[103] When we have purpose, we are more engaged and socially connected, which provides stimulus. And, curiously (or maybe not), the meta-analysis also discovered that individuals with purpose were more likely to maintain other healthy behaviours and experience a lower risk of depression.

How you find a new (or renewed) sense of purpose beyond work is entirely up to you. For example, you could think about new types of physical activity you might want to try. Or explore where you can build new social networks—through groups or classes—or reignite old ones by reconnecting with friends and family. And, speaking of reigniting old activities, how about reading a book or even joining a book club? Reading is associated with a lower risk of cognitive decline, and book clubs offer increased well-being through reflection on the material as well as supporting connections with new people and friends.[104] For the pursuit of cognitive function and headroom to be sustainable, you need to have a reason to do it. For most of us, this will involve other people, especially given our need for relatedness. It also underlines the idea that we should not do this all alone. As humans, we need to have a place where we belong and where all our hard work building headroom feels worth it.

It is also important, as you approach retirement, to consider your preconceived notions about ageing itself. As discussed in part 1, if we think getting older automatically means a slow decline and loss of function, we'll stop engaging in the activities that help to *maintain* function in the first place, and those expectations will come true. But, equally, there is probably some benefit to welcoming certain inevitable parts of getting older.

This last point is important because I think trying to actively *avoid* ageing may eventually result in some unexpected (and potentially negative) cognitive effects. In the past few years there has been an explosion of focus on longevity—extending our lifespans for as many years as possible. Thankfully, the focus on longevity also usually comes with the more holistic idea of *healthspan*—the number of healthy years we have—rather than just the total number of years we're alive. This is an important distinction, as gains in healthspan seem to be achievable by focusing on the same core risk factors that influence most chronic diseases as well as our risk of developing dementia.

Unfortunately, at the extremes of the focus on longevity is an inherent assumption that ageing is *bad*, even though there's no avoiding it (at least right now). As a result, I think those who push the hardest against the forces of ageing might end up experiencing quite a bit of distress when that ageing process continues its march forward regardless of their efforts. The stress of worrying about ageing might then become a factor that further *accelerates* aging.

One way that scientists assess somebody's approach to ageing is to examine their perceptions. In the Ohio Longitudinal Study of Ageing and Retirement, adults fifty years and older were tested on their perceptions of getting older by seeing how much they agreed with statements like "As you get older, you are less useful." Participants were followed for more than twenty years, and those who had a more positive perception of ageing were found to live on average 7.5 years longer.[105] Of course, some of this could be due to changes in health that make people feel gloomier about ageing as well as increasing their risk of death, but the study found that self-perceptions of ageing had more of an impact on survival than sex, socioeconomic status, health, or loneliness.

Considering what we know about how our thoughts can influence our physiology, the notion that a concerted battle against ageing might end up being counterproductive is certainly something to ponder.

In addition to holding a more positive attitude about aging, optimism also appears to be a factor associated with living a longer and healthier life.[106] The best and most balanced approach I can suggest is this: avoid the processes that accelerate ageing by minimising mismatch. Be optimistic that you can continue to have an important and purposeful place in the world and seek a wide range of stimuli. At the same time, it's worth appreciating that there are *benefits* to aging, such as wisdom, as well as the opportunity to gain more control over our time and try new things. With this mindset, you can make the most of what you're capable of, enjoy the fruits of your labours, and benefit from all your current brain function now, as well as your continued cognitive function in the future.

THE STIMULATED MIND

In many ways, the brain is like a muscle. From the moment we're born (and probably even before that), the brain is becoming attuned to the environment in order to help us adapt to and survive the world around us. As a result, our brains are shaped by the skills and knowledge that ultimately determine their function. Though it's absolutely critical that we support the core biology of the brain with physical activity, nutrition, and adequate rest (more on that coming soon), the primary driver of our brain function is the stimulus our brains are exposed to—that is, the number of mental bicep curls we do across our lifetimes.

Our trajectory of cognitive function is therefore driven by activities that *enhance* function—education, skill learning, and other cognitively stimulating activities. We also have to *maintain* the inputs the brain has adapted to, be that skills we practise or sensory inputs to our brains, so that the underlying structure is maintained. But there is another piece to this puzzle: engaging with a social environment. And that too provides critical inputs that can help to build headroom and future-proof the brain.

CHAPTER 10

CONNECT

In part 1, when I asked what's so special about the human brain, I mentioned that our social environment is thought to be a major reason humans developed their large and complex brains. However, it turns out that's not quite enough to explain it. For example, there are small birds and fish who live in (relatively) complex social groups despite having teeny tiny brains.[1] Access to enough calories and certain nutrients such as omega-3s have also been proposed as being critical supporters of human brain evolution, and this no doubt played a role as well.[2]

But the real driver of human brain evolution may have been something that Charles Darwin himself was fascinated by: compassion. In 1871, twelve years after the publication of *On the Origin of Species,* which is considered the foundation of evolutionary theory and the idea of "survival of the fittest," Darwin wrote *The Descent of Man* about human evolution in particular. He had come to realise that an every-animal-for-themselves approach to evolution couldn't explain some of the core aspects of human behaviour. Instead, he theorised that "those communities which included the greatest number of the most sympathetic members, would flourish best and rear the greatest number of offspring."

What Darwin called sympathy is what we might now call empathy or compassion. Instead of the strongest or fittest winning out, it was the individual or group of individuals who best cared for one another who were most likely to survive and reproduce. This idea eventually became known as *survival of the kindest,* often attributed to (and at least popularised by) psychologist Dacher Keltner.[3] This idea underpins one of the essential rules of the brain game: *Don't go it alone.*

Survival of the kindest is particularly critical for humans, who need to be cared for by others for years (or maybe even decades) before they become fully self-sufficient. It's therefore the combination of societal complexity, prosocial behaviour, and the passing on of cultural information from older adults in the community to the next generation that is thought to explain the unique evolution of the human brain.[4] It might come as no surprise, then, that our social environment plays a key role in our long-term physical health, brain health, and cognitive function.

SOCIAL HEADROOM

Shortly after Josh Turknett and I published our paper on cognitive decline as a natural response to decreases in stimulus with age, I was in London for a conference and met my friend Julian Abel for breakfast. Julian is a retired palliative care physician famous for his work building compassionate communities. As I described our idea of stimulus-driven cognitive function, Julian looked at me and said: "I'm sure this is right, but the benefit of cognitive stimulus is *really* driven by our biological need for social connection."

Between 2013 and 2017 Julian led a project to build a compassionate community within Frome, a small town in the southwest of England. The goal was to bring social networks to local individuals, especially those living with chronic disease. Each patient was allocated a "community connector" who helped them set goals and determine their desired level of support. Based on their personal situation and interests, patients were connected with one or more of several hundred local professional, volunteer, and community groups. If new groups were needed, they were established. The people in those groups actively worked to become the patient's social network. Over the course of four years, emergency room admissions in the area decreased by 14 percent while those in all the surrounding areas *increased* by 28 percent.[5] This result has since been replicated in other towns, and is now being implemented in several countries around the world.[6]

The importance of social connection and compassion, which is rooted in human evolution, can also help to explain the biology of many chronic diseases, including cognitive decline and dementia. Recently, Julian and I edited a collection of scientific papers on the many ways community can affect health, written by world experts on the topic.[7]

This included Julianne Holt-Lunstad, a psychologist and neuroscientist who led the U.S. surgeon general's report *Our Epidemic of Loneliness and Isolation*.[8] In 2010, she published a paper showing that loneliness was one of the biggest risk factors for death, outcompeting smoking, obesity, and physical inactivity.[9] These findings on the importance of having strong social connections as a protection against mortality risk have been replicated in multiple large studies since.[10] Another paper in the collection, written by George Slavich and Steven Cole from UCLA, detailed in physiological terms exactly how the absence of social connection can affect our long-term health. They showed that loneliness is linked to increases in stress, inflammation, and other health issues directly associated with long-term cognitive decline and dementia.[11]

At first glance, you may wonder how social isolation can have such a dramatic impact on brain health. But when you consider human evolution, it makes quite a bit of sense. Imagine that you're one of your distant ancestors, living in a non-industrialised environment as part of a group of a few dozen people. For me this might involve grass-roofed huts on a freezing mossy hillside in Iceland. When we're in close proximity to others, our nervous system and immune system respond accordingly. People in close and supportive social groups tend to have lower baseline levels of stress and higher activation of the parasympathetic nervous system—especially the vagus nerve.[12] For example, prosocial and compassionate thoughts and behaviour have been shown to activate the vagus nerve, which is responsible for coordinating a more restful state throughout the body. As part of the baseline physiological changes associated with being in a group, our immune systems shift toward being better at dealing with respiratory viruses like colds or flus, which we are more likely to be exposed to when we're surrounded by other people.

However, if you suddenly got separated from the group, wandering lost and alone on the lava fields of Iceland, your body would adapt. Either due to the loss of the stress-relieving aspects of social connection or the heightened stress of being alone (or a bit of both), a low-level fight-or-flight response would be activated. As part of this response, your immune system would shift away from focusing on antiviral processes and instead increase your readiness to deal with an injury. After all, there's nobody to expose you to the flu, but also nobody to help you if you fall over and cut your leg. This survival response increases the speed of wound healing but comes with an increased baseline level of inflammation.[13]

In the short term, the stress response driven by isolation would help to keep you alive until you rejoin your tribe. But if it is activated for years or decades because you're isolated and don't have social support or opportunities to provide compassion to others, this chronic increase in stress and inflammation can result in anxiety, depression, and accelerated aging. You can even measure the relationship between loneliness and inflammation as it happens. For example, a study of more than forty thousand people found nearly two hundred proteins in the blood linked to social isolation, which were then associated with heart disease, depression, stroke, dementia, and death.[14] One particular loneliness-related protein, adrenomedullin, was strongly correlated with markers of inflammation, including C-reactive protein and GlycA, and seemed to drive at least some of the relationship between loneliness and the risk of dementia.

The benefits of being caring and compassionate to others—as well as the broad range of cognitive stimuli involved—might explain an interesting conundrum when it comes to the brain regarding parenting. On the face of it, becoming a parent should be a disaster for your brain health. Kids tend to come with years of sleep deprivation, multiple types of stress, and less time to focus on eating or exercising. But they also come with a lot of love, inspire prosocial and caring behaviour, and provide a fair amount of stimulus and joy. These latter factors probably tip the balance when it comes to the effect kids can have on our brains. In a study of more than thirty-five thousand parents in the UK—a similar number of males and females—the number of children an individual had was positively associated with function in certain networks in the brain that tend to deteriorate with age. So, it's quite possible that, despite how it might feel sometimes, having kids could actually make your brain *younger*![15]

ISOLATION VERSUS LONELINESS

When thinking about our social relationships, studies often focus on two separate but related ideas: isolation and loneliness. Isolation is more about the *quantity* of social contacts—how many people you're frequently connected to—whereas loneliness is more about *quality*. You can feel lonely while seeing lots of people every day, and you can also see very few people but have such good relationships with them that you never feel alone. In a given situation, different people can also feel different levels of isolation and loneliness based on their personality. But both extroverts and introverts need social support, with quality generally being much more important than quantity. (I'm looking at you, social media!)[16]

The difference between isolation and loneliness is important when it comes to our brain health in particular because it can be difficult to untangle cause and effect. For example, if somebody has depression they might pull away from their social contacts and become isolated, but it wasn't the isolation that *caused* the depression. This means that some of the relationship between social isolation and dementia might be driven by other factors that affect both our health and our desire to socialise with others. However, it seems that loneliness and isolation (probably because it increases loneliness) have a two-way relationship with depression symptoms, both causing depression and being caused by depression.[17] This is important both for our day-to-day mental health but also because of the relationship between depression and dementia. Studies show us that depression increases the risk of dementia, and dementia also increases the risk of depression.[18] This second bidirectional relationship could be due to a number of possible reasons, including changes in stimulus and social connection as well as common causes related to ways that loneliness might increase stress and inflammation.

Because of the intimate relationship between social connection and brain health, a lack of social relationships can be directly seen in our brains and cognitive function.[19] Evidence of this comes from some fascinating research looking at how humans might deal with long periods of isolation during spaceflight. For example, one study—MARS-500—confined people to a simulated Martian habitat for 520 days, which resulted in chronic increases in the stress hormone cortisol and decreased global brain activity.[20] In a similar experiment, conducted by NASA, people who were confined for just thirty days also showed higher levels of cortisol and decreased brain activity due to what the scientists called "a neural adaptation to less external stimuli."

When the results from these studies are combined with others such as one looking at the brains of people before and after polar expeditions, an interesting pattern emerges. The major areas of the brain most affected by isolation seem to be the *same* brain regions that develop after birth and are tied to our most complex cognitive (and social) functions—which, as we've seen, are the brain regions that are most at risk when we age.[21] So not only does social activity drive the development and function of our brains, but social isolation and loneliness may accelerate brain ageing later in life too.

This idea is supported by at least two studies that found that social connection later in life is associated with greater brain reserve. In a group of nearly nine thousand Japanese adults over sixty-five, more frequent social contact was associated with higher brain volumes and less age-related white matter injury.[22] In a similar study in Germany, both low initial social connection and decreases in social connection over time were associated with smaller hippocampi and worse memory, processing speed, and executive function. Large meta-analyses have found that having a strong social network and feeling supported are protective against dementia.[23] Therefore, the stimulus, support, and interaction we receive from our social contacts and relationships provides headroom—bigger brain volumes, better cognitive function, and a lower long-term risk of dementia.

The research converges to demonstrate that having a strong social environment to engage with is a critical part of long-term brain health. Not only that but, as Julian Abel suggested to me, our social relationships drive many other brain-supporting factors as well. Our social activities provide a range of stimuli for the brain, and they can also influence lifestyle, including how we eat and move. For example, the 2025 World Happiness Report found that across 142 countries, one of the strongest predictors of well-being was the number of meals per week that people share with others.[24] And fascinating new research is finding that our brains have entire separate networks and connectivity patterns specifically for social coordination, which become activated when we do social activities like dancing.[25]

COMBATING LONELINESS

The most studied direct intervention to stave off the effects of social isolation is exercise.[26] Exercise can of course be done alone, but, like with dancing, it can also be an excellent way to extend your social group. I benefited from this myself right at the end of my time in medical school. After final exams but before graduation and being thrust into the world as a junior doctor, medical students in the UK spend a couple of months doing an "elective." This is usually a chance to travel and experience medicine somewhere else in the world. For my elective, I received a scholarship to spend some time doing sports medicine at the University of Iowa (Go, Hawkeyes!). I then spent time travelling to various cities around the United States sightseeing and visiting family and friends. By the end of three months, I had figured out a routine. On my first day in a new city, I would take a trip to the local CrossFit gym and sign up. CrossFit as a company and a sport has had its ups and downs, but they have always championed the benefit of community. Whenever I showed up at a new gym, I left an hour later with at least five new friends. I took part in charity events and even did some travelling with people I had met at the gym just a few weeks earlier.

I mention this personal example because we have to acknowledge that maintaining a healthy level of social connection can be difficult at times. I can't just sit here and tell you to go out and make some more friends, because the world doesn't really work like that. But joining groups that already exist and revolve around a theme or topic that you're interested in is a great place to start. This could be an exercise, dance, language, or music class. It could also be unrelated to any of those and just involve a personal interest, or volunteering with a group that is working toward solving a problem or reaching a common goal.[27]

In order to distinguish whether cognitive engagement actually stimulates cognitive function or if people who have better cognitive function happen to seek out more engaging activities, researchers at the University of Illinois Urbana-Champaign randomly assigned adults aged fifty-eight to ninety-three to either a control group or a cognitive-enrichment programme built around team problem-solving.

Teams in the problem-solving group met for twenty weekly sessions to develop a presentation for a competition. Problems included building a structure of balsa wood that would bear as much weight as possible, and presenting a performance that reinterpreted a classical piece of literature or a historical event. With no perfect solution or plan, participants were encouraged to take risks in suggesting solutions and to piggyback on one another's ideas in a way that included coordination, spatial processing, language processing, and memory. After the intervention, those who had been a part of a problem-solving team saw improvements in cognitive functions like processing speed and reasoning compared to the control group.[28] This shows that cognitively stimulating social activities have the potential to directly improve cognitive function.

While people who are more socially active tend to have lower dementia risk, bigger brains, and better cognitive function overall, and while *any* kind of supportive or stimulating social interaction has the potential to increase headroom and improve health, volunteering seems to be particularly beneficial.[29] One study of British households found that frequent volunteer work was associated with improved mental health, especially as people got into their forties and beyond. Another study of more than four hundred married couples in Detroit found that, in particular, *providing* social support was associated with a lower risk of death. The researchers thought this might be because acts of compassion and prosocial behaviour improve health and overall well-being.[30]

In the Harvard Study of Adult Development, which started in 1938—the longest-running study of human happiness—higher attachment and feelings of security in elderly couples was associated with better mood and lower likelihood of cognitive deficits.[31] The combination of prosocial behaviour and social connection again seems to explain this. However, there's an argument to be made about making sure you're not volunteering or looking after your spouse just to benefit your own brain or health, because that's technically neither altruistic nor compassionate. Altruism and compassion aren't just activities; they're also feelings. So maybe you should just go out and do some good in the world without overthinking it too much. Focus on the relationships and activities that really mean something to you.

As you read this, you may be thinking that some people are just naturally more social than others. Certainly, the many interconnected aspects of health, social connection, stimulus, and dementia risk probably explain some of the fascinating results seen in a recent large meta-analysis of personality traits and dementia risk. Using patient data from over forty-four thousand people followed for up to twenty-one years, in eight different studies across three continents and five countries, researchers found that those with higher levels of personality traits associated with engagement and prosocial behaviour—conscientiousness, extraversion, openness to experience, and agreeableness—tended to have a lower risk of dementia.[32] The signal was strongest for conscientiousness, which is associated with being organised, reliable, and goal oriented.[33] At the same time, those who had higher levels of neuroticism had a consistently higher risk of later dementia. As these traits make up core parts of personality but also change over time and are affected by our age and health, the authors suggested that the relationship between neuroticism and dementia may be at least partly due to stress and inflammatory conditions that increase both neuroticism and dementia risk.[34] By comparison, one could at least hypothesise that the other personality traits might make somebody more likely to engage in activities that increase both cognitive stimulus and social connection, therefore increasing headroom.

Interestingly, there's nothing to suggest that your prosocial behaviour or connection has to be purely human focused.[35] In studies exploring the relationship between social isolation and dementia, any living situation that doesn't involve living alone seems to be beneficial. For example, one study found that prolonged pet ownership was associated with better memory function in adults over sixty-five.[36] In English adults living alone, pet ownership was also found to be associated with better retention of memory and language skills over time, so being a pet parent may provide similar benefits to raising human children.[37] This may be because of the benefits and stimulus that come from looking after another living being, or because of other effects that we're still just starting to learn about. For example, the heart rate variability—a measure of vagus nerve activity—of dogs and their owners are correlated.[38] Outside of the direct pet-owner bond, it's also thought that social connection—either with animals or other humans—may be beneficial because it helps us create a more diverse microbiome (the bacteria and other various small things that live on and inside us).[39] Having a pet also increases your contact with other humans; if I ever want to hear "Who's a handsome boy?" I just have to take our boxer, Morgan, for a walk around the block.[40]

FINDING WAYS TO CONNECT

Our level of social connection and support directly influences our cognitive and physical health, but this can be a daunting topic to think about when we don't feel well connected or supported. Though none of these is a perfect solution on its own, below are some starting points for ways to build social connections and prosocial behaviour.

Join a Group

Seeking out people with similar interests or engaging in new skills is a great way to connect with others. This could be literally anything, but groups or classes that also include some kind of movement (many of the open-skill sports mentioned in chapter 7 are inherently social), cognitive stimulus (like a book club), or opportunity to eat nourishing food (potluck with colleagues, cooking classes) would be a bonus.

Touch Somebody

Or have them touch you. (With their full and unwavering consent, of course.) Compassionate and loving touch decreases stress and counteracts many of the physiological responses to loneliness.[41] If preferred, similar results have also been seen with pets, as well as from a professional massage.[42]

Volunteer

A special version of joining a group. Dedicating your time in the service of others seems to be particularly beneficial when it comes to our long-term brain health. And though the direct health benefits are debated, blood donation has also been associated with improvements in blood pressure and well-being.[43] Either way, at the end of the day you've done some good in the world. Win-win!

Go to the Library

In many cities, libraries are both social hubs and great places to read and find out what's going on in the community, including events and groups you might like to join.

Phone a Friend

Instead of sending an email or a text (or a message on social media), call a loved one. As one study put it when summarising the results of three different experiments involving nearly a thousand people, "Engaging in as little as one communication behaviour with one friend in a day can improve daily well-being."[44]

CONNECTION IN THE DIGITAL AGE

Direct social contact with other humans and our pets seems to provide a host of health benefits and positive cognitive stimuli, but what about social interactions that occur online?

I distinctly remember the halcyon days of social media. In March 2005, during my first year as an undergraduate student, Facebook expanded to the first three universities outside the United States, and Cambridge was one of them. I initially resisted, despite some mild peer pressure, but a period of procrastination during exam preparation led me to sign up. Back then Facebook was pretty basic; this was before you could even post status updates or message people, and most of what you did on Facebook was upload photos and "poke" your friends.

Facebook as it existed more than two decades ago held a lot of promise in terms of bolstering our social connection virtually. In many ways, I think some of that promise is still available to us. The problem is that successive iterations of social media have become less and less about connection and sharing with friends and family and more about content creation and consumption. This leaves us vulnerable to situations that foster feelings of loneliness and social isolation while providing fewer of the potential benefits of online social connection.

Soon after Facebook became more widely accessible, people started researching the impact of Facebook groups on various aspects of health, especially for those struggling with chronic health conditions. Though there were of course cases where these groups fostered an us-versus-them mentality, in general, individuals found them to be beneficial in terms of peer support, practical advice, self-efficacy, and the opportunity to share personal experiences.[45] In addition to disease-specific groups, online support groups can be places to meet and learn from people on any number of topics—from cruciferous recipes in the Broccoli Bros group to expert tips for your next dance class. My colleague Josh Turknett even has a Facebook group specifically to teach others about the wonderful world of banjos. These types of groups—which are also increasingly moving away from traditional social media to other content platforms like Substack and Discord—can be a great way to connect with new people over shared interests or to navigate new lifestyle changes.

As with social connection in real life, it's the *quality* of virtual interactions that seems to determine their overall effect, where they fit in the context of your other social relationships. Multiple studies have investigated the use of virtual communication through Facebook, video calls, and messaging apps as a way for older adults to decrease feelings of loneliness and improve social connection.[46] Giving people tools to connect with loved ones virtually tends to decrease feelings of loneliness and improve some aspects of memory—potentially due to the added benefit of stimulus from using a novel technology.[47] Interaction over video calls in particular can elicit some of the synchrony and alignment that people experience when they interact in person.

Importantly, however, there's a big difference between using online platforms to provide a new method of communication—where you're more likely to expect benefit because of the net *increase* in stimulus and social contact—and a reliance on social media as a primary form of social connection. The latter is what often happens to those who have grown up with these technologies and use them every day. Some of the best examples of this discrepancy came from shifts in contact and connection during Covid-19.

Though studies differ in their methods and conclusions, in general, the more direct methods of virtual connection—like calls and messages—seem to buffer some of the negative effects of social isolation.[48] However, virtual connection is not an adequate replacement for in-person connection.[49] One study of nearly a thousand adults explored the relationship between different levels of in-person and online social interaction and mood during Covid-19 lockdowns.[50] They found that messages and calls improved feelings of social connection, but posting and commenting on social media did not. When it came to mood, though, only face-to-face interaction was associated with people feeling more content. More time spent browsing content on social media was associated with feeling *less* content (though, to be fair, most online content was pretty depressing at the time). As a result, there seems to be a sliding scale of effects of virtual connection, with direct contact with friends and family on one end and passively consuming social media content at the other.

Perhaps the largest study on social media use during the pandemic leveraged UK data from four longitudinal cohorts who were in different age groups during lockdown—the Millennium Cohort Study whose participants were nineteen to twenty-one years old, Next Steps who were thirty-one and thirty-two, the British Cohort Study who were fifty and fifty-one, and the National Child Development Study, who were sixty-two and sixty-three. What they found was that both in-person visits and video or voice calls were associated with less anxiety and depression, and greater social media use was associated with higher anxiety and depression, and these effects were greatest in the youngest group.[51] When comparing to data from before the pandemic, an increase in social media use during lockdown was associated with worse anxiety and depression scores. Another study in multiple countries also found different effects of social media use during the pandemic by age group—higher social media use was associated with lower loneliness in the older age groups (forty and above) but higher loneliness in the youngest group (eighteen to thirty-nine).[52]

While these studies can't prove that social media use worsens mental health *directly,* they support an increasing body of literature suggesting that a high volume of social media use is at least partly responsible for the worsening mental health of younger generations (though worsening mental health may also drive people to use more social media instead of having in-person interactions).

Some of the most compelling explanations for the relationship between social media and well-being stem from the negative effects social media can have on our physiology. Many of the interactions we have online appear to trigger the same physiological responses that our bodies experience when we become socially isolated. This is because social isolation fits into a broader category of social *stress,* which is what social media seems to excel at. For example, social media is well known to be a breeding ground for FOMO (fear of missing out), where seeing your supposed friends or other people like you having fun without you triggers feelings of rejection. You might also experience direct feelings of rejection if you post something and you don't get many likes or views, or if people respond with negative comments.

Due to the importance that the human brain assigns to social cues, even these relatively minor and brief online interactions can have outsized effects. This is because the human brain interprets social rejection very similarly to physical pain, with areas of the brain that are critical for processing physical pain also triggered by "social pain."[53]

Another important source of social stress is the way that we see ourselves compared to others—what we might think of as our self-perceived social "rank." We saw in chapter 6 that comparing our own health behaviours to others', which is one way we determine our own rank in the world, may alter how much we benefit from those behaviours. By consuming a lot of social media content of people who are more jacked, more beautiful, more successful, and richer than we are, we lower our perceptions of ourselves. This internal demotion in social rank triggers some of the same stress responses we see when people are socially isolated, which, as outlined above, are associated with increased risk for several chronic diseases as well as depression, cognitive decline, and dementia.[54]

But if social media is such a torrid breeding ground for self-loathing, why do we keep returning to it? Again, at least part of this stems from our nature as social animals, which means that we're wired to seek out information that helps us navigate the social environment. We prioritise gathering information that is PRIME—Prestigious, Ingroup (e.g., based on cliques or your own social bubble), Moral, or Emotional.[55] The fact that we're *primed* to seek this type of information as part of our desire for learning is specifically leveraged by social media algorithms in order to capture our attention.

Dopamine is involved in many processes in the brain related to memory and mood, as well as motivation and learning, all of which are relevant to how we interact with social media. The human brain has evolved dopamine networks that seem to underpin unique aspects of learning as well as reflection and overall intelligence.[56] One of the best-known functions of dopamine is in reward pathways, with dopamine driving motivation to seek a given reward. When a reward is uncertain—the number of likes you'll get on your Instagram post, for example—your brain releases larger amounts of dopamine. When a reward is particularly good—your post suddenly goes viral—you get an even *bigger* bump of dopamine due to the reward being better than you expected. The brain then uses these bumps of dopamine to help it learn what set of factors or elements of the post caused it to perform so well.

But when it comes to learning, more dopamine isn't necessarily better. Decreases in dopamine also help us learn and occur especially during the detection of errors and mistakes, as we saw in chapter 9.[57] In general, larger dopamine changes in either direction drive larger learning responses. This dopamine-related learning also tends to be greater in social contexts because of the importance we place on PRIME information and learning from others. This means that social media is well positioned to regularly drive large dopamine responses—larger dopamine bumps if the TikTok videos are highly novel and engaging or a lot of people like our posts, and larger dopamine dips if we're exposed to unexpected politicised or emotional information that makes us mad, or if people are mean about our thoughts on the latest hot restaurant in the neighbourhood.

As a result of all these dopamine swings, social media represents the ultimate social mismatch. The reason we prioritise PRIME information is that it should help us learn about our social environment in order to maximise connectedness and safety. Social media takes advantage of our desire for this kind of information while offering us the opposite—isolation. But we keep going back because our brains are constantly wondering whether the *next* time might be different. Unfortunately, unless we're very careful about how we craft our social media experience, the sheer volume of people we're exposed to can make that very difficult.

While hopefully everybody can agree that being exposed to and interacting with a wide variety of people with differing experiences and opinions can be beneficial (and stimulating), the downside of having more of these opportunities online is that you end up exposed to a *lot* of opinions. This, again, is not necessarily something that we're adept at handling. Before the advent of social media, we might meet a few thousand people over our lifetime and be well connected to hundreds. But now, the average person can interact with or be exposed to the thoughts of thousands of people in a single day. This means that we're exposed to a lot more jerks in a given day than we would have had to deal with just a couple of decades ago. The combination of our natural negativity bias and our focus on interactions that cause an emotional response leaves a greater emotional drain on us, even if the vast majority of our daily interactions are positive.

Where does that leave us with respect to virtual connection and social media? For individuals who increase their number of close social contacts or their connection to friends and family (and learn a skill by adopting a new technology or platform), this is probably going to be beneficial. Being able to spend time with those closest to you will foster deeper connection, building more headroom. However, if virtual connections or social media are being used as a replacement for face-to-face human connection, this is likely to have the opposite effect. So, as ever, the greater context is important. For example, one large Austrian study during Covid-19 found that social media use had little overall relationship with well-being, which was much more tightly connected to physical health, exercise, and socioeconomic factors.[58] So, overall, spending time in the virtual world can be fine, as long as you avoid some of the obvious pitfalls and make sure it's balanced with time spent with others in real life.

NAVIGATING SOCIAL MEDIA

Many of us feel that our time on social media isn't serving us in the best possible way. If that's the case for you, here are some tips for ways to better navigate the online world.

Go Cold Turkey
Sometimes it's easiest to just cut the cord. But if you do this, it might be tricky initially. For the first couple of weeks, going without social media can either be stressful—almost like constant FOMO—or have a minimal overall effect.[59] This is probably related to what people do instead of spending time on social media, or the reasons they used social media in the first place. So context always matters. But in studies where people quit social media for at least four weeks, they tend to see improvements in happiness, well-being, and mood as a result, especially if they also increase time spent with friends and family.[60]

Go Old-School
It's still possible to primarily use social media for its original intended purpose: meaningfully connecting with others in a way that you wouldn't be able to do in person. Focus on joining groups and spending more time sharing with friends and family rather than unknown strangers whose opinions you probably shouldn't care about anyway.

Unfollow

Think carefully about the people you follow and remove those that don't add anything—especially if you find yourself consuming their content and feeling like you're not doing enough or that you're not successful or attractive enough. Unless it's benefitting you in some other way, this kind of content is only eroding your self-worth. Unfollowing can also help you to avoid the minority of people who cause most of the conflict online. In one analysis, 74 percent of conflict on the social media platform Reddit was instigated by just 1 percent of users.[61]

Add Time Limits

Social media isn't inherently *bad* as long as it's not interfering with real life or triggering social stress. Like puzzles and crosswords, social media can provide a calming break that requires some focus without being too cognitively demanding. It's fine to consume content in this way, but use it as a defined mental break rather than reaching for it frequently to stimulate or distract yourself.

Diversify Your Inputs

Very heavy social media use displays some of the elements of addiction, and we know from addiction research that consistently receiving dopamine-related inputs from a single source decreases the reward we get from other sources.[62] One way to combat the pull of social media is to engage in other stimulating activities that are fun and drive learning.

Sleep

When we're sleep-deprived or stressed, our dopamine signaling changes so that we become more focused on *now* rewards rather than *later* rewards.[63] As a result, we might reach for social media rather than engaging with work or exercising. Just knowing that our physiological state might change our likelihood of engaging with social media can help us to understand why we're reaching for it and what we might do instead.

THE SOCIAL BRAIN

Social isolation and loneliness are mismatches that can negatively affect our biology and long-term cognitive function. While social connection can be challenging territory, it has consistently been found to be critical to our physical and cognitive health, probably because it is so intimately linked to our development as a species. Luckily, we can develop meaningful social connections in a number of ways that best suit our own living situation, interests, and personality. These social interactions can then provide the environment we need to build and express our skills as humans. Call a loved one. Take care of them. Or join a local dance troupe.

Engaging with the environment around us, especially by connecting with the people within it, helps to make the brain more resilient in the face of aging. This builds headroom and provides us with the physical, emotional, and cognitive buffers we need to better future-proof our brains. Embracing more real-world social connections therefore provides us with yet another way to hone cognition and reduce stress, adding to our arsenal of tools to help prevent age-related decline.

CHAPTER 11
ADAPT

Early on in my career as a coach I was primarily focused on how stimulus (training) affected performance. But over time I had to accept that every day I was seeing how those pesky *other* parts of life were also playing a huge role in the performance and well-being of the athletes I worked with.

I distinctly remember the first time I stood back in a one-on-one coaching interaction and tried to take in the full picture of an athlete's health. We were working with a runner who had come to us with the goal of improving his performance. He felt the work he was doing during training wasn't translating into the race times he knew he was capable of. In fact, over the previous year or so, his race performances had been going backwards in terms of both his time and how he ranked in the field. He was fatigued, with hormone levels and some other indicators suggesting that he was experiencing low energy availability. And though he competed at a high level, he was not a professional athlete; he had a job and family commitments in addition to his schedule of training at least two or three hours per day and competing every couple of months. Many of these races required long-distance or international travel. After taking in all this information, the first thing I told him was: "If you continue your current approach, all I can guarantee you is a high likelihood of getting a divorce."

Though my comment was slightly tongue-in-cheek, the sentiment was very real, because there's only so much that a body and brain can handle. As we saw in chapters 7 and 9, the function and health of our brain and body are dependent on the challenge or stimulus we expose them to. This drives adaptation mechanisms that result in increased capacity and slower aging. But a critical part of this process is that we provide only as much challenge as the body can handle and make sure we have the necessary time and support for recovery and adaptation to occur.

At a certain point, if the accumulated challenges we're exposed to are too great or we don't provide enough time for adaptation, we end up triggering chronic stress processes that can negatively affect our brain health and cognitive function. Nowadays, we tend to use the word *stress* to mean one specific type of stress—psychological stress that momentarily or chronically overwhelms us. But physiologically, stress can come from any of a number of stimuli that challenge our biology and function, and the body has a standardised set of responses to these stressors, regardless of their source. As a result, the pathways that cause feelings of frustration when we make a mistake during piano practice are essentially identical to those that make us lean on the horn when somebody pulls out in front of us on the motorway without indicating.

This all-purpose response to stimulus means that there can be a fine line between adaptation and chronic stress because there are overlapping biochemical processes that underlie both. The brain is ultimately the place where all the stimuli we're exposed to—physical, psychological, and cognitive—are integrated, and when we're exposed to too many stressors at once, the brain can lose sight of the stimulus we should be directing our attention to.

One classic response to stress is something called *attentional narrowing*, which has a literal meaning but also a broader and more abstract one. When we're acutely stressed, our vision physically narrows as a result of the action of adrenaline, diverting our attention to what is right in front of us and filtering out what's going on in the periphery.[1] This makes sure that we primarily focus on the cause of the stress so that we can deal with it. Throughout the brain, the release of hormones like cortisol also diverts our cognitive processes to focus on storing information related to the stressor while suppressing other information that might cause interference.[2] Just as our body triages nutrients and calories based on the most important functions we need to maintain for short-term survival, sometimes at the expense of long-term function, our brain triages attentional resources in the face of significant stress, focusing on the *now*. This results in us defaulting to ingrained patterns of behaviour instead of looking at the bigger picture of our goals and plans.[3] Simply put, because of all the cognitive effort we're putting into dealing with a stressor or stressors, we shift from thinking to *doing*.[4]

These coordinated responses to stress were really typified by what we saw with the runner mentioned above. On the surface, he was doing everything right from a training standpoint, but because of the accumulated stress of his other commitments—including his work, family, and travel schedule—his body couldn't adapt to the training he was doing. Not only that, but his brain was so busy trying to manage the fact that he was overdoing it that he didn't even have the time or headspace to make sure he was eating enough food to fuel his workouts. His attention also narrowed so that he became singularly focused on training—a habit that he turned to during times of stress—even if that didn't best support the overall picture of his long-term plans (which presumably involved staying married).

I think all of us can identify with parts of this picture. When faced with stress on multiple fronts, we default to patterns of behaviour that we know don't necessarily serve our long-term interests, but they're all our brain can handle at that moment in time. This is completely normal. As the brain is largely responsible for integrating and coordinating our response to multiple stressors, stress from multiple causes can add up and prevent us from being able to focus on long-term goals or cause us to ignore other factors that are important for long-term brain health.

As we're all going to be exposed to stressors and occasionally feel stressed, it can be useful to have strategies to help us benefit from stress and maximise adaptation. These include removing *unnecessary* stressors, increasing our headroom in both the short and long term so that we have more cognitive capacity to function even when stressed, and learning to better understand and manage our stress responses in the moment. This will allow us to direct our resources, focus, and attention toward engaging in activities that best support our health or cognitive function and will make sure we're more likely to benefit from them when we do.

STRESS IS REQUIRED FOR ADAPTATION

The physiological effects of stress were famously first explored by endocrinologist Hans Selye, who documented how rodents responded to cold, excessive exercise, injury, and various drugs.[5] As a result of his experiments, Selye developed the idea of the *general adaptation syndrome* to describe how the body responds to stressors.[6] Though the terminology and how we think about stress as an overarching concept have changed since, the original definition of general adaptation had three phases that can still be helpful in framing the idea of adaptation. The first is the *alarm* or *shock* phase in which some physiological or psychological disturbance is detected—either through increased demand or because of some kind of damage. This original terminology was perhaps a little misleading (and potentially *alarming*), because we now know that increased demand is something we need in order to maintain health and function—physical and cognitive demands drive many beneficial physiological adaptations. But even though a mistake during French class or falling over during your yoga practice can (and should) feel uncomfortable, it doesn't need to be *shocking* to have the desired effect. So perhaps Selye was being a bit hyperbolic with his original terminology.

The next phase of general adaptation syndrome was what Selye called the *resistance* phase, in which the body responds, drawing on greater resources in order to maintain or increase function. But this response is fairly *general*, as the name implies. What I mean is that any important stimulus triggers a version of a stress response. This is a good thing. The general stress response is there to help you take notice of something important and direct the necessary resources to respond to it. It helps drive adaptation, which maximises our functional capacity and the likelihood of survival.

If you took blood samples from somebody during intense exercise and after they cut their hand and needed a few stitches, both scenarios would result in similar increases in adrenaline and cortisol. During exercise, adrenaline and cortisol stimulate the release of glucose and fatty acids into the bloodstream as an energy source for the muscles, and adrenaline increases heart rate and muscle contraction so that we can work harder and move faster. When we're injured or have an infection, adrenaline and cortisol do the same thing but for the immune system—

stimulating immune function to repair the wound or eliminate an invader, increasing the available energy for the immune system to do that job.

When you think about it, the stress response is the body reacting to the internal or external environment when it notices that something needs to change. It then kicks off the processes required to create that change, resulting in adaptation. Maybe the required change is your fitness, or the removal of a bacteria from a wound. The need could also be more immediate, like changing where you're standing when you encounter a bear in the woods (and doing so very quickly).

In all these ways, stress is a good thing. Even experiences that are overwhelmingly stressful at the time can be significant drivers of growth and change, and it's common for people to reflect on very stressful life experiences and think about the beneficial consequences that emerged during or afterwards. Looking back on my fairly horrific snakebite experience in the Costa Rican jungle, there are a huge number of positives that came out of it.

Don't get me wrong—that snakebite *sucked* and was very stressful for me and several other people. But you can acknowledge the positives of a stressful experience without diminishing or downplaying the negative aspects of it. For instance, my jungle adventure gave me an opportunity for reflection. I quit a job that was making me unhappy, which allowed me to change my career in ways that made me feel much more satisfied with my work. My savior on the day, and in the days afterwards—Ben House, whom I had met only a couple of days earlier—has become a close friend and colleague, which might not have happened under less exciting circumstances. And, most importantly, all the photos we took of my leg as it recovered has provided my wife with endless fodder to make fun of how skinny my calves are.

When you hear people talk about stress, and dealing with stress, it's clear that there's a tension between what stress is *for*—integrating information that suggests our biology (or location) needs to change and orchestrating the necessary adaptation—and how we think about stress as a concept. In particular, we tend to characterise stress as uniformly bad. Hans Selye himself said that stress was "a scientific concept which has received the mixed blessing of being too well known and too little understood."

I think Selye needs to take some of the blame here. This is because the third phase of his general adaptation syndrome was the *exhaustion* phase, in which ongoing stress leads to overwhelm of the body's resources and an eventual loss of health and function. This idea that stress will eventually overcome us has led to the framing that stress is inherently bad and that we should avoid it as much as possible. However, in reality, the exhaustion phase Selye promoted doesn't happen exactly as described.

This doesn't mean that stress can't have negative effects, or that there isn't a point where we will feel exhausted due to everything we have to deal with—or that we shouldn't take this seriously. Chronic exposure to stress has been linked to increased risk of multiple diseases, including heart disease, autoimmune disease, and dementia. Though acute stress can help direct our focus and attention to an important task, a large overall stress burden and the related anxiety can also increase our cognitive load, decreasing the mental resources we have for more complex thought processes like problem-solving and planning.[7]

When a stress response is first initiated, though, it's not inherently harmful—it's there to do a specific job or get you out of trouble. This general response to stress does include "stress" hormones like cortisol and adrenaline, but you also release other hormones that act to counterbalance the stress. For example, during exercise you release hormones like IGF-1 that support growth and repair. High-stress periods can also increase production of neurotrophic factors like BDNF, probably to help direct neurological resources as part of adaptation.[8] It's the balance of these different processes over time that determines how well we adapt to the situation we find ourselves in—either improving overall health and cognitive function or contributing to long-term risk of cognitive decline.

WHAT DOESN'T KILL YOU MAKES YOU STRONGER

Physiologist Walter Bradford Cannon coined the term *fight or flight* for the rapid initial response to stress that makes us want to, for example, either escape a bear or (aggressively) face down that offending driver who cuts in front of us. He also developed the theory of *homeostasis*, which he defined as "the maintenance of relatively constant conditions in the body by physiological processes that act to counter any departure from the normal." Homeostasis makes up the vast majority of what we spend our energy on, like making sure our body temperature remains somewhere near 98.6 degrees, regardless of how hot or cold it is outside.

What homeostasis doesn't do, though, is help us adapt to challenge. While I would like my body to stay the same temperature regardless of whether I'm visiting family in Iceland or wandering through the jungle in Costa Rica, I don't want my body or brain to stay the same when I do Pilates or learn some new Spanish verbs. Otherwise, what would be the point?

The process of adapting to challenge is better described by the more recent concept of *allostasis*, which has a definition that I love: "achieving stability through change."[9] This idea encompasses the fact that the initial response to stress is supposed to protect the body and drive some form of adaptation. In the face of an ever-changing world and an unknown number of stressors, the combination of adaptation and stability is what we're all ultimately looking for—improving and then maintaining stable health and cognitive function, regardless of what life might throw at us. And our ability to do this comes from adapting to challenges, be they psychological, physical, or cognitive. The opposite is also true; the more we have adapted to challenges, the more headroom we have to withstand future challenges and maintain stability when it's most needed.

If you'll allow me one more physiology word, we should also mention *hormesis*. Hormesis is essentially the scientific term for the cliché, "What doesn't kill you makes you stronger." Though *hormesis* as a word wasn't coined until the 1940s, the idea of hormesis has been around for more than two thousand years—since King Mithridates VI supposedly ingested small amounts of poison in an attempt to make himself immune to assassination attempts.[10] The idea was that exposure to smaller doses of poison would increase his ability to survive if somebody slipped a larger dose into his tea.

While the story of Mithridates might be based more in mythology than fact, using small doses of a stressor to improve function is exactly the right formula for anything we might want to get better at. Think back to part 1 when we discussed getting stronger by lifting weights as a way to build physical headroom. Just as Mithridates couldn't tolerate a large dose of poison immediately, without any kind of training you might get pinned under a sofa in the stairwell while trying to help your friend

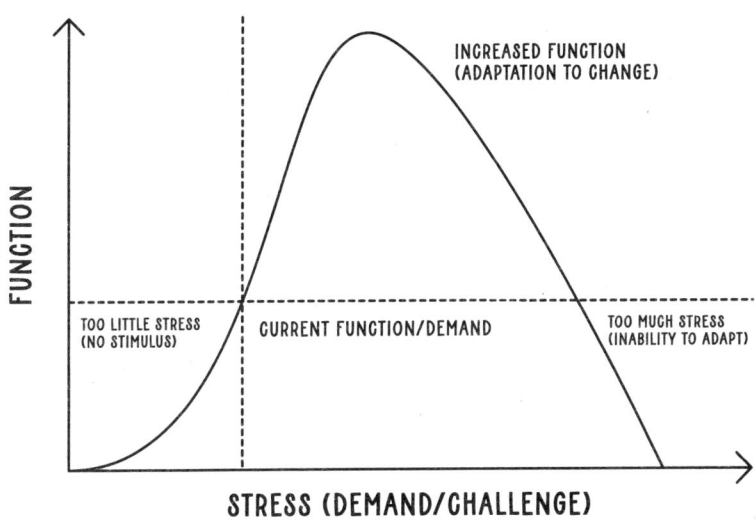

FIGURE 1. Hormesis and adaptation. The dotted lines show our starting level of demand and function. In order to get stronger, we need to provide a stimulus or stress (increase demand), but we also need to make sure that we don't push beyond our ability to adapt, because that can decrease function. Similarly, if we don't place enough demands on ourselves, function decreases.

move their furniture. But with a little hormesis—a few drops of poison or a few sessions in the gym—function improves over time.

In most cases, stress and function have a bell-shaped relationship (figure 1). At the top end, you can be exposed to more stress than you can handle, resulting in fatal poisoning or a sofa-induced chiropractic adjustment. But if you don't receive *any* exposure, function in that area will decrease, as the process of allostasis also ensures that we're continually matching capacity to need. Allostasis explains why retirement results in a decrease in cognitive function and why continued stimulation is so critical. After all, why would our body spend energy on a big and complex brain if we're not using it to its full capacity?

It's clear that at least *some* stress is needed to both maintain function and provide a stimulus for positive adaptation. In fact, Hans Selye himself even described the idea of *hypostress*—a condition where stress on a given system is too low to enable optimal health and functioning. But a critical part of adaptation means that each successive challenge of the same type—doing a bicep curl with ten pounds, for instance—will generate less of a stress response over time as your body gets stronger. That means that you also need to keep upping the stimulus as you get stronger and more skilled.

But just like with our runner at the start of the chapter, when you're applying a stimulus, you also have to consider the bigger picture. At any given time, we're dealing with—and adapting to—multiple stressors and stimuli, as well as balancing multiple lifestyle factors like nutrition and relationships, all of which can influence our body's and brain's ability to adapt. If we're dealing with too many stressors or don't give ourselves enough time to adapt and recover, we'll struggle to get stronger no matter how many reps we do in the gym. Neuroendocrinologist Bruce McEwan called the total sum of everything we're exposed to and our ability to adapt to and cope with it our *allostatic load*. Over time, if it is too high, our allostatic load can cause wear and tear on our brain; several studies have shown that a high allostatic load—a level of stress that we don't have the resources or time to adapt to—increases the risk of cognitive decline and dementia.[11]

Our capacity to handle and respond to stress or a higher allostatic load is a core component of headroom. This is easier to see and feel when it comes to strength—some time spent in the gym increases our capacity and ability to move furniture—but the same is true for the brain. Lifestyle factors that lead to increases in headroom—higher educational and occupational attainment, cognitively stimulating work, and physical and social activity—are associated with higher cognitive performance, faster information processing in the brain, and greater efficiency of the networks involved in cognitively demanding tasks.[12] As we've seen several times, these same lifestyle factors are also associated with lower long-term risk of cognitive decline and dementia.[13]

When we expose ourselves to various stimuli and adapt to them accordingly, our brains increase both their capacity and their efficiency. As a result, we're more likely to maintain cognitive function in the face of acute stress, just like carrying shopping is easier after a few months in the gym. However, none of us has unlimited physiological or cognitive resources. That's why we need to find a balance between stimulus and adaptation in a way that helps us push ourselves and continue to build capacity and headroom over time.

First, we'll cover ways to make sure we can manage our allostatic load, so that we aren't inadvertently overburdening our capacity to adapt to stimuli, like the runner burning his training candle at both ends. Then, in the next chapter, we'll discuss how to promote recovery from stressors in a way that builds headroom and future-proofs the brain.

GETTING IN THE ZONE

Hopefully, by now, you appreciate that the stress response can be a good thing. That feeling of agitation or stress we feel when we make a mistake while learning a complex skill, for example, is our brain initiating the processes of neuroplasticity. This initial stress response can also help our focus and concentration. However, sometimes an acute stress response can lead to a less-than-desirable outcome. The amount of stress or anxiety that somebody experiences in a given situation—like an exam or an athletic competition—might be the difference between them experiencing a boost in performance or choking under pressure.[14] This is why the word *freeze* was eventually added to the standard *fight or flight* line as another common response to acute stress.

The stress response we have can also be disproportionate to the stressor. If you encounter a bear in the woods, a large increase in adrenaline and an urge to flee is very appropriate. But some of us will experience a very similar response if we find ourselves late to an important meeting—a surge of adrenaline and a corresponding urge to fight all the other drivers in rush hour traffic, which is perhaps less appropriate. Therefore, being able to regulate our responses in the moment can help us perform better and think more clearly while reducing our overall allostatic load.

In the world of sports, ensuring a good performance requires having the right level of arousal. In this setting, "arousal" is just a more performance-focused way of talking about the general stress response outlined above. And, as you no doubt know, arousal is important for *many* things. So, if we want to better manage how we work and perform on a day-to-day basis, we could all do with thinking about our arousal a little more. Of course, hopefully it goes without saying that if you want to perform you need to be aroused. But depending on the activity (or how quickly or slowly that activity is progressing), the ideal level of arousal will differ.

Think about watching athletes in an Olympic final. If you're anything like me, you'll be picturing a track event like the 100-metre or 400-metre sprint. The athletes at the starting blocks of those events need to be *very* aroused. And by that I mean they need to have all their stress systems firing and heart and muscles ready to immediately move at maximum speed. Compare this to the Olympic archery final that might be happening one arena over. Those athletes also need to be focused, but they have to stay a lot more relaxed than the sprinters next door.

In fact, before the mid-eighties when they were banned, athletes in shooting sports like archery used to take beta-blockers—drugs that block the effect of adrenaline that causes your heart to beat faster and your hands to tremble—because they counteracted stress and improved accuracy. But giving beta-blockers to a sprinter would be a disaster because they wouldn't be able to get their heart rate up to supply blood to their muscles. So, in different sports, even the very best in the world need very different levels of stress (arousal) to perform at their best.

Just as in sports performance, for most activities that involve complex skills, learning, and focus, the relationship between arousal and performance looks like a bell curve (figure 2). Arousal increases performance—but only up to a point. Once you cross a certain threshold, more arousal is not so helpful and is likely to decrease performance as you become increasingly anxious. The trick is learning the difference so you can find the right level of arousal for your particular needs. In fact, this is one reason that exposing yourself to stressors can increase your headroom: you become better at managing your physiological responses and are less likely to become overanxious in stressful situations.

The curve describing the relationship between arousal and performance is named after Robert Yerkes and John Dodson, who actually had nothing to do with athletes but instead performed their experiments on mice.[15] These mice were trained on tasks of different degrees of difficulty, and during the process of learning, they were stimulated with small electric shocks through the floor of a maze. Nothing painful—just that weird squirmy feeling you might have experienced if you've ever touched an electric fence.

What Yerkes and Dodson found was that for simple tasks, the more stimulated the mice were, the faster they learned. But for a more complex task, medium-sized stimulation was best. Too little and there wasn't

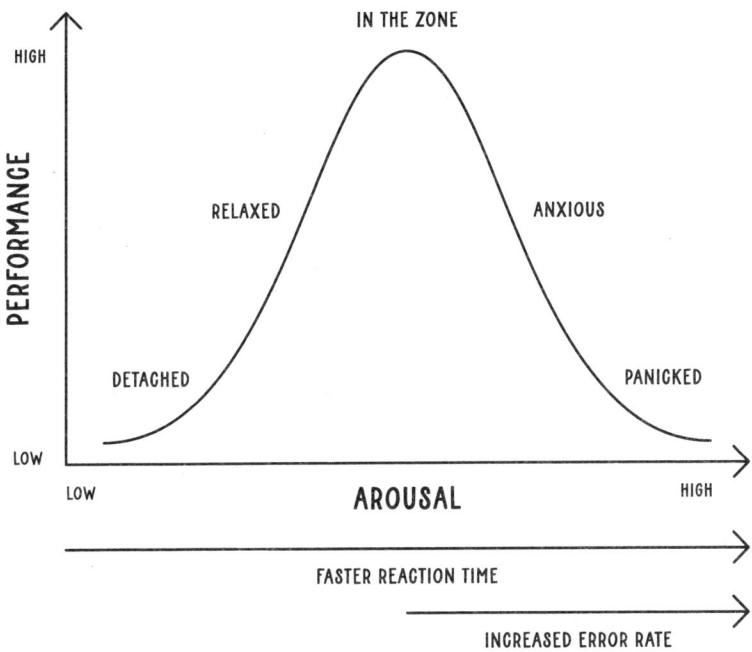

FIGURE 2. The arousal curve. For any type of performance—whether in the boardroom or the bedroom—there is an optimal amount of arousal. Too little and we're not engaged with the process and haven't committed the necessary cognitive and bodily resources to make sure we can perform well. As arousal starts to increase, performance as well as basic functions such as reaction time tend to speed up. But too much arousal and we can become sweaty and panicked, making more mistakes and decreasing our performance.

an increase in the arousal that helps to drive learning. Too much and the mice became anxious and didn't remember as well. Just in case it's not clear, this is not a recommended technique to improve learning. Though it might be tempting, employing electric shocks to motivate learning in colleagues, undergraduates, or spouses is generally frowned upon. Nonetheless, these results and ideas carry over to humans surprisingly well.

A regular part of my work in Formula 1 is helping drivers and their coaches put together strategies to help manage arousal before a race. Just as experiences of stress and stressors are very different from person to person, arousal is also very personal. All drivers go through exercises and drills to warm up before the race, most of which help to increase arousal and get them toward the top of the Yerkes-Dodson curve. This might include reflex drills or even juggling with balls. Other drivers may practise start sequences to get their reaction times firing, or brief bursts of body-weight exercises that reliably increase heart rate. But depending on the situation, it's also common for drivers to get nervous. And because driving a Formula 1 car requires performing a number of very complex skills at high speed, getting the right amount of arousal in the car tends to require a fine balance. Not enough, and reaction time might be a little slower than normal. But too much and a driver's errors in the car can increase, sometimes with loud and expensive consequences. For this reason, some drivers might spend time before a race doing some breathing exercises to help regulate their heart rate or listening to music that calms them down rather than pumping them up. It's all about getting to the right point on the curve for them.

It's worth remembering that it's completely normal to experience some level of anxiety any time we have to perform, even if it's something we've done hundreds or thousands of times before. Actors, public speakers, and athletes all get the jitters. We should welcome this feeling any time we experience it, because it's a good thing. Being nervous shows that we care, and this stress response is all part of increasing arousal so we can focus and complete the necessary task at hand. But, as you can see from the arousal curve, too much stress or anxiety will end up making us too anxious or panicked to perform at our best.

The experience of being overly aroused in the moment might manifest itself in many different ways. Broadly speaking, overactivation of our stress response can decrease activity in parts of the prefrontal cortex of the brain that are involved in decision-making and deliberation.[16] As a result, people under stress often do what makes them feel better in the short term—or they gravitate toward an activity that requires minimal decision-making. For instance, we might reflexively say something (or shout something) we don't really mean because we don't take a moment to reconsider it. Or we might interpret somebody else's actions as more negative or more of a threat than we would have if we were feeling calmer. When we give an important presentation, too much arousal may result in forgetting what we're supposed to say, or feeling rushed so we make mistakes. Elevated stress or anxiety may even prevent us from engaging with the task entirely, resulting in procrastination.

STRESS, AROUSAL, AND PROCRASTINATION

Sometimes we're supposed to be doing something and find ourselves doing literally *anything* else. All of a sudden, cleaning the house, raiding the snack cupboard, opening up a social media app, or even going to the gym becomes far more appealing than it might be otherwise. While we all frequently experience procrastination,[17] there seem to be a number of reasons that people procrastinate, many of which can relate to our overall headroom and level of arousal. We might procrastinate, for instance, because we're actively avoiding the work, because our mind is wandering, or because we're just naturally more distractible. These different states can give us some insight into how to get back on task when we need to.

Too Much Arousal or Stress

Procrastination can be a direct response to stress. When we're stressed, we're less likely to engage in cognitively demanding tasks.[18] Stress can also make us feel less positive about a given situation, resulting in avoidant procrastination because we feel like the outcome won't change regardless of the work we put in.[19] Avoidant procrastination can also be a way to manage feelings of stress—we avoid working on something difficult because it helps us manage our emotions in the short term, even though it might cause even *more* stress later on.[20] Stress is also a cause of cognitive failure, which includes becoming more distractible or failing to maintain attention to a task.[21] In situations like this, finding ways to reframe the stress or decrease the current level of stress can help provide a better mental state so we can get back to work.

Too Little Arousal or Stress

There is a group of people who seem to procrastinate because they aren't aroused *enough*. Either the task is too boring or they know they have enough time to get it done so they put it off. Some people may even feel a thrill from doing clutch work at the last minute.[22] This kind of procrastination may (consciously or unconsciously) be a way to help increase arousal and motivation to complete the task. For instance, we know that the tension of having unfinished tasks can increase feelings of stress (also known as the *Zeigarnik effect,* after psychologist Bluma Zeigarnik), and that interrupting a task midway through can increase feelings of time pressure.[23] People who experience this type of procrastination may benefit from a brief activity that increases their arousal, like exercise. (Or maybe a mild electric shock?)

Too Little Sleep

Inadequate sleep is one of the most common reasons that we experience low arousal and performance. Sleep deprivation can make it harder for us to pay attention and stay on task.[24] A wandering mind is also more common when we need sleep, and at least some of that is because our brain takes microbreaks that look a lot like sleep, resulting in lapses in attention.[25] While the obvious answer would be to take a nap if possible, some of this can also be overcome in the short term by increasing arousal through exercise, breathwork, bright lighting, or exposure to cold.

Too Little Headroom

As we get older, there appears to be a shift in the way arousal changes our level of focus. In younger people, arousal activates a network in the brain centred on the locus coeruleus—one of the main areas where noradrenaline, the brain's version of adrenaline, is released—that helps to direct attention and filter out distractions.[26] However, in older adults, a shift in the network makes it harder for distractions to be filtered out during arousal. As we know that brain ageing and the function of brain networks are determined by how we use and support our brains, it seems reasonable to hypothesise that building headroom provides a long-term strategy to decrease distractibility and procrastination as we get older by maintaining the brain networks responsible for attention.

Too Little Planning

Not all procrastination is a bad thing. In fact, it might be telling you something or helping you achieve your end goal. Computer scientist and productivity expert Cal Newport has suggested that procrastination may be an evolutionarily hardwired signal from the brain telling us it's not convinced by our plan, and that maybe an alternative approach (or spending your time on something else entirely) would be better.[27] Procrastination can also be an opportunity to boost creativity: letting your mind wander or disengaging from a task momentarily may be a way for your brain to make new connections. Procrastination in this context might help your brain solve the problem at hand, making it easier to do the work when you return to it.[28] In these scenarios, allowing a little procrastination could actually be the best approach.

Over long periods of time, regulating stress in the moment can help to decrease our allostatic load—the total burden of stress that generates wear and tear on the brain and body. Studies continue to show that a high allostatic load is associated with lower psychological resilience, higher inflammation and stress markers in the blood, and worse metabolic and cardiovascular health.[29] And a persistently high allostatic load is associated with brain volume loss, increased accumulation of pathology in the brain, and a higher dementia risk.[30]

When we experience stress responses, we want to make sure that we can use them to our advantage—allowing them to improve our performance and drive adaptation. But in order to manage our performance and cognitive function in the moment—as well as to decrease our overall stress burden and allostatic load over the long term—it can be helpful to have a set of tools to bring us back toward the top of the arousal curve when our stress or anxiety had pushed us too far past that point.

MANAGING AROUSAL

When I think about arousal, I think about Pauly DiTuro. Don't worry, my wife already knows. This is not only because Pauly is an expert in arousal management, but also because he exudes an incredible level of calm—beyond what I've seen in any other human. He and I first met at a meeting of experts to discuss the problem of overtraining in special forces soldiers. In a room full of bluster, Pauly's clear and levelheaded thinking made him probably the only person that *everybody* listened to.

I often call Pauly the most interesting person I've ever met. Having been a graduate student in quantum physics helping to search for the Higgs boson at the Fermi National Accelerator Laboratory while also competing at two U.S. Olympic trials in boxing and playing rugby professionally, Pauly then spent more than a decade as a special operations medic. He is now the guy that elite sporting, academic, and government organizations call when they have problems that need solving. He's played important roles in the creation of entirely new molecules in the lab, developing therapies for traumatic brain injury, and figuring out how to help athletes gain that 0.01 percent of extra performance they need to break world records. You probably don't know it, but Pauly is behind many of the health strategies you hear about on the top health podcasts, as well as some of the most incredible human feats of performance you've seen on TV or social media. Particularly relevant to our purposes here, Pauly has excelled in some of the most stressful environments that humans have ever had to perform in and, as a result, has become a sought-after expert for helping others do the same.

One time, while working in an understaffed ER, Pauly had to run triage when a truck full of people from Guatemala collided with the car of a family from Russia. Over the course of a few minutes, he somehow placed multiple IV lines, reinflated collapsed lungs, and performed a cricothyrotomy (that procedure medical dramas love where you have to cut open the patient's trachea to restore their airway), all while calmly and seamlessly switching between three languages so that he could direct staff and communicate with the patients being treated.

And then there was the time Pauly was big-wave surfing in Fiji and was thrown against a reef and dragged underwater by a rip current. This first part is maybe not a huge surprise because he's a terrible surfer. But while concussed and having already gone for longer without a breath than most others would be able to survive, Pauly had the presence of mind to swim *down*—deeper into the water and away from the shore—to get away from the current.

As the go-to guy for surefire ways to regulate responses to stressful situations, Pauly has graciously shared his four-point tool kit for regulating stress responses in the moment (no cricothyrotomy required). You can use one of them or all of them as needed—it's just about figuring out what works well for you. Because finding ways to downregulate stress, and adapt to any situation at hand, is a key tool in developing headroom and playing the brain game.

BREATHE. When the stress response is activated to the point where we're overly anxious, our physiology can start to override our brain function. And once we're in this state, it becomes challenging to wish or think ourselves into being calmer. The rational parts of our brain are too busy getting dunked in adrenaline to listen. Instead, we can come from the other direction and use our physiology to bring back a sense of calm and clarity. One of the easiest ways to do this is by changing the way we breathe—specifically, using types of breathing that involve breathing out for longer than we breathe in. When we exhale, the heart responds to the movement of our diaphragm and lungs by slowing down how fast it's beating. This is done by activating the vagus nerve, which controls many of the relaxation-related activities in the body. By spending more time exhaling than inhaling, we can start to override some of the stress we're experiencing. And by slowing and controlling our breath, we can begin to experience a greater degree of calm and access better cognitive function.[31]

> ## DOWNREGULATING WITH BREATH
>
> There are an increasing number of studies showing that we can use our breath to change our physiology and arousal, including a meta-analysis that found that breathwork was a potential strategy to improve stress and mental health.[32] When it comes to decreasing arousal and emotional reactivity, slow-paced breathing techniques that focus on a prolonged exhale help to activate the vagus nerve and decrease stress responses.[33]
>
> ### Pursed Lips
> The easiest way to slow your exhale is to breathe out through pursed lips. The extra resistance means that it takes longer to get the breath out. There are no hard rules in terms of the number of seconds breathing in and out—it should feel comfortable and relaxed.
>
> ### Nasal Breathing
> Like pursing your lips, forcing yourself to think about breathing in and out only through your nose will automatically slow things down and give you a moment to relax. Again, think about breathing comfortably with the exhale lasting longer than the inhale.
>
> ### 3:7 and 4-7-8 Breathing
> For those who like numbers, breathing with a three-second inhale and seven-second exhale has been shown to increase heart rate variability—a measure of vagus nerve activity—and improve sleep. In a group of people with insomnia, twenty minutes of 3:7 breathing before bed cut the time it took them to fall asleep by almost two-thirds.[34] A similar approach is 4-7-8 breathing, where you breathe in for four seconds, hold for seven, and breathe out for eight.
>
> ### Physiological Sigh
> This involves taking a deep breath in through your nose (although through your mouth is fine too), holding it for a brief moment before taking one final small breath through the nose to really fill the lungs, and then doing a long, slow exhale through the mouth. Doing this type of breathing for just five minutes a day has been shown to improve some aspects of mood,[35] but even just a few breaths like this at a moment of stress can help calm

you down and bring you back to a level of arousal that can help rather than hinder your brain function.

UPREGULATING WITH BREATH

Sometimes you feel sluggish and want to get yourself amped up—moving up toward the top of the arousal curve from the relaxed side. As you might imagine, this involves the opposite of downregulation breathwork—fast breaths with a short exhale.[36]

High-Ventilation Breathwork
Thirty to sixty seconds of a full breath in through the mouth or nose (about one second) and fast and forceful breath out through the mouth (one second or less) increases heart rate, noradrenaline release, and arousal.

4-6-8 Ramp
The 4-6-8 ramp is an easy-to-remember protocol to quickly increase arousal if you need it. Take four paced breaths in and out through the nose, about four seconds each on the inhale and exhale (sixteen seconds total). Then take six high-ventilation breaths—in through the nose and out through the mouth. Finish with eight high-ventilation breaths, this time in and out through the mouth, moving the air as quickly and forcefully as you can.

PRIORITISE. If we suddenly face a stressful situation or feel the accumulation of a period of stress overwhelming us, decision-making can become harder.[37] This was common during the Covid-19 pandemic, when the total burden of stress left many people struggling to make basic day-to-day decisions.[38] One of the main reasons for this—and a common contributor to stressful situations—is uncertainty.[39] Not knowing what's going to happen, or imagining a range of terrible outcomes, is often stressful enough to prevent us from taking action. One way to combat stress-induced indecision is to prioritise. Think about the *one* thing you need to do next. When I speak publicly on science or health, I usually insert a joke somewhere around the second or third slide. When I get nervous before the start of my talk, I just focus on getting to and delivering the joke. Even if it doesn't land as well as I hoped, I know that once I get to that point, I'll be fine afterwards. Similarly, when I arrive at my desk in the morning and my to-do list feels overwhelming, I just pick one thing to do that day. Even if it's a small task, I know that once I've done *something* I can pick one more thing to do. I can also immediately feel better about having done the most important thing I had to do that day. This is the secret power of prioritization: it gives you something to focus on, and also a quick win that the next thing can flow from.

CHANGE WHAT YOU SEE. Just like our breath, our eyes (and, in fact, all our senses) are an important window into the brain and our physiology when we're stressed. As vision is one of the primary ways that stressors are detected, Pauly recommends simply closing your eyes when you feel stressed or overwhelmed. This can also give you a moment to breathe or prioritise. Closing our eyes decreases the amount of information we have to process, freeing up cognitive resources. Some studies also suggest that the activation of stress response networks in the brain decreases when we close our eyes.[40] This is why closing our eyes may boost creative thinking and improve memory, including when under stress.[41] Alternatively, step back and take in the bigger picture. Because focus requires at least a small amount of arousal or stress, we can decrease that by purposefully broadening our visual fields. The opportunity to use our full field of vision and spend less time focusing on one specific target (like a phone or computer screen) is one of the reasons being outside in nature can decrease stress and rumination.[42] Amazingly, the benefits of viewing green, natural environments when stressed even seems to work when those environments are in virtual reality.[43] However, spending time in *real* nature seems to have some unique benefits, triggering stress reduction and cognitive restoration through movement as well as multiple senses, including hearing the sounds of wildlife and smelling volatile organic compounds, like terpenes—hydrocarbons released by trees and plants.[44] But even if you can't take a break for a walk in the park, simply looking up or away from the current source of your stress and thinking about broadening your vision can help to decrease arousal in the moment.

LEVERAGING YOUR SENSES

Experimental psychologist Ethan Kross is director of the Emotion and Self-Control Lab at the University of Michigan. His research shows that sensation and emotion are inextricably linked, and that strategically activating each of the five major senses can help us to regulate our emotions.[45] His lab has also found that, because each of us is different and responds differently to stress, we need a toolbox of emotional-regulation strategies so we can pick what works for us.[46]

Sound

Athletes use music to increase focus and arousal before an event, and nostalgic music can activate reward and memory pathways in the brain.[47] Calming music can also be used to decrease stress responses, so pick some songs to have on standby that make you feel less stressed. If you don't know where to start, you can have my personal go-to destressing song—"I Giorni" by Ludovico Einaudi.

Smell

Several smells have been found to reduce feelings of stress, including the smells of nature (like pine and cedar, or petrichor—that smell right when it rains) and essential oils like orange, lavender, and rose.[48] Smelling clothes worn by a romantic partner can also reduce responses to stress.[49]

Touch

An obvious example is touch from a loved one, which can improve multiple aspects of well-being.[50] This isn't always possible in the moment, but touching pets or soft objects, like a teddy bear, also works, as does self-touch. No, not (necessarily) like that. Gently touching your own face on the chin or temples activates brain networks related to emotion and attention and can be soothing, potentially as a way of self-grounding.[51] Interestingly, due to the asymmetrical nature of emotion control in the brain, clenching the right hand (in most people) can improve mood—whereas clenching the left hand can exacerbate negative emotions.[52]

Taste

What we eat also targets several emotional pathways, so any food you enjoy might help you regulate your emotions in the moment. However, the general approach in chapter 8 ("Nourish") still applies, so when you're stressed, perhaps try a small amount of dark chocolate rather than several brownies.[53]

The Quiet Eye

Closing your eyes isn't always an option. I'd certainly lose some credibility if I told a professional racing driver to close their eyes if they got anxious during a race—their vision is so critical that they even control their blinks in a very specific pattern to make sure they don't miss vital inputs. If we're in a stressful situation where our vision is an important input, as in many sports, anxiety can make our eye movements and attention more erratic.[54] Consciously using very controlled eye movements and specifically focusing on your target or goal can override this and improve accuracy or performance. One version of this is called the *quiet eye*, where somebody purposefully focuses on their target right before they initiate an action. Across fields like shooting sports, basketball, and surgery, using the quiet eye before executing a movement improves performance, especially when under stress.[55]

CHANGE THE NARRATIVE. One of the biggest impacts we can have on our response to stress is to mentally reframe the stress itself. Though it's not always the case, often we're stressed because we are juggling a number of things that are simultaneously difficult and exciting. As a result, Pauly reminds us, stress often comes from an opportunity to do something cool or impactful. This might be a musical performance for friends and loved ones, or an important presentation. The stakes might also be very high—for instance, in scenarios where members of the military or first responders have to save or protect their lives and the lives of others. Changing the narrative around stress is important because it reminds us that the stress response is important—it helps you focus and perform, and becomes activated when something important is happening. That doesn't minimise the stakes or the feelings of anxiety we might have, but it allows us to remember the important reasons we're in that situation in the first place. Reframing a stressful event can directly change how our body responds to it. In one study, participants watched short videos on the effects of stress before undergoing a stressful test. One group was told about the "bad" effects of stress on the body, and the other group was told about how stress can enhance performance, health, and growth. After exposure to stress, both groups saw an increase in the stress hormone cortisol. However, the group that was told about the beneficial and enhancing effects of stress also had increased levels of a growth-related hormone (dehydroepiandrosterone, or DHEA) that can offset some of the downsides of cortisol and help to promote resilience.[56] Other studies show that people who release more DHEA when stressed perform better and make better decisions.[57] Therefore, just acknowledging that a sudden increase in stress can be beneficial may help us make better decisions and perform when we need to.

Sometimes it's helpful to regulate how we respond to stress in the moment, but the goal isn't to eliminate or avoid stress, because it is critical to improving our performance. By using some of Pauly's guidance we can manage a feeling of overwhelm or overstimulation to get ourselves back in the zone of being aroused—in all the right ways. And that, ultimately, is going to provide the kind of cognitive buffer that minimises the long-term impact of stress on brain health and allows us to maximise our headroom.

BUILDING STRESS TOLERANCE

Though the general impression that stress is bad has continued to dominate how most of us think about it, new research has provided a range of ways to understand stress, reframe it, and change how we respond to it. One important aspect of this is knowing that stress is incredibly personal, and each of us will have different responses to different situations (or even the same situation) based on our own past experiences and the current context.[58] This is one reason that we might want to regulate our arousal and stress level in the moment. But long-term stress and the compounding effects of multiple stressors can also take their toll. For example, more stress in one area might make you less able to tolerate stress in another.

Shortly after his initial work on general adaptation, Hans Selye described the idea of *adaptation energy,* showing that adding a second stressor (food restriction) on top of stress caused by large amounts of exercise decreased tolerance to the first stressor and accelerated the onset of exhaustion. This is the idea that eventually led to the definition of allostatic load. Not only can multiple stressors influence our total stress burden and allostatic load, but, as we saw in chapter 10, prolonged stress responses from a single source like social isolation can start to impair our long-term brain health. Therefore, it is helpful to have another set of tools for building our ability to resist stress. In the short term, this helps us to maintain headroom and cognitive capacity in the face of stressors. In the long term, this can help to avoid having lots of small stressors contributing to a high allostatic load that increases the risk of neurodegeneration and dementia.

Though stress can have many different effects, in general, stress causes an increase in the activation of many parts of the brain.[59] This is what helps to drive adaptation. However, that can have downsides if activated for long periods—stress needs to switch off for beneficial adaptation to occur. Responding to stress also takes a lot of energy. So, if it doesn't get switched off, stress can act as a drain.

This type of ongoing stress or high allostatic load is kind of like running on a treadmill where you can't adjust the speed. You've jumped on for a nice leisurely jog, but then you notice the buttons stop working and you're forced to keep running or risk being thrown backwards into a gym full of people in a comical (for them at least) manner. Initially it's fine, because you're comfortable with the pace and you know you can take it. But over time, while waiting for a fortuitous power cut or for a helpful gym manager to walk by and rescue you, you start to get tired. Then, all of a sudden, just like when life throws another curveball that you have to deal with—additional tasks, deadlines, and demands on your time—the malfunction spreads and the incline suddenly starts to increase. Though we can deal with a lot, if we're always operating right near the limit of our capacity, a speed that felt tough but doable suddenly becomes completely untenable.

Over time, this level of stress does have the potential to harm the brain. Prolonged elevation of cortisol seems to negatively impact the hippocampus in particular, impairing functions like working memory—the ability to quickly store and manipulate information. In the short term this might impact academic or work performance, but over time, a high allostatic load is associated with a faster decrease in the size of the hippocampus in adults as they age.[60] As the hippocampus is one of the regions of the brain most susceptible to both ageing and dementias like Alzheimer's disease, finding ways to minimise the impact of stressors can help you maintain extra headroom.

Psychological stress from work or other difficult or traumatic events (the death of a spouse or child, divorce, financial problems, health problems) is associated with an increased risk of dementia as well as depression.[61] What's particularly interesting, though, is that the *experience* of feeling chronically stressed is also associated with an increased risk of later dementia, regardless of the exact cause of that stress. This suggests that the long-term impact of a stressor is largely driven by how we respond to it, which allows us to have some control over the situation by managing both our stressors and our response to those stressors.

The importance of control is shown in multiple studies looking at work stress and its relationship with dementia and depression. In those who have very demanding jobs, the stimulus that the job involves can be protective for the brain and decrease the risk of dementia, as we saw in chapter 9. The catch is that this is only true if the individual has control over those demands.[62] We need to be challenged, but we also have to be able to control the intensity of the stimulus and be able to back off when needed.

Instead of the demon uncontrollable treadmill, you can think of successful management of daily stressors as something like running outside on hilly terrain. It's not easy (and we don't necessarily want it to be—we're going running, after all), but we can put in extra effort when the hills get steep and also control our speed if we need a break to recover. Luckily, depending on our own preferences and the challenges we face, there are a whole host of tools we can use to expand our ability to handle stress and minimise its impact. These strategies can help us keep stress at a manageable level—and, as an added bonus, protect our brains.

MOVE. The ability to maintain function under duress is often called resilience. Sometimes resilience is sold as being able to just suck it up and continue no matter what, but simply plowing ahead under stressful conditions does not necessarily change the situation or how it might affect you. True resilience is more about being able to make sure a stressful situation drains you less than it otherwise might. One of the best ways to do this is with exercise—partly because exercise activates stress responses. By training these stress responses, we also train our ability to tolerate other sources of stress—sometimes referred to as cross-stressor adaptation. For example, one study enrolled sedentary university students in an aerobic exercise training programme that started with walking and gradually increased in intensity, eventually adding some sprints (a nice example of progressing through the "propel" and "sprint" levels in the movement funnel). A few months later, during an exam period, students who were doing the exercise programme had lower stress responses compared to a group that hadn't been exercising.[63] Regular exercise also seems to rewire the brain, making the amygdala—a part of the brain that controls our responses to fear and stress, including the fight, flight, and freeze responses—more likely to suppress fear and increase happiness when we're doing some kind of physical activity.[64] This might be one way that exercise significantly improves mood over time—those who exercise regularly (more than once per week) have been found to experience smaller negative changes in mood when stressed.[65] Even one exercise session might be enough, because stress responses are decreased in the hour or two after exercise.[66] Therefore, not only does movement improve overall brain health and cognitive function and reduce dementia risk, but it can help you be resilient to other stressors. You can even use movement to provide an extra buffer before an event that you might find stressful. Over time, regular movement directly increases headroom and decreases the negative effect of stressors that interfere with optimal cognitive function, providing a double whammy for future-proofing your brain long term.

REFRAME. Besides being important for regulating our response to stress in the moment, how we think about the demands placed on us can also make a difference more broadly. Some of the best research on how to handle stress focuses on an idea called *stress optimization*. By acknowledging both the potential benefits of stress as well as the downside of long-term unchecked stress, people can actively engage with stress on their own terms and lean into it when needed.[67] This process includes thinking about ways that stress is enhancing—acknowledging the good and bad of stress but welcoming and utilising it when it arrives—as well as appreciating stress as a functional response that helps us cope and adapt. University students who were taught to think about stress in this way had less anxiety and performed better on exams,[68] while a similar intervention in people working for a large financial institution resulted in greater performance at work as well as improved employee health.[69] This "stress is enhancing" mindset even predicts the likelihood that Navy SEAL recruits will complete their training,[70] and it fits well with the growth mindset—the idea that our abilities aren't fixed and can be improved with effort (literally, the topic of the entire previous chapter). In a very large study in the United States, training students in both the stress-is-enhancing and growth mindsets resulted in improved cognitive and cortisol responses to stress, improved psychological well-being, and decreased anxiety.[71] With all that said, it can still be hard to convince people that stress is a good thing when it is much more common to hear the opposite. This is important because we know that our mindset—whether or not it is grounded in truth—can become self-fulfilling. For instance, one study found that for people who felt they were under a lot of stress, their stress was only associated with worse physical and mental health if they *also* believed that stress negatively impacts health.[72]

We know stress is unavoidable, so it's counterproductive to try to avoid it. The process of actively avoiding stress can even be detrimental, for two reasons: firstly, because we'll miss out on a number of opportunities for challenge and growth, and secondly, because avoiding stress can potentially *increase* stress in the long term as all the stressful things we're avoiding build up. Instead, by rethinking stress, we can leverage its benefits and be happier and perform better, without ignoring the importance of stress on our long-term health.

REFRAMING STRESS

Psychologist Alia Crum is a world expert in the way stress-is-enhancing mindsets can improve performance and well-being in the face of stressors. Through her work, she has developed a three-step thought process for reframing stress.[73] Her studies also provide some other tools and thought processes we can use, according to personal preference.

Three-Step Approach
In times of stress or in preparation for a stressful event, Crum suggests we do three things. The first is to welcome the stress because inherent in that stress is something you care about. Once you've done that, you can ask yourself, "What is it that I care about here?" Finally, think about how you can actively use the stress to achieve the thing you care about.

Thinking About the Benefits of Stress

In their research, Crum's team often uses videos that remind people of the benefits of stress or of people who have performed while under significant stress. We can use these examples ourselves—like thinking about how the stress of exercise makes us fitter and stronger. Participants are also reminded that stress can lead to skilled performance at risky moments—athletes succeeding in clutch moments or doctors performing life-saving surgery—and the same can be true for us. Similarly, there are the historical leaders who have made remarkable decisions and actions in the face of stress such as Lincoln, Churchill, and Sully Sullenberger, the pilot who safely landed a disabled passenger jet on the Hudson River.[74] To try this idea out, think about some of the benefits of stress—or performances in clutch moments—in a way that speaks to your own experience.

Assess Your Stress Mindset

The Stress Mindset Measure is used to determine how people approach stress and can be a good way to take an inventory of our thoughts about stress and apply reframing measures if we need to. To assess your mindset, simply think about how much you agree with the statements. The statements in bold can even make good mantras to use to remind ourselves of the potential benefits of stress when we feel overwhelmed:

1. The effects of stress are negative and should be avoided.
2. **Experiencing stress facilitates my learning and growth.**
3. Experiencing stress depletes my health and vitality.
4. **Experiencing stress enhances my performance and productivity.**
5. Experiencing stress inhibits my learning and growth.
6. **Experiencing stress improves my health and vitality.**
7. Experiencing stress debilitates my performance and productivity.
8. **The effects of stress are positive and should be utilised.**

CHANGING PERSPECTIVE

In his book *Shift*, Ethan Kross provides some ways to reframe our perspective to provide emotional relief in a stressful situation. These can be used in the moment but are also helpful when trying to navigate a bigger picture of our stress burden over time.[75]

Mental Time Travel
Ask yourself, "How will I feel about this in a week? How about a year, or five years?" This helps you create emotional distance and see how your current situation fits into a bigger picture, which can decrease the emotional impact it's having right now.

Reflect on Past Challenges
Remind yourself of times when you've overcome a challenge or stressful situation. This helps us remember that most situations are temporary, and that we have the tools we need to deal with them.

Third-Person Self-Talk
Another way to create some distance is to talk to yourself in the third person. Rather than saying, "I'm stressed," I could ask, "Why is Tommy stressed?" and then, "What can Tommy do to manage the situation?" Studies by Kross show that this kind of linguistic reframing can help with emotional regulation without requiring additional cognitive resources.[76]

WRITE. One of the ways having a significant burden of tasks, responsibilities, and stressful events wears on us is that it can leave us without much time to really process everything that's going on. This includes not being able to express or understand the various feelings that roll through us on a daily basis. One tool that has consistently been shown to help people navigate stressful situations or negative feelings is to write about them. Expressive writing, where participants write about a stressful event or topic, has been shown to decrease anger and distress and improve life satisfaction, cognitive function, and maybe even some aspects of immune function.[77] The benefits of writing tend to be higher when people have a higher burden of stress or physical health issues, meaning that it works better for people who need it more. In general, improvements are seen with relatively short interventions—fifteen minutes of writing repeated a few times over one to four weeks. Perhaps the most important aspect is being able to write freely, without fear of judgment. Your writing is for you only, and you don't need to worry about spelling or grammar, just bringing out your thoughts on the topic or event. The goal is simply to get the words out, because putting feelings into words can help to moderate their impact. Processing thoughts in this way—

simply getting them out of your head—can then free your mind to relax and unwind, which is critical to replenishing our cognitive and physical resources. For example, one study found that having women write about body concerns in three fifteen-minute sessions over two weeks decreased negative comparisons of themselves to others and improved sleep.[78]

Even simpler writing tasks can also improve sleep. If you find yourself worrying about everything you need to get done, studies show that completing a to-do list before bed allows your brain to relax, decreasing the time it takes to fall asleep.[79] The goal of using writing to offload our thoughts and worries, or to process stressful situations, is to decrease our cognitive and allostatic load, making it easier for us to switch off the stress signal and take time to rest and adapt. This frees up headroom, directly decreasing the negative effects of chronic stress on the brain, but also giving us more capacity in the moment to deal with stressors and perform high-quality work when we need to.

THERAPEUTIC WRITING

The best-studied writing intervention was developed by James Pennebaker.[80] His therapeutic writing protocol has been shown to have wide-ranging benefits in terms of helping deal with stressful or difficult situations, improving mood and health as a result. Typically, people are asked to write for fifteen minutes on four consecutive days, but less frequent writing (one or two times per week) can also work. The protocol below is taken from his website and lightly edited for brevity.

Preparation
Find a time and place where you won't be disturbed. Promise yourself that you will write for a minimum of fifteen minutes a day for at least three or four consecutive days. Once you begin writing, don't stop until the time is up. Don't worry about spelling or grammar. If you run out of things to write about, just repeat what you have already written. You can write by hand or type on a computer. You can also record yourself talking.

The Topic(s)
Write about something that you are thinking or worrying about too much. Something that you are dreaming about. Something that you feel is affecting your life in an unhealthy way. Something that you have been avoiding for days, weeks, or years.

The Prompt

Write about your deepest emotions and thoughts about the most upsetting experience in your life. If there isn't one specific experience you want to write about, think about major conflicts or stressors that have been weighing on you. Really let go and explore your feelings and thoughts about these experiences. In your writing, you might tie experiences to your childhood, your relationship with your parents, people you have loved or love now, or even your career. How are these things related to who you would like to become, who you have been in the past, or who you are now? You can write about the same issue every day or a series of different issues. Whatever you choose to write about, however, it is critical that you really let go and explore your very deepest emotions and thoughts.

What to Do with Your Words Afterwards

Burn them. Erase them. Shred them. Flush them. Tear them into little pieces and toss them into the ocean or let the wind take them away. Eat them (not recommended). The writing is for you, and for you only—the purpose is for you to be completely honest with yourself. Some people keep their samples and edit them, but whether you keep them or destroy them is really up to you.

A Final Note

Pennebaker does warn that people sometimes feel sad or depressed after their writing session. He says that, like a reaction to seeing a sad movie, this typically goes away in a couple of hours. But if you find that you are getting extremely upset about a writing topic, simply stop writing or change topics.

MENTAL OFFLOADING

Having incomplete tasks in the back of your mind can prevent you from focusing on another task, or make it harder to fall asleep, because some mental energy is being used to remember those tasks or thoughts so we can deal with them later.[81] Simply getting the thoughts out of your head or formulating a plan for how to address problems or tasks can help to decrease stress and rumination. If that feels familiar, try this prompt from a study that showed writing to-do lists before bed can improve sleep:

> We'd like for you to spend the next five minutes writing down everything you have to remember to do tomorrow and over the next few days. You can write these in paragraph form or in bullet points. Use all five minutes to think and write about tasks you have to complete tomorrow and in the near future, even if few are coming to you.
>
> Some people use a similar approach to offload other thoughts or concerns (in addition to tasks) before bed, which can help them stop ruminating about those worries in the knowledge that they can pick them up again in the morning if needed. One of the easiest ways to do all this is to keep a small notebook and pen with you or beside your bed.

SYNC. Another collection of tools to consider are those that can give us a better overall sense of well-being and the ability to navigate longer periods of increased stress. Many of these tools come under the umbrella of "meditation." From my own experiences in coaching, I've seen that meditation can be hard to sell—either due to some notion people have in their heads of what meditation involves or because of the time and preparation they think it will take. For many people—myself included—meditation and mindfulness have become another thing we're all supposed to do but don't have time for. So I'm going to risk going a bit rogue and suggest that I don't think it really matters exactly *what* you do. There are a whole range of techniques that have shown benefit in terms of mental health and cognitive function, and I want you to choose the one that suits you.

Meditation itself does seem to have some interesting effects on the brain. When people who have never meditated before are exposed to a meditation programme over a few weeks, changes in the white- and grey-matter structures of the brain are seen in areas related to memory, emotion, and emotional regulation.[82] Mindfulness-based interventions focusing on breath, thoughts, and sensations have been found to improve some aspects of cognitive function and lead to lower stress and greater well-being.[83] Loving-kindness meditation, which cultivates thoughts of kindness to ourselves and others, can improve self-compassion and mood.[84] One fascinating recent study from the Icahn School of Medicine at Mount Sinai took advantage of electrical recording devices implanted into the brains of patients with epilepsy to show that loving-kindness meditation changes activity in emotional regulation centres of the brain, including the amygdala.[85] Transcendental meditation, which involves silently repeating a mantra, may improve blood pressure, stress responses, anxiety, and feelings of burnout.[86] Other tools that can fit into this broad category include breathwork, like doing a few minutes of the physiological sigh, which was mentioned earlier. Gratitude practices that involve either journaling or reflection can also improve multiple aspects of well-being, even if done only once a week.[87]

If any of these practices appeal to you, it's worth finding one that feels right and that you're willing to regularly engage in because I'm not sure there's any evidence to say one approach is better than the others. Just like with writing and reframing, these tools help offload some of the negative effects of chronic stress, improve overall mood and well-being, and/or (with practice) build insight and resilience, all of which can improve cognitive function and prevent cognitive decline. Nowadays there are an endless number of good apps that can provide guided meditation and mindfulness sessions of multiple types for as little as five or ten minutes at a time.

So when I talk about meditation and mindfulness, it's not that I think we all need to spend several hours a day in silent contemplation. Though that may well be helpful for some people, for most of us something much shorter is probably enough—as well as being more practical. In fact, some of the benefit probably comes simply from consistently setting aside a few minutes in your day to step away and take a moment to look after yourself—decompressing, and focusing on the moment, something positive, or nothing at all.

WAYS TO SYNC

There are a whole host of related techniques that have been shown to improve mood and well-being and decrease stress. Many have also been shown to improve brain structure and cognitive function, which might be either because they act as a novel stimulus or because they decrease the burden of stress that can negatively impact brain structure and function. Note that sitting still with our thoughts or leaning into gratitude can feel a little uncomfortable to start with, which probably means it's working.

While there's currently no strong evidence that these activities directly help to prevent cognitive decline and decrease dementia risk, their mechanisms of action, such as decreasing cortisol levels with regular mindfulness and meditation practice, would support the idea.[88] The worst-case scenario is that you make a habit of taking some time to yourself, which provides an opportunity for relaxation and recovery.

Gratitude

Meta-analyses suggest gratitude is beneficial if done at least once per week.[89] Prompts include:

- List five things you are grateful for and why you are grateful for them.
- Spend five minutes writing about somebody you are grateful for.
- Write a letter to somebody you are grateful for.
- Write about one aspect of your life that you take for granted and imagine it is no longer present.
- Spend five minutes writing about a past experience you are grateful for.
- During the day, try to notice and be grateful for at least three things.

Transcendental Meditation

Transcendental meditation has been found to decrease blood pressure, anxiety, and cortisol levels.[90] Generally performed for ten to twenty minutes per day, it involves silently repeating a mantra in your head. There are many mantras that you could use, but the first one taught to me by ordained Zen Buddhist teacher Kim House, which I still use to this day, is: "Gate gate paragate parasamgate bodhi swaha." Known as the Heart-Calming Mantra, you pronounce it something like "gah-tay gah-tay pah-rah-gah-tay pah-rah-sahm-gah-tay boh-dee swah-hah." Though these mantras are not supposed to have direct meaning for the meditator, it roughly translates to "Gone beyond the beyond to enlightenment."[91]

Loving-Kindness Meditation

Loving-kindness meditation can decrease anxiety and stress, increase self-compassion, and improve mood.[92] The mantras can be directed at yourself, loved ones, friends, or even difficult acquaintances. Start by closing your eyes and imagining yourself sitting with the person in front of you. You begin by wishing them well and thinking: "May you be safe and protected from danger. May you be happy and peaceful. May you be healthy and strong. May you have ease and well-being." And as you say these words, have a sense of letting this loving kindness come from you and reach out to them.

> **Mindfulness**
>
> A large body of literature suggests that mindfulness practices decrease stress and can result in improved attentional control as well as associated changes to the structure of the brain, including in the hippocampus.[93] One technique is a body scan—lying down with closed eyes and slowly and deliberately bringing your attention to all your digits, joints, and limbs, starting at one foot, going up one side of the body and then down the other—noticing any sensations like heat or cold, moisture, tingling, numbness, or anything else you might be feeling. Another technique is bringing your awareness to your breath—for instance, during box breathing (four seconds in, four seconds hold, four seconds out, four seconds hold).

BE BRAVE. The story that stress is bad for us can make us actively avoid situations that have the potential to be uncomfortable or that include some risk. Of course, this might seem very sensible in the moment. If you already feel like your capacity for more stress is low, it doesn't really make sense to dive headfirst into a new career in public speaking or have arguments with people whose politics you disagree with. But by engaging with, and overcoming, difficult or stressful situations, we can both directly improve our well-being and improve our ability to deal with stressful situations in the future by building headroom. In children, for instance, engaging in risky or adventurous play is associated with better mental health and skill development, as well as a better ability to assess and handle future risk.[94] Of course, there's a difference between risk and *danger*. Risk in this context is play that comes with the possibility of minor injury, such as running or climbing, or getting lost. These are the kinds of activities that allow kids to find and understand their limits and overcome challenges in a way that requires control, concentration, and determination. As adults, we can think about doing difficult things as a way to enhance our competence—one of the three core aspects of self-determination theory we encountered in chapter 8—in stressful situations. Knowing that we have overcome difficult things—physical challenges, hard conversations, unexpected setbacks—we feel more comfortable when faced with something similar in the future. This is also important because the opposite approach—actively avoiding conflict or difficult situations—has been shown to be associated with worse mental health in the long term. By actively *choosing* to engage in activities that have the potential to be stressful, and gaining some control over our stressors, we increase our autonomy and benefit from the positive feelings that come from having prevailed through significant effort.[95]

This combination of factors—engaging with challenging situations and using those as opportunities to bolster autonomy and competence—seems to be an important part of what athletes call *mental toughness*. Of course, when somebody mentions toughness, you might imagine being yelled at by some macho drill sergeant. But that's not what I mean by toughness. Mental toughness is a collection of personal characteristics that allow individuals to regularly attain and sustain performances at the upper limits of their abilities.[96] In this context it just means engaging with, overcoming, and learning from physical or psychological challenges to build confidence in our ability to deal with difficulties when they arise. Maybe that's an event like a 5K race or jumping into a cold plunge. Or maybe it's signing up to give a presentation or performance in a forum that's new to you, or joining a class to learn about something in which you're a complete novice. Or perhaps it's choosing to (respectfully) engage with information or people whose ideas are different from yours. All of these can help bolster your toughness in a safe but challenging way—and help your brain build headroom and foster greater resilience against stress.

FINDING ADAPTATION

The core idea behind having a stimulated mind is that by exposing ourselves and our brains to challenges, we drive adaptations that increase function—enhancing skills or cognitive processes, and building physical and functional headroom that helps protect our brains against ageing and neurodegeneration. However, in order to do that, we need to make sure that the total burden of our everyday and ongoing stressors doesn't impair our ability to adapt or perform in the moment, and several studies show that allostatic load increases the risk of dementia both directly (through the effects of chronic cortisol elevation on the brain) and indirectly (by increasing inflammation, worsening metabolic health, and making us less likely to engage in cognitively difficult tasks because we already feel exhausted).

It helps to have a set of tools for dealing with stress or emotions in the moment or minimising the effects of ongoing stressors. For our runner at the start of the chapter, improving his adaptation involved removing unnecessary races and training so he could spend more time reconnecting with his wife. He decreased his total load and kept the bigger picture in mind, and by the next season he was consistently and considerably faster (not to mention happier) as a result.

Remember that nobody is expected to use all the tools in this chapter, so just pick one or two to try out, and experiment to see what works for you. Building a bigger stress tolerance doesn't always require a ton of time and work—it might just involve reframing stress as an important part of the adaptation process, which allows us to welcome and leverage times that we're challenged. It can also be helpful to think about what you're *already* doing that fits into this category, and to diversify if you can. For instance, many people use exercise to offload or manage stress, but if you are already very active, exercising *more* might have the opposite effect—all that extra stimulus could add to your overall allostatic load. Instead, think about some breathwork or a writing practice that might have a complementary effect rather than doing too much of one thing. The goal really is to make sure that you're most likely to adapt to and benefit from the challenges you face—which also, conveniently, sets you up for the next phase of that process: recovery.

BE PREPARED FOR UPS AND DOWNS

American boxer Mike Tyson is famous for saying that "everyone has a plan until they get punched in the face." While it's very important to plan new activities and goals to help build and support headroom, it's equally important to prepare for times when even our well-ingrained health habits are challenged. Because it's a fact of life that—metaphorically at least—at some point we're going to get punched in the face. Life will get busy or stressful (or both), and we'll find ourselves short on cognitive capacity, patience, and time. That's when all those new healthy habits tend to go by the wayside. Having a plan for this scenario makes it more likely that we can maintain some of those habits (and our headroom) while under duress.

My favourite way to plan for periods of increased load is to use the traffic light system invented by Simon Marshall. Simon was a performance psychologist with incredibly keen insights into human behaviour. His book *The Brave Athlete*, which he wrote with his wife—multiple offroad triathlon world champion Lesley Paterson—is a fantastic resource for anybody trying to understand their brain, whether they're an athlete or not. Many of the people Simon worked with were trying to juggle hectic work and family schedules. And just like the rest of us, when these people didn't have time to exercise, eat, or sleep the way they'd like to, their inclination was to give up entirely. To combat this reaction, Simon instead had people classify their actions according to a green/yellow/red system.

Green is what you do when everything is going well—you have time to eat, sleep, exercise, meditate, and stimulate your brain in the ways that you want to. This list can include activities you've done for a long time as well as new habits you're trying to develop.

Yellow is what you shift to when things get busy. Maybe you're travelling and you don't have time to do the activities you normally would. Perhaps you are on a tight deadline and everything else needs to be put on pause. Rather than just winging it (or getting more stressed because you can't fit in your daily workout), you can create a predefined plan for yellow activities during these times. Decide what things you are likely to drop when you're busy and just eliminate them entirely. Any remaining activities can stay the same or be modified as needed. For example, if it feels like there's no time for your full exercise regimen at the gym, do a shortened workout or do some movement at home. Remember that not doing something and then worrying about not doing it is the worst of both worlds. Instead, acknowledge that some things probably won't happen and have a plan to do the rest.

Red is for the (hopefully) rare times when you're stretched to maximum capacity. Maybe a project means you're having to work fourteen-hour days, or somebody in the family is sick so you're sleeping less and spending a lot of time at the hospital. When you are in this red category, select one or two non-negotiable things that give you an anchor in your day. This could be just five minutes of movement or some breathwork to reduce stress—whatever you can fit in that will help you feel good. Then let everything else go so you can focus on what you need to do to get through this tough period.

An example of a yellow adjustment is my wife's approach to physical activity. When she's had a long day and is unable to do the movement she had initially planned to do, she's aware that *everything counts* (because she's heard me harping on that for years). So she defaults to a few minutes of any kind of movement that requires no preparation. Maybe a walk or some squats in the living room. When I'm in the midst of a red period, my focus is usually sleep. If I can get enough sleep, I know I can survive well enough even if I'm not eating the healthiest foods or moving as much as I'd like. If sleep is an issue due to work or travel (especially jet lag), I instead default to a short period of exercise (maybe just some push-ups and squats) to give me a boost when I need it. Not only does this help my cognitive function and mood, I know I will still see benefits from even occasional workouts or catch-up sleep when life becomes overwhelmingly busy.[97]

Having the green, yellow, and red plans in place prevents you from needing to make decisions when you're busy or stressed. Instead, you can spare that brain power for the tasks in front of you. Because these shifts are part of the plan, you also don't have to feel guilty if you miss a workout or skip a meditation session. You can feel grateful for the headroom they build when you have more time, and know you're well set up to get through this tough period by focusing on the things you *can* do.

CHAPTER 12
RECOVER

One of my first jobs as a doctor was as the orthopedic intern on the foot-and-ankle service. I was the only junior member of my team, and my days largely involved handing out crutches and pain medications to patients after bunion surgery. However, as we were a small team and rarely dealt with emergencies, I also had time to have long conversations with my bosses, either during surgery or in follow-up clinic. As we saw a lot of athletes, we frequently talked about sports and training. I vividly remember one day in clinic when a runner came in with a stress fracture in one of their metatarsals—the bones in your feet that connect to your toes. Stress fractures are small breaks in the bones that are caused by overuse and are very common in runners. After the consultation, my boss looked at me, rolled his eyes, and said, "Only amateurs get stress fractures."

I later learned this isn't true—there are a number of factors that may make an athlete more or less susceptible to stress fractures, which occur even in experienced runners. But the implication was clear—amateur athletes are more likely to get themselves into a situation where stress fractures happen. While most professional athletes follow balanced and purposeful training programmes, amateurs often think that training should always be hard, and they push themselves toward a higher risk of illness or injury.

When you're training for fitness or athletic performance, it's easy to assume that a lack of progress, or even loss of progress, is because you're not doing *enough*. This is especially true for people who are trying to fit training around their job, family, and other commitments. Therefore, they think that the difference between them and more successful athletes is the amount of time they train. But often it's less about how somebody is training and more about what they're doing the other twentysomething hours out of the day. One of the biggest differences between an amateur and a professional is knowing when you need to do more, when you've done enough, and when you should do less. Most importantly, the best athletes know that if they want to adapt, they must make time to recover.

Throughout the majority of our history as a species, our productivity was focused on harvesting food, building shelter, and caring for one another. But, while our ancestors lived hard (and often very dangerous) lives, we also know that they spent a lot of time resting.[1] They worked hard but usually had ample time to recover from their efforts. Today, many of us rely on our brains rather than physical toil as the primary source of our productivity, and the nature of the modern work and social environments means we are now cognitively the equivalent of amateur athletes who spend hours and hours running every day without attending to their recovery. And yet we wonder why the cognitive versions of stress fractures—high allostatic load, stress, and burnout—are the only things we have to show for all that effort.

While the brain-dependent nature of many modern jobs has given rise to the term *knowledge workers,* I instead like to think of us as cognitive athletes. I would also say that all humans fit into this category, regardless of our specific jobs. The word *athlete* is derived from a Greek word meaning to "compete for a prize." So, if the prize of the brain game is more headroom and prolonged brain health, we should all consider ourselves cognitive athletes and treat our brains the way the best athletes treat their bodies. Recall the successful athletes over forty discussed in part 1. The one thing that seems to be consistent across all of them is a focus only on doing the training (stimulus) they really need and spending more time supporting adaptation and maintenance through nutrition and recovery.

It may seem counterintuitive, but recovery is the time when all your hard work starts to pay off. You don't get stronger in the gym—you get stronger in the hours and days after you leave the gym as your body adapts to the challenge you exposed it to. Whether it's building your muscle fibres and tendons to be able to lift a heavier weight, improving the function of the mitochondria in your heart so you can run faster for a longer period of time, or building and maintaining synapses in the brain to retain and express new memories and skills, this all happens during the recovery period *after* you've done the hard work.

By now, I'm sure you can see where I'm going with this. Just as the brain responds to challenge in a similar way to how our guns respond to bicep curls, our brains also get bigger and stronger during rest. The problem is that we often tend to continually ask more and more from our brains without ever resting, which has the opposite effect. The drive to do *something* is one that most of us experience every day, though it's not always the best use of our time. To quote Mark Manson, one of my favourite sources of practical modern psychology, "Sometimes the most useful thing you can do ... is nothing. Coincidentally, this is usually also the hardest thing to do."

This is a lesson that my friend and colleague Greg Bennett knows well. Greg and his wife Laura Bennett are former professional triathletes who, between them, made four trips to the Olympics. When they were competing, more than one media outlet dubbed them "the world's fittest couple." In 2008, Greg was ranked as the number-one triathlete in the world and competing in a multirace competition called the Lifetime Fitness Series. It all came down to the final race in Dallas. If he won that race, he'd win the series and have a significant six-figure payday. If he didn't, the whole season would be a bust (by his high standards, at least).

The pressure was massive. In the weeks leading up to Dallas, he made the classic mistake that so many athletes—even some professionals—make. He started grinding harder. He increased his training load even though he was already fatigued. His brain was constantly racing, and he was both mentally and physically fried. Losing sight of the bigger goal, he continued to push himself harder but went slower, still convincing himself that the answer was to do *more*.

Greg will tell you himself that he has an ego to match the size of his athletic accomplishments. Having always been self-coached—to great success—he equated control with confidence and performance. But, in a rare moment of insight before the big race in Dallas, he realised that he didn't have the clarity needed to get his preparation right. So he turned to Laura and said, "You listen to your body better than I do. I want you to take over my training."

Laura did exactly what any of our loved ones would want to do for us when they see we are overextended. For his last few weeks of training, she slashed Greg's workouts by 75 percent. Sessions that he had originally programmed as fifteen-mile high-intensity runs were now three-mile jogs and an easy swim.

As you might expect, Greg was terrified. He questioned every session and thought he was going to lose fitness. But he stuck with it, and just four days before the race he suddenly felt alive, rested, and clear-headed. His mind had stopped racing, and his cognitive and emotional bandwidth returned. He noticed for the first time in a long time that he was actually *excited* to race.

When the gun went off in Dallas, Greg immediately knew he had made the right choice. The nerves were there, but they were the good kind—that slight increase in stress that gets you to the top of the arousal curve and drives performance. He went on to win both the race and the series. Reflecting back on the story later, he told me that what stuck with him so much more than the win was the lesson he learned in those final weeks. He'd been willing to step back and realise that he was pushing himself too hard, and that's when he truly benefitted from all the hard work he had put in and was able to unlock his potential.

ALLOSTATIC OVERLOAD OR UNDER-RECOVERY?

In the world of sports performance, there's an age-old debate about whether a lack of performance when training demands are high is due to overtraining or under-recovery. Sometimes there's a clear explanation, such as low energy availability because the athlete isn't eating enough calories to recover from their training. But the rest of the time, and especially when we relate these ideas to cognitive function and brain health, stimulus and recovery are two sides of the same coin. Because when you're doing more of one, you have less time for the other. Balancing the two is the key to bolstering our brain's headroom and resilience over the long term, as well as being able to perform at a high level when it really counts.

The cognitive effects of inadequate recovery during prolonged periods of high allostatic load are what most people would refer to as *burnout,* although others have used terms like *vital exhaustion*.[2] The symptoms are basically the same—physical and mental decline indicating that we're at the limits of our headroom, because we're asking for too much from our brains without giving them the rest that they need.

> ## SYMPTOMS OF OVERLOAD
>
> In a recent large study of burnout, Gordon Parker explored the wide range of symptoms experienced by those who are cognitively, psychologically, and physically overloaded. These are provided below in order of how common they were in his study. While many of these symptoms can have a range of causes, if they map to an extended period of high strain, they could be signs that you need to decrease the number of plates you're trying to juggle, increase dedicated time to recovery, or both.[3]
>
> **Exhaustion**
> Feeling exhausted, fatigued, tired, drained, or lethargic.
>
> **Anxiety and Stress**
> Feeling anxious, stressed, overwhelmed, unable to relax or switch off, ruminating over or worrying about work when not there, having a sense of dread, or feeling more fidgety or restless.
>
> **Indifference**
> Lack of empathy, a lack of interest or pleasure in work or leisure activities, apathy, disengagement, or a feeling of "just going through the motions."
>
> **Depression**
> Low mood, sadness, hopelessness or helplessness, a drop in confidence or self-esteem, self-doubt, feelings of worthlessness or guilt, or suicidal thoughts.
>
> **Irritability and Anger**
> Feeling frustration, anger, or resentment, or being irritable, impatient, or easily agitated.
>
> **Sleep Disturbances**
> Experiencing insomnia or excessive sleepiness, or an increased frequency of nightmares.
>
> **Lack of Motivation or Passion**
> Decreased motivation, drive, passion, or satisfaction with life or work. Feeling as though you're not making a difference or that your work has no purpose.

Changes in Executive Function
Problems with concentration, attention, or memory. Brain fog or confusion. Racing or disorganised thoughts, or difficulty planning or making decisions.

Reduced Performance
Reduced performance or quality of output cognitively or physically, lower productivity, procrastination, avoiding responsibilities, or making more frequent mistakes.

Withdrawal
Less desire to spend time with or engage with family, friends, colleagues, or clients/patients.

Physical Symptoms
Aches and pains, headaches, eating or appetite changes (either increased or decreased), increased alcohol use or smoking, nausea, or low libido.

Emotional Lability
Feeling fragile or more sensitive. Experiencing emotional outbursts or more crying or tearfulness.

MARKERS OF OVERLOAD

Several studies have looked for clinical markers and blood test values that indicate high allostatic load. In general, the picture is very similar to what we see in the setting of excess energy availability—an increase in waist circumference, high blood pressure, high blood sugar, high triglycerides, high total cholesterol, or low HDL cholesterol.[4] This is likely due to the fact that persistent increases in stress hormones and inflammation associated with high allostatic load impair metabolic health, and that in some people, higher stress can increase the likelihood of energy excess due to increased appetite and decreased physical activity.

The most consistent marker of allostatic overload seems to be high inflammation as measured by C-reactive protein (CRP). Though it differs according to the study, a level above the 3–5 mg/L range is often used as a cutoff for evidence of high allostatic load.[5] Other markers include low vitamin D (stress susceptibility increases when vitamin D levels are low), and

> low albumin (a protein made by the liver that decreases with inflammation).[6] Perhaps unsurprisingly, physical activity is associated with a lower allostatic load, while high alcohol intake and smoking are associated with higher allostatic loads—either because they decrease stress tolerance or because people who are very stressed are less likely to jog and more likely to smoke and drink.

Taking the long view of recovery as it fits into the bigger picture of cognitive decline and dementia, I think it's important to tie together several ideas to map the route from allostatic overload and burnout to recovery, adaptation, and improved cognitive function—and to show why we're even talking about those things in the context of long-term brain health.

The first idea is that prolonged burnout is probably associated with an increased risk of dementia. I say "probably" because burnout wasn't defined until the 1980s or widely studied until much later. However, in addition to the studies mentioned in the previous chapter, we see signals of a connection between burnout and dementia risk in several longitudinal cohort studies. For example, a study of nearly seventy thousand people in Finland that began in the 1970s found that psychological distress (stress or exhaustion) was associated with an increased risk of dementia over the following twenty-five years.[7] Similar results have been found in studies where allostatic overload was defined as midlife stress-related exhaustion and vital exhaustion.[8]

Regardless of what name is used in the research, symptoms outlined in the Symptoms of Overload box above all seem to stem from chronic stress: experiencing demands beyond our current capacity, a lack of time or resources to recover from those demands, or a bit of both. Knowing this, it's imperative that we consider how we might be contributing to this and where to best intervene. Some stressors are harder to control—for instance, those that stem from socioeconomic disadvantage, which is strongly linked to increased dementia risk.[9] But for those stressors that we *do* have control over, finding ways to increase our headroom or minimise the drain they place on our overall cognitive capacity is important. To do that, we *must* allow ourselves to rest and recover.

EXTEND YOURSELF SOME COMPASSION

In chapter 6, I mentioned that when we think about all the things we *could* be doing to support our health, we're subconsciously creating a mental list of the ways that we're failing by not doing them. You might even interpret the information in the previous chapters as a catalogue of all the ways you're failing your brain because of the things you're not doing. This is also why there's almost a catch-22 around writing about stress. When you tell people about all the ways stress can negatively affect their health, they then begin to stress about their *stress*.

Hopefully, by this point, you realise that this doesn't need to be the case. As I've mentioned before, I truly believe every person is doing the best they can, and the reality is that there's a *reason* we're doing (or not doing) certain things at any given moment in time. The fact that there are so many ways to support our brains, and a long period of time over which we can influence our cognitive health, means that we have a lot more capacity and time to change trajectory once the right opportunities arise.

Some of the problems with setting ourselves overly ambitious health goals (and beating ourselves up if we don't meet them) can be solved by reframing the information and acknowledging that health-related targets aren't set in stone. You already know that, when it comes to exercise, *everything counts,* and if you're not exercising frequently, you'll benefit from pretty much any additional movement you do. Incremental improvements also make a big difference when it comes to nutrition, stimulus, and sleep. The goal is less about getting some perfect amount of sleep or exercise and more about using those targets as waypoints on the journey to the brain-filled life you want to lead. Yes, we can always do a bit better, but we're more likely to engage with and maintain activities and habits that align with some bigger purpose or outcome we hope to achieve.

By acknowledging this, we can loosen our expectations slightly if we need to. This has the double-whammy effect of increasing the likelihood we will engage in a certain health behaviour—even if the way we do that isn't "perfect"—while decreasing perfectionism-related stress that could erode the benefit we get from that behaviour. For example, setting lower exercise goals with a broader definition of what counts as exercise—as we did in chapter 7—makes it more likely that people will actually stick with it, which also improves how they feel about their health.[10] Similarly, those who have a more flexible approach to their diet (rather than being very strict or rigid with themselves) are more likely to feel like they have control and remain engaged with their nutrition-related goal, even if they lapse.[11]

Many studies also show that self-compassion improves both health behaviours and health outcomes. Self-compassion includes self-kindness (responding to failures with understanding, patience, and acceptance rather than with self-criticism), common humanity (the recognition that all people are imperfect, make mistakes, and experience failure), and mindfulness (nonjudgmental awareness of thoughts and feelings).[12] In this way, self-compassion essentially allows us to treat ourselves the way we would hope to treat others: with understanding and support, even when things get difficult, or we fail to live up to our own expectations.

Those who are more self-compassionate tend to experience lower levels of anxiety and stress and are more likely to engage in physical activity, eat healthily, and quit smoking.[13] As a result, people who have more self-compassion tend to have better health outcomes.[14] For example, a self-compassion intervention in individuals with diabetes resulted in a significant improvement in blood sugar control over a period of three months.[15]

As you know by now, this doesn't mean you shouldn't work hard. Hard work is important. But one part of working hard on something is understanding that we will fail sometimes, and we should acknowledge those failures with compassion. Doing so will make it more likely that we continue to engage with activities that will help to build headroom and future-proof our brains, while decreasing the allostatic load that can do the opposite.

MAKING ROOM FOR RECOVERY AND SELF-COMPASSION

Psychologist Kristin Neff is perhaps the world's foremost authority on self-compassion, having created many of the techniques used in studies and written several impactful papers on the topic. Her work has busted myths around self-compassion and shown that it increases mental strength and motivation, improves health, and allows us to be better at caring for others.[16] If you feel like you struggle to find the time for yourself, beat yourself up when you fail, or feel guilty for allowing yourself to rest, you might benefit from exercises in self-compassion.

A typical course in self-compassion involves multiple sessions including mindfulness-based practices like body scans and internally focused loving-kindness meditation, as mentioned in chapter 11. But Dr. Neff has also developed some shorter self-compassion exercises that are a great place to start.[17]

Self-Compassion Break

Think of a situation in your life that is difficult or that is causing you stress. See if you can actually feel the stress and emotional discomfort in your body. Starting with the mindful part of self-compassion and acknowledge the stress by telling yourself, "This is a moment of suffering." Then add some common humanity by reminding yourself that other people feel this way, or that all of us struggle sometimes. Then express self-kindness by asking, "What do I need to hear right now to be kind to myself?" This could be a specific example or situation where you hope you can be more kind to yourself, or a more general phrase like "May I learn to accept myself as I am" or "May I forgive myself."

Self-Compassion Journaling

Write down anything that you've felt bad about or judged yourself for. Write how you felt—sad, ashamed, frightened, stressed, etc. Write down the ways this experience connects to the larger human experience. Maybe acknowledge that being human means being imperfect, making mistakes, and having painful experiences (e.g., "Everyone overreacts sometimes, it's only human."). Then write yourself some kind, understanding words of comfort (e.g., "It's OK. You messed up, but it wasn't the end of the world. You can learn from this and do things differently next time.").

Redirecting Motivation

Do you use self-criticism as a motivator? For example, is there a personal trait that you criticise yourself for (too overweight, too lazy) because you think being hard on yourself will help you change? If so, think about and acknowledge the pain and the experience of being judged in that way. Then think of the words a loving friend would say to you if they heard that somebody else had spoken to you like that, and how they might support and encourage you to make a change that's in line with your desire to have a healthy and happy brain. Go through this process again any time you catch yourself falling into a pattern of self-criticism, focusing on how you might be more likely to achieve your goals with self-talk that is more encouraging and supportive.

One of the most interesting things about self-compassion is that it is associated with both mental toughness and resilience.[18] This means that self-compassion directly increases headroom—increasing our ability to function well during periods of stress. By giving ourselves a break when we need it and being compassionate with ourselves when we make mistakes, we boost our mood and improve our ability to deal with tough times. Self-compassion and targeted recovery also provide space for adaptation so that we have the capacity to work hard and push ourselves when it really matters. Sometimes it seems like everything we've ever been told—or told ourselves—about needing to toughen up by pushing through the pain is the complete *opposite* of how the brain actually builds resilience and headroom.

One reason toughness isn't just about sucking it up and pushing through is that engaging with and overcoming challenges is more beneficial when we have control or agency over that process. As mentioned in chapter 11, when you look at both dementia and depression risk, having high demands put on you (or even having periods of high stress) can be a good thing, but only if you also have control over those demands. For this reason, being kind to yourself also includes knowing when to say no, or to take something off your plate. Of course, sometimes it isn't possible to say no, and sometimes we have to do things we don't want to. This is where we can rely on the headroom we've built up over time to help regulate stress in the moment. But this process also involves exercising some control over what you choose to engage with and knowing when to push yourself and when to pull back. This is because those who exhibit allostatic overload or burnout often disengage from health-supporting behaviours, making it even harder to preserve cognitive function in the long term.

BRAIN-FOCUSED RECOVERY

While sleep is a foundational component of brain recovery and function, both in the short and long terms, there are other techniques we can use during the day to bolster our recovery when allostatic load is high, when we have a particular need to boost performance in the short term, or if we didn't get the chance to sleep as much as we wanted to in the day(s) previously.

Meditate and Breathe

Many of the relaxation-focused meditation and breathing strategies mentioned in chapter 11 can make for good restorative mental breaks to support overall brain health and cognitive function when we're feeling stressed or overwhelmed. One type of meditation that boosts mental recovery, as well as being helpful for learning and sleep, is yoga nidra. Yoga nidra includes elements of body scanning, breath awareness, and visualization, which, as we've seen, have been found to decrease levels of stress hormones and improve blood pressure and mood.[19] One study that had participants perform yoga nidra for twenty minutes per day for two weeks using a recording on YouTube reported improvements in sleep, learning, and working memory.[20] When the electrical signals in the brains of people performing yoga nidra are measured, changes are often seen that are similar to what happens with sleep, even though participants are still awake.[21] This has resulted in yoga nidra being included in a group of meditation strategies called non-sleep deep rest (NSDR), which can be easily found in apps and online.

Rote Activities

Gloria Mark is a psychologist who studies how we use our attention, and ways to improve focus while minimising the likelihood of stress and burnout. In her book *Attention Span*, Dr. Mark describes four main cognitive states based on how engaged and challenged we are.[22] *Focus* is when we do hard work and really stimulate our brains by being both engaged and challenged. The two low-engagement states are *bored* (low engagement, low challenge) and *frustrated* (low engagement, high challenge). The fourth category is *rote* attention, which is when we're engaged but not challenged. When people do rote activities, they tend to feel good, and their stress decreases. These activities include crosswords or other puzzles, simple but engaging games (like *Angry Birds* or *Candy Crush*) and scrolling on social media (assuming you're avoiding the posts that get you riled up). The key here is to use these rote activities as short (maybe ten-minute) planned mental breaks after periods of intense focus or work or when we feel stressed, rather than going down the TikTok rabbit hole for two hours and telling ourselves it's good for our mental health.

Find the Familiar

There's evidence that when we're stressed or have exerted a lot of cognitive effort, we can recharge by entering familiar fictional worlds. In two different experiments, participants who exerted a lot of cognitive effort had decreased cognitive function in a test that involved finding a pattern in words, as well as more negative moods. However, their function and mood were restored by engaging in reading a familiar book or watching a rerun of a favourite TV show.[23] Re-experiencing something familiar seems to increase feelings of belongingness and restore a sense of self-control. It turns out that there's a reason that we feel less stressed after watching that episode of *Friends* for the seventeenth time.

Take a Walk (Reality Encouraged but Optional)

Taking a walk is one of the best ways to combine a brief mental break with a movement snack, and to perhaps experience the benefits of nature for stress reduction at the same time (see chapter 11). For example, several studies have found that just fifteen minutes of walking in nature (sometimes as part of the Japanese practice of connecting with nature through forest bathing, or *shinrin-yoku*) improves mood and physiological measures of stress like cortisol and heart-rate variability (a measure of increased relaxation due to vagus nerve activity), as well as supporting creativity in ways that are similar to the benefits of sleep.[24] Interestingly, some of the same benefits seem to be attainable using virtual reality (VR). The immersive quality of modern VR, available through headsets you can buy to use at home, is increasingly impressive, and several studies have found that taking VR nature walks or meditating in a relaxing virtual environment can have some of the same benefits as doing those activities in more traditional ways.[25] Though interaction with the real world is so critical to long-term cognitive function that it should be our main ongoing daily priority, VR could be a great option for those who don't have easy access to nature for brief breaks during the day or who like the idea of a more immersive approach to a meditation practice at home.

Garden

Like walks in nature, gardening provides an opportunity for light movement, exposure to nature, and repetitive and meditative work. Gardening and spending time in gardens has been associated with better cognitive function across a wide range of ages, as well as reduced pain and stress and improved attention.[26]

Nap

I'm cheating a little bit with this one because this box is about non-sleep recovery. But during periods when you have a greater sleep need or haven't been able to get as much sleep as you need at night, napping can be a useful way to increase alertness and improve performance. Napping can help you retain newly learned information or a new skill and can also improve cognitive function in the hours afterwards.[27] So, if you have the time to nap, a quick snooze can help boost performance for a critical event. In pro-

> fessional athletes training multiple times per day, napping during the day can improve performance and decrease exertion and fatigue.[28] However, it's best to avoid napping late in the day in case it affects your ability to sleep that night by decreasing sleep pressure. So, if possible, nap in the late morning or early afternoon.

YOU CAN'T JUST SLEEP WHEN YOU'RE DEAD

On our quest for better brain health, we've arrived at the final major stop: the critical importance of *stopping*. As I've alluded to a few times, every good athlete knows that the process of getting fitter and stronger requires a balance of two major components: stimulus and recovery. Sleep, in particular, is where we adapt to the stimuli we've received during the day and replenish our cognitive resources to go again and learn and adapt some more. Sleep is also when the brain takes out the rubbish—clearing out metabolites that build up during the day and resetting the system so that we can receive, process, and integrate information the next day. Sleep also indirectly supports multiple aspects of the game of brain health. For example, when we don't sleep well, we're less likely to socialise, move, or choose a nourishing meal.[29] A good night of sleep, on the other hand, makes it more likely that we'll engage with the world in a way that supports headroom and cognitive function, and lowers our long-term risk of dementia.

Luckily, now that we're more than two decades into the twenty-first century, we've seen a shift in terms of how society views sleep. When I was younger, it felt like society was permeated by the "sleep when you're dead" mentality. But now we've started to appreciate that if we don't sleep enough, our biology will make sure we reach that final endpoint sooner rather than later. Not only does sleep provide the necessary time for adaptation and learning to occur, it allows us to build the maximum possible headroom. Sleep also grants us *access* to our headroom, knowledge, and function when we most need it. (Though I should admit that it took me a *long* time to absorb this lesson, mostly learning it the hard way: forgetting it and then having to learn it all over again.)

One of the most vivid memories I have from my time as an undergraduate student is from the final weeks of my last year. The exam and grading schedules at Cambridge were particularly brutal—there was no partial credit, very little coursework, and no accumulation of exam marks over time. The sum of three years of learning and work essentially came down to a barrage of exams, each lasting three hours, at the end of the final year. Though the name is thankfully just a very dark inside joke, there's a reason that the last day of the final exam week at Cambridge has long been referred to as "Suicide Sunday."

In this particular memory, I'm sitting in a study room surrounded by other students, staring at a huge stack of biochemistry lecture notes. It's a few days before exams start, and the sun is blazing outside while I slowly begin to panic. At this point I have already realised that I won't be able to study all the material, so I have to decide which topics I have time to cover. I'm reading some notes about chromatin (a structure that our cells use to keep DNA organised) when I suddenly feel overwhelmed by the futility of the task ahead of me. I get up, walk out of the room, go into the bathroom next door, and break down into an uncontrollable flood of tears. To this day, I'm still amazed by how well I remember this scene, because I was so exhausted that it's a wonder my memory was functioning at all.

Of course, all of this was self-inflicted. I hadn't done a good job of staying on top of the material in the previous months, and I left it all to do with a couple of weeks to go. So I started to cut my sleeping hours in half to make up for lost time. The night before my breakdown, I found myself so tired that I couldn't concentrate but with so much coffee running through my veins that I couldn't sleep. That week I calculated my peak caffeine consumption at the equivalent of around twenty-five espressos in a single day.

Luckily, much like Greg (or, rather, his wife, Laura), I was capable of enough insight at this point to realise that I needed to give myself some time over the next couple of days to get some sleep. There are huge bodies of research that show how not getting enough sleep makes us anxious and impairs both learning and memory, so by not sleeping I was impairing my ability to benefit from the studying I *was* doing while also making myself feel much worse about what I *wasn't* doing. In learning and many other aspects of cognitive performance, you're also much more efficient when you get enough sleep; you can engage with material better and remember more of it, so you have to spend less time doing work to get the same benefit. As I sit here writing this book with a reasonable academic track record behind me, you know that this strategic switch in approach (less cramming, more sleep) did enough to help me survive those exams.

Though it's not always easy to do—and I've still occasionally struggled to take my own advice at busy times or when I become singularly focused on a task—it's clear that sleep is the lynchpin that allows our brains to have the incredible capacity that they have. But that also means we need to be mindful of our sleep—and other related recovery strategies—so that we are able to reach and maintain our full cognitive potential.

SLEEP AND THE BRAIN

World-renowned sleep expert Matthew Walker, who in many ways has popularised the importance of sleep through his research and his book *Why We Sleep,* calls sleep "the price we pay for wakefulness." Thinking back to our brain-as-a-car analogy in part 1, simply the act of driving our brains around all day results in some wear and tear. This is because our brains are energetically expensive, and just like burning fuel in an engine, the process of generating and using energy in cells can cause damage like a buildup of oxidative stress and inflammation. In addition to this, the process of constantly receiving, interpreting, and responding to information from our environment is inherently stressful (in a good way), and we need a time when we're *not* doing that in order to finish processing all of those inputs.

For the brain, like most of the body, sleep is the time when most maintenance and repair is scheduled to happen. If we didn't give the brain a chance to sleep, trying to carry out repairs would be like having your poor mechanic clinging to the underside of your car while you're speeding down the road because you're late for work. The repair process is much less treacherous if you can put the car in the shop for the night and let the mechanic take a look in a slightly more controlled manner.

The critical nature of sleep is highlighted by the fact that if we could do without it, evolution would have eliminated it at some point. Not only is spending a third of your day completely unconscious (and defenseless) risky from a survival standpoint, but that's also a lot of time that could be spent doing *other* things related to survival, like finding food and procreating. So sleep is clearly essential. And as we have all probably experienced at some point, productivity in pretty much any area goes out the window when we don't get enough sleep. This is due to the overall effect of sleep but also the ways that specific parts of sleep support different cognitive functions.

Sleep occurs in multiple stages that we cycle through during the night, completing one full cycle approximately every ninety minutes (figure 1). There are two broad stages of sleep—REM (rapid eye movement) sleep, and non-REM (NREM) sleep, both of which are critical but have slightly different effects on the brain. Deep sleep (also called slow-wave sleep) occurs in the later stages of NREM sleep and is critical for saving memories accumulated during the day before. Deep sleep and the other parts of NREM sleep that occur before deep sleep are used to reset synapses—the connections between neurons—so that the brain is refreshed and ready to receive new information.[30]

REM sleep is when we tend to dream. Like deep sleep, it plays an important part in memory storage, but it is also a time when new connections are made between different collections of unrelated memories and pieces of information that help with creativity, problem-solving, and building a bigger picture of our knowledge. REM sleep is also critical for processing emotions and preparing us to respond to and deal with emotionally challenging situations or experiences.

While all animals experience some form of sleep, only NREM is thought to be evolutionarily conserved across all species. The distinct cycling between NREM and REM sleep is generally only seen in mammals and birds and is thought to underlie some of our most important cognitive functions. For a long time, sleep experts thought this meant that REM sleep was so important to complex cognitive function that it evolved twice—in mammals and birds separately. However, more recent studies measuring sleep in lizards, mollusks, and fish (who says scientists don't know how to have a good time?) suggest that these animals also have two sleep states that they cycle through. So it's possible that REM sleep has an ancient common evolutionary origin.[31]

The balance of these different stages changes as we go through four or five sleep cycles in one night. At the start of the night, we spend more time in deep sleep, whereas later in the night we spend more time in

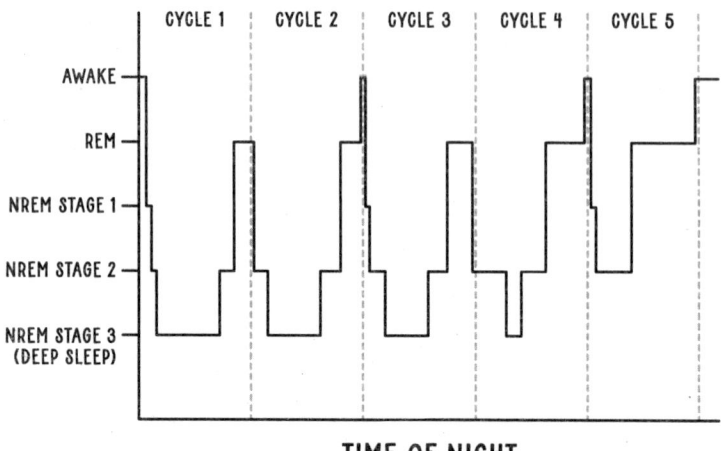

FIGURE 1. Sleep has four main stages that we cycle through—first through stages 1–3 of non-REM (NREM) sleep as sleep becomes deeper (NREM stage 3 is deep or "slow-wave" sleep), followed by REM sleep. Over the night, we spend less time in deep sleep and more time in REM sleep.

REM sleep, which helps us prepare for new learning the next day. As the different stages of sleep have different effects on the brain, it makes sense that an important part of getting enough sleep to support cognition and long-term brain health is cycling through all the sleep stages enough times to be refreshed and replenished the next day. In fact, the effects of the different sleep stages synergise and work together to support learning and cognitive function.

For example, studies in mice learning a new motor skill have shown that the neurons activated during learning are *reactivated* during NREM sleep, creating new connections related to that skill or memory. If the animals are allowed to have REM sleep but not deep sleep, or if reactivation of the skill-related neurons during deep sleep is prevented, learning doesn't occur. But while NREM sleep is critical for developing the new brain connections involved in learning, the REM sleep that comes afterwards is required to make those new connections as efficient as possible—removing new synapses that are unnecessary and cementing those that are needed to retain what has been learned.[32]

This synergistic effect of NREM and REM sleep on memory is thought to be one reason that we're less able to learn the night after poor sleep—we haven't yet processed and cemented the previous day's memories properly, which leaves us with less capacity to learn more new things. This also probably explains a very common complaint: that annoying feeling we get when a certain fact (or somebody's name) is just out of reach, even though we *know* we know it. Often, particularly as we get older, we worry that these minor lapses are a sign that our faculties are on the decline and that Alzheimer's might be on the horizon. Luckily, this usually isn't the case, and though the effects of long-term sleep deprivation are definitely linked to an increased risk of dementia, most of the time these experiences are more likely due to the shorter-term (and reversible) effects of sleep loss on memory.

In addition to supporting memory, REM sleep plays a role in integrating disparate information to drive creative thinking. In a classic paper by a team from Lübeck, Germany, called "Sleep Inspires Insight,"[33] participants were trained and then tested on a task that involved converting a string of numbers into another string of numbers by applying some simple rules—kind of like deciphering a message written in code, one letter at a time. However, unbeknownst to them initially, there was a more complex rule that could allow them to skip several steps and complete the task much faster. Two groups were trained at 11 P.M. and tested at 7 A.M. the next day, with half allowed to sleep and half staying awake. A third group trained at 11 A.M. and was tested at 7 P.M. to test the effect of staying awake but not experiencing sleep deprivation.

Compared to the two groups who stayed awake, more than twice as many people in the sleep group experienced a "eureka" moment and figured out the complex rule that allowed them to complete the task quickly. A later study did something similar using word associations but this time either allowed participants to nap or not between the training and testing session. By studying the brainwaves of the nap group, the researchers found that it was the presence of REM sleep during the nap that allowed participants to generate more creative solutions to the problem.[34] As a result of experiments like these, it's thought that REM sleep in particular is what allows us to process experiences in a way that supports creativity and helps us generate insight. REM sleep is also critical for processing emotional experiences—almost like your brain's own built-in process of therapy.[35]

Several studies have manipulated the sleep of participants—either one night of complete sleep deprivation or a few nights of only four or five hours per night—to see how sleep influences the way people remember or respond to emotional information. We know that REM sleep is particularly critical to remembering information that elicits an emotional response, such as remembering that you've already seen a cute photo of fluffy kittens that a bunch of neuroscience nerds showed you several hours ago. But while remembering cute photos of kittens can be important (for instance, when sharing memes on Instagram), what happens to our emotional responses when we're sleep-deprived is *particularly* important when we think about how our emotions influence our engagement with the world and other people.

When we're sleep-deprived, the part of our brain responsible for rapid negative emotional responses like anxiety and fear—the amygdala—has higher levels of activation.[36] Activity in the connection between the prefrontal cortex and the amygdala also decreases. The prefrontal cortex is where a lot of decision-making happens; it tells your amygdala that the dog that suddenly jumps in front of you doesn't have nefarious intentions and is in fact a cute, overexcitable puppy that wants to lick your face.

But when we're sleep-deprived, that short-term control of our emotional responses is weakened. We're still able to notice and respond to stimuli that elicit positive emotions, but, on average, we respond more negatively.[37] In ambiguous situations, for example, we're more likely to interpret a neutral image, comment, or facial expression as a negative one. This can have big consequences for how we see the world and interact with others, as well as small consequences that accumulate over time.

We all know how it feels to be sleep-deprived. Our tempers are a little shorter, and in general we're more likely to respond negatively or impulsively in a given moment.[38] This is the real-life version of what the studies on sleep deprivation above show. Studies have also found that when we're sleep-deprived, we feel less social overall,[39] which can make us less inclined to socialise and interact with other people. Over time, our more negative mood or reactions and less sociable demeanor due to poor sleep might then affect our ability to maintain close relationships with loved ones or colleagues, increasing difficulties at work and making us more likely to become isolated as we get older.

So, while we might notice the immediate impacts of sleep loss on our mood, when it comes to maintaining headroom and supporting long-term cognitive function, it's clear that sleep plays a critical role that can evolve over time. Every day we have new experiences and interactions, and learn new information, that must be integrated into the decades of knowledge we have already accumulated. NREM sleep helps to solidify the synapses generated by experiences from the previous day, and then REM sleep makes those connections as efficient as possible, integrating new information into our own bigger picture. In this way, many aspects of brain function are reset, refreshing the metaphorical page for the next day so that we can continue to beneficially interact with and learn from others. In fact, it's this overnight refresh that increasingly seems to be the overarching role that sleep plays in supporting brain health and cognitive function.

WIPING THE SLATE CLEAN

Regardless of how old you are, using your brain is hard work. And, just like your real car (assuming it isn't fully electric), your brain car releases exhaust when it's running—molecules and proteins that accumulate as a result of all that cognitive driving. But unlike your car exhaust, which disappears into the atmosphere so that you can conveniently forget about it, a lot of your brain exhaust just sits outside the cells, accumulating during the day. This accumulation of brain exhaust is what helps create the "sleep pressure" that makes us sleepy in the evening and initiates the processes of sleep. In fact, one of the reasons we experience lapses in attention after being awake for a long time is that the metabolites produced by all our hard cognitive work can lead to sleep-like processes in certain areas of the brain, even while we're still technically awake.[40]

The most common neurotransmitter in the brain is glutamate. Glutamate is an *excitatory* neurotransmitter, meaning that when it binds to receptors at the synapse of a neuron, it gets that neuron aroused and more likely to become activated. Recent studies have found that the buildup of molecules like glutamate during a day of high cognitive load contributes to mental fatigue. In an attempt to simulate different types of workdays, a team of scientists in Paris had participants do more than six hours of cognitive tests.[41] Half the participants did hard tasks that required a lot of cognitive shifting and memorization. The other half got easy tasks that were much less complex. The hard-task group had a bigger accumulation of glutamate in a part of the prefrontal cortex involved with cognitive control, which was then associated with more impulsive choices during decision-making. Similar studies have found that cognitive effort also results in increases in other metabolites, like aspartate (another excitatory neurotransmitter) and lactate (as if your brain had been doing some sprints or heavy bicep curls), and when these increase over time, that means we're more likely to avoid additional cognitive or physical effort.[42]

You know when you've had a long day at work, filled with a ton of decisions, and all of a sudden, the idea of stopping at the gym for your workout just feels impossible? Or maybe, even though you have a fridge full of healthy food ready to cook, you choose to pick up takeaway on the way home? This is why. And it underlies the importance of mental breaks during the day if we want to consistently feel sharp and ready to engage in our work (not to mention the behaviours that support our long-term brain health). But it also shows why sleep is so important for getting ready to perform the next day. People who are sleep-deprived are less likely to engage in cognitively challenging tasks (like learning new skills) as well as other behaviours that help build brain function and, ultimately, headroom. I'm not saying that occasionally skipping a workout or getting some Thai takeaway is a bad thing. But if you continue to do these things over weeks, months, and years, it can add up to a lot less stimulus and adaptation that our brains could be benefitting from.

One reason an accumulation of certain metabolites might increase mental fatigue after cognitive work is that many neurotransmitters—like glutamate—are released into synapses alongside ATP, the main energy currency of our cells. In this setting, ATP acts as a neuromodulator, manipulating the effect of the neurotransmitter it's being released alongside. This ATP is then broken down into adenosine, which builds up during the day. Adenosine acts to decrease the metabolism and activity of the cells in the brain that it binds to, eventually helping to trigger the transition into NREM sleep.[43] During sleep, the activity of the enzyme that breaks down adenosine increases, resetting everything for the next day.[44]

This process is what Matthew Walker is referring to when he says that sleep is the price we have to pay for wakefulness. Using our brains results in the slow buildup of metabolites like adenosine, but also neurotransmitters and inflammatory cytokines, all of which trigger the brain to sleep and are then removed while we slumber. This reminds us that the processes of stimulus and recovery are linked—the more you use your brain, the more it needs to sleep the following night. It also explains why we feel groggy when we don't sleep enough—we haven't yet cleared out all the sleep-promoting metabolites like adenosine. By failing to clear out the inflammatory cytokines that build up during the day, long-term sleep loss can also increase inflammation, which is one way poor sleep is thought to contribute to an increased risk of dementia.[45] And while some metabolites have specific mechanisms for clearance, like adenosine, the brain also relies on a large-scale overnight sweeping operation—much like what happens in the streets of any major city—to make sure it's ready to go the next day.

Shortly after I started my PhD, one of the first blog posts I wrote was about a discovery that has since taken the sleep- and brain-health worlds by storm. In 2012, a team led by Maiken Nedergaard at the University of Rochester discovered a system that washes away proteins and molecules that accumulate outside the cells of the brain during the day. They called it the *glymphatic* system because it involved glial cells (specifically astroglia or astrocytes) moving debris into the lymph nodes, the body's waste-management system. One of the scientists on that team was Erlend Nagelhus, a professor at the University of Oslo whose lab was directly below mine at the time. The first author of the paper—usually the one who does most of the work and writes the paper—was Jeff Iliff, who now happens to be my colleague at the University of Washington.

Using an imaging technique called two-photon microscopy that allows you to watch what's happening in the brains of mice in real time, Jeff showed that there was a fluid system that surrounded the blood vessels in the brain. The coordinated effects of astrocytes, which control fluid flow through pores in their star-like projections, and pulses of blood flow in arteries with each heartbeat, push fluid through the spaces between cells in the brain, clearing out the waste. In a subsequent study, Nedergaard's team showed that the glymphatic system expands specifically during sleep, increasing fluid flow through the brain to clear out all the brain exhaust that has accumulated during the day.[46] In particular, they found that the glymphatic system was responsible for clearing out amyloid protein that had accumulated during the day as a result of neuronal activity—just one of many metabolites and proteins that are flushed by the glymphatic system during sleep.

While most of this work was done in mice and is tricky to replicate in humans (because it generally involves doing multiple MRI scans after injecting a tracer directly into a person's spinal canal), all the evidence so far suggests that glymphatic function is critical to the benefits we experience from sleep, with significantly delayed clearance of waste products if we don't sleep well or for long enough.[47] In fact, one fascinating study that took MRI scans of one person's brain every twelve to twenty-four hours for thirty consecutive days found that the fluid spaces in the brain expanded in the evening as it prepared for sleep, seemingly making room for the glial cells to start their cleanup duties.[48]

Several studies have found that it doesn't take much sleep loss for exhaust to build up in the brain. For example, a study performed at the National Institutes of Health showed that one night of sleep deprivation was associated with an increase in amyloid signal in the brain, and those who accumulated more amyloid had worse moods the next day.[49] Remember that amyloid isn't the whole story of brain function and dementia, but in studies like this one it acts as a marker for everything that accumulates in the brain during the day and needs to be cleared out during sleep. While one night of sleep deprivation is unlikely to have a big long-term impact, both the amount we sleep each night and the quality of that sleep are associated with amyloid accumulation in the brain, again suggesting that if the brain isn't getting enough time to clean out the exhaust, it will have trouble recovering from its daily activities.

Luckily, this effect seems to be reversible. In a study from Matthew Walker's lab, people whose sleep improved over time—regardless of whether it was in their fifties, sixties, or seventies—had fewer signs of Alzheimer's disease–related changes in their brains.[50] This suggests that it's never too late to benefit from a good night's sleep.

The critical importance of the glymphatic system as an overnight metabolic reset during sleep has led to the suggestion that many neurodegenerative disorders may be driven by failures of the glymphatic system or inadequate deep sleep, during which the glymphatic system is most active.[51] For example, in older adults whose brains were scanned more than thirteen years after having their sleep assessed, several parts of the brain were smaller in those who experienced less deep sleep.[52] Relatedly, in a subset of the Framingham study, those who experienced the least deep sleep had the highest risk of later dementia.[53] And recent work by Jeff Iliff has found that military personnel exposed to blasts have altered function of the glymphatic system, which seemed to be worsened by poor sleep.[54] This is thought to be due to injury to the astrocytes in the brain, which affects their ability to regulate fluid flow through the glymphatic system. As glymphatic function during sleep is clearly critical to cognitive function both day-to-day and long term, these changes could explain at least part of the cognitive decline and increased dementia risk seen in those exposed to brain trauma.

In the near future, glymphatic dysfunction might be something that we can overcome with technological advances. There are several promising stimulation technologies that may be able to enhance the effects of sleep in those with either insomnia or brain injury, or in situations where sleep is in short supply and performance could be affected, like on certain military missions. In my role as a visiting scientist at the Institute for Human and Machine Cognition in Florida, I am part of a group working to build a device that supports both REM sleep and glymphatic function in those who are unable to get a full night of rest. Though there are plenty of kinks to work out—like how to time a stimulus to certain brainwaves to get a specific effect—there are several companies and groups of researchers using a variety of sounds, lights, and electrical signals to improve sleep through specific stimuli, and this is an exciting area of future research that I look forward to seeing develop.[55]

In addition to brain trauma, many other risk factors for dementia also seem to coalesce around the glymphatic system, highlighting the critical importance of sleep to support brain health and cognition. For instance, we know that slight expansions of the blood vessels with each heartbeat are an important driver of waste clearance in the brain by creating waves of fluid that move through the glymphatic system.[56] But as we get older, our blood vessels become more stiff and less stretchy, which means that these waves of flow are lost. This can also be compounded by other risk factors related to physical health. Not only do physical activity and blood sugar control directly improve brain health, as we saw in chapters 7 and 8, but being sedentary and having high blood sugar—as well as other cardiovascular disease risk factors like high blood pressure or smoking—can indirectly increase dementia risk by worsening the function of our blood vessels. This, in turn, impairs the ability of the glymphatic system to take out the rubbish each night.

This may help explain why vascular disease and Alzheimer's disease are so commonly found together.

THE BASICS ALWAYS MATTER

If you weren't already convinced before reading this chapter, by now you've hopefully realised that giving our brains time to rest and recover—primarily through sleep but also other types of cognitive downtime—determines how our brains perform each day. Sleep also plays a big role in our long-term dementia risk. This, then, raises the question of how much sleep we need to get in order to reap all of its benefits. In a practical sense, that is actually a difficult question to answer, for two main reasons.

First, while it's relatively easy to have somebody sleep *less*—for instance, in sleep-deprivation studies in the lab—it's hard to make somebody sleep *more* unless their body is amenable to that plan. So we're left with research that estimates how much people are sleeping and then follows their long-term brain-health-related outcomes. Though informative, this type of research can also be hard to interpret. Correlation does not equal causality, and one person may simply need more sleep than another, for a number of reasons.

The second reason that it's hard to give an estimate of how much sleep we need is that our sleep needs change all the time. For instance, we've all experienced the need for more sleep if we're sick. This is one reason sleeping for very long periods (more than nine hours per night) is often associated with worse health outcomes in the general population. It's not that more sleep is bad for you; people who are sicker tend to sleep more. Athletes also have a higher sleep need to recover from all their training, and this is important for both their health and their performance. And sleep is affected by stress, which increases our need for sleep while simultaneously making it harder for us to get to or stay asleep. In fact, one way that we might think about whether stress is "chronic" and tipping over from being beneficial to potentially being problematic is if it regularly interferes with sleep.

There are plenty of studies that show that, as we age, the number of hours we sleep decreases. Though some of this is due to changes in the brain's ability to truly "switch off" during sleep—leading to lighter and more fragmented sleep as people age[57]—I've often wondered whether these sleep changes are partly the result of older adults spending less time engaging in two of the main activities that help to drive the processes of sleep—physical activity and cognitive challenge. This hypothesis comes from looking at how sleep changes as children age. Newborns, who spend every waking hour stimulating their brains to help them grow and adapt to their environment, spend two-thirds of the day sleeping. This amount steadily decreases until adulthood, when humans, on average, spend one-third of the day asleep. Teenage sleep time is somewhere in the middle, because their developing brains still require a lot of sleep. With that said, it's also likely that most teens aren't getting enough quality sleep. For example, in the Sleepmore in Seattle study, the Seattle school district delayed school start time by an hour from 7:50 to 8:45 A.M. during the 2016–17 academic year. Using tracking technology, researchers found that students slept around thirty minutes more on average, and as a result, attendance, graduation, and exam results all increased.[58]

Because performance is so tightly linked to sleep, strategies to support sleep have received a lot of attention over the past decade or two, especially in professional sports. Today, high-profile athletes might completely overhaul hotel rooms to minimise light and noise, or even travel with specific mattresses and pillows to make their sleep environment as constant as possible. These strategies can definitely provide a lot of benefit, and many of the Formula 1 drivers I work with take this approach. But I also think that this kind of hyperfocus on sleep optimization has often been oversold to the rest of us.

When we sleep in a new environment, we tend to sleep less well—a phenomenon called the *first-night effect*.[59] If you're a professional athlete and travelling to games or races all the time, almost every night could induce a first-night effect. Therefore, manipulating your hotel room to make it as similar to home as possible can be of benefit. For the rest of us, though, it's not that we need to necessarily deck out our bedrooms in the latest sleep-supporting technology or follow all the procedures that professional athletes do. Instead, most of us just need to go back to the basics.

I remember once being sent a whole load of sleep-tracking data by a professional athlete. They were using a wearable device that monitored time in bed and attempted to provide a breakdown of the various sleep stages. For most of these devices, despite what their marketing materials might say, the quality of the sleep data they provide can be quite poor. For instance, they're usually not very good at determining exactly how long you're spending in each different phase of sleep.[60] But these devices can be useful for looking at trends, and the trend that concerned this particular athlete was the fact that they never seemed to get any REM sleep.

Though it's very unlikely that they weren't getting *any* REM sleep—part of it was probably an error on the part of the device—a quick glance at the data made it clear what the issue was. Every night, the athlete would spend five or six hours in bed before getting up. We know that REM sleep tends to happen toward the end of the night, so if you don't spend long enough in bed and therefore miss the last couple of sleep cycles, when most of the REM sleep happens, you're automatically going to get less REM sleep—and that will have an impact on your brain over time.

I should point out that this athlete is very successful in their sport. They were operating at an incredibly high level while routinely getting much less sleep than we're told we need to get. But in the search for that extra and ongoing edge, the answer to improving sleep was fairly simple: spend more time in bed. Because being in bed (or any place that's suitable for restful sleep) is the first and most important determinant of how much and how well we sleep. As I said, usually we just need to start with the basics.

Even people whose whole lives revolve around enhancing performance have the same struggles that you or I might have when it comes to embracing the factors that support brain health. But this athlete reminded me that the core requirements for quality sleep are the same for all of us. While this athlete's physical training might look very different from yours because of the requirements of their specific sport, the same sleep principles apply. In particular, if we're trying to build a framework around the type and amount of sleep that will be most likely to help us build headroom to protect our brains for decades to come, there are three main components of sleep to consider.

The first component of good sleep is *quantity*. Having had to point this out dozens of times as a coach, I will (again) state what I originally thought was obvious: if you want to sleep more, you need to make sure that you have enough of what the sleep nerds call "sleep opportunity." Translation: just like the athlete in this example, you need to spend more time in bed. With that bombshell dropped, consistent evidence suggests that most people do best with around seven to nine hours of sleep per night.[61] Getting enough sleep is important for that balance of NREM and REM sleep—shorter nights usually mean less REM sleep and therefore less opportunity to optimise new connections in the brain and process complex and emotional information and experiences.

A recommendation of seven to nine hours of sleep provides a fairly broad range, but considering how different and individual our sleep needs truly are, a range of six to ten hours might be even more appropriate. However, the seven-to-nine-hour range seems to provide the most consistent benefit when measuring brain-related outcomes like mental health, cognitive function, and dementia risk. We can usually do just fine after the occasional night of short sleep, but as the Sleepmore study demonstrated, having additional sleep opportunity makes a substantial difference in how well our brains function over time. Similarly, in a study where university students maximised their sleep opportunity, their reaction times improved, as did their moods.[62] University basketball players who increased their sleep opportunity to ten hours each night in another study slept for nearly two additional hours, and over a period of a few weeks their reaction times, sprint speed, and free throw and three-point-shot accuracy all significantly improved.[63] This shows that giving our brains and bodies the opportunity to sleep as much as they need can result in impressive improvements in cognitive function and proficiency in complex skills.

In addition to quantity, our sleep *quality* matters. People who report more disturbances during the night, or who say they have poor sleep, tend to have a higher risk of dementia later in life.[64] This is probably because interrupted sleep means that we're missing the natural cycling of sleep stages, which synergise to support learning, memory, and our willingness to socialise and engage in cognitively difficult tasks. Again, I don't think that the occasional restless night is going to have too much of an effect, but if it is a consistent problem, it is worth doing something about it.

One of the reasons sleep quality has become so important is because of how people respond when they're not sleeping well—by medicating. In fact, one of the ways sleep quality is measured in studies examining sleep and dementia is by asking people whether they take something in order to sleep. This might be antihistamines like Benadryl, alcohol, or prescription sleep medications. When used for sleep, most of these medications (either prescription medication or self-medication) are associated with worse cognitive function.[65] Part of this may be because of whatever is causing sleep problems in the first place—stress, allostatic overload, or too little physical and cognitive stimulus—but we also know that these sleep "aids" change the quality of our sleep. For instance, both antihistamines and alcohol can make us drowsy, but they tend to reduce the amount of time spent in REM sleep.[66] This leaves us with a REM sleep debt even if we manage to get the recommended seven to nine hours.[67] In animal studies, sleep medications like Zolpidem can also impair neuroplasticity and glymphatic functions in the brain.[68] So, while the mechanisms may differ from one drug to another, they are not necessarily helping you sleep *better*, despite rendering you unconscious.

The final core principle of good sleep is *regularity*. Our bodies run on an internal clock that resets every twenty-four hours based on the inputs we provide it. This clock—often called our circadian rhythm—controls how most of the processes in our body change over the course of the day. This includes everything from how we metabolise food to our hormone levels and body temperature.[69] How well our sleep lines up with our internal clock seems to play a role in the benefits it provides to our brains, with the ideal scenario being that we go to sleep and wake up at approximately the same time each night.

Discovery of the genes and proteins that regulate circadian rhythm resulted in geneticists Jeffrey Hall, Michael Rosbash, and Michael Young receiving the Nobel Prize in medicine in 2017. They found that the expression of thousands of genes, and levels of the associated proteins, cycle up and down during the day,[70] controlling the activity of the majority of metabolic processes in the body in predictable fashion. The upshot of this is that your body is constantly trying to match its function to the activities it expects you to be engaging in at that particular time of day. For example, the glymphatic system expands and contracts to time our nightly clear-out with the time our brains expect us to be asleep.⁷¹ A misalignment between circadian rhythm and sleep is likely why deep sleep is less restorative when we nap during the day rather than during the night.⁷² The balance of sleep stages is also governed by circadian rhythm rather than the number of hours you've been asleep—with more NREM sleep earlier in the night and more REM sleep later. Keeping a regular balance of sleep stages is easiest when you keep to a regular bedtime.

There is another factor to consider when you are trying to line up your sleep with your internal clock. The primary input that controls our circadian rhythm (known as a *zeitgeber*, from "time-giver," in German) is light. Thanks to Thomas Edison's commercialization of the lightbulb, there is now a mismatch between the environment we evolved in and what our brains experience during the nighttime hours. We spend most of our days inside with artificial light, meaning we're exposed to too little sunlight during the day and too much artificial light during the night.⁷³ As a result, daily fluctuations in our light exposure are much smaller than they would be if we were exposed to natural light fluctuations due to the sun, which may make it harder for our body to create robust circadian rhythms that support us feeling alert and awake in the morning and sleepy and ready for bed at night.

Though each of us has a different circadian rhythm, based partly on our genes but largely on our unique daily routines, if we're exposed to natural light, our circadian rhythms will tend to align with the sun. This was shown in two fascinating studies by Kenneth Wright Jr. at the University of Colorado. Participants were taken camping in both the summer and the winter, and each time, within a week, their circadian rhythms had shifted according to the environment's natural light and dark cycles.⁷⁴ As you might expect, the cycles were different in the summer and the winter depending on the length of time it was dark each night.

The power of light over our biology is strong enough that light exposure also seems to influence our risk of cognitive decline and dementia. For example, a study of more than 350,000 people in the UK found that those who spent one to two hours per day in outdoor light—which kickstarts our circadian rhythm each day—had the lowest risk of dementia.⁷⁵ Though it only looked at population patterns, which means the results are by no means definitive, another study that looked at data across the whole of the United States found that dementia was most common in areas where light pollution from artificial light was highest during nighttime hours. In fact, artificial light levels at night were more closely related to dementia risk than local levels of alcohol abuse, chronic kidney disease, depression, heart failure, or obesity.[76] And because light and dark are two sides of the same coin, you probably won't be surprised to hear that a study that tracked individual light exposure in nearly ninety thousand people found that those who were exposed to less light during the day and more light at night had an increased overall risk of death.[77]

One major way that light exposure is tied to long-term brain health is through sleep. As glymphatic function and the balance of NREM and REM sleep are controlled by our circadian rhythm—and therefore our light exposure—more consistent timing of sleep allows you to sleep in tandem with your natural rhythms to better support cognitive function. For example, one study in medical students showed that the more regular their sleep was, the better their exam marks.[78] Another large study found that people who have a more regular sleep schedule have a lower risk of dementia, as well as larger brain volumes—suggesting that a regular sleep schedule helps to build and maintain both functional and physical headroom.[79] Studies even suggest that sleep regularity (going to bed and waking up at around the same time every day) may be more important than sleep duration when it comes to overall risk of death.[80] The risk is most pronounced in those whose sleep is completely unpredictable, so, once again, I don't think having the odd late night or sleeping late on the occasional morning is going to cause any issues. But equally, it might mean that it's worth getting up at your normal wake-up time even if you went to bed late, because that will keep your clock on schedule (not to mention make it easier for you to get back on track the next night).

CONSTRUCTING A BETTER NIGHT'S SLEEP FOR BRAIN HEALTH

For each of the primary components of sleep—quantity, quality, and regularity—there are multiple aspects of our daily routine and our environment that we can leverage or manipulate in order to improve our sleep. Many of these ideas were recently summarised in a review paper written by me and some colleagues—led by circadian biologist Greg Potter—on how we can improve our sleep environment.[81]

Light and Dark

Light is the primary input to our brain's circadian clock, regulating hormones like melatonin that help to initiate sleep in the evening. The best way to help set up this rhythm is to expose yourself to bright light in the morning. Even just ten to fifteen minutes outdoors on a cloudy day is enough to help keep the clock ticking. Lights inside don't tend to be bright enough, so if you struggle to get outside in the morning, specialised bright lamps (the type often sold for seasonal affective disorder) can do the job too. The other side of light is the need for darkness in the evening. As you approach bedtime, turn down lights and the brightness of screens, as even normal room lighting can suppress the production of melatonin. Kids are particularly susceptible to this effect of bright light in the evening, but it affects adults as well.[82] And for both kids and adults, stimulating activities involving screens (games, certain movies and TV shows, or social media use) can provide a double whammy of bright light plus getting you wired when you want to be winding down. In the bedroom, if there are bright streetlights outside or lights on elsewhere in the house, you can put up blackout curtains or wear a sleep mask. Sleep masks have been shown to increase cognitive function and alertness the next day when there's light from outside that can impact sleep.[83] By comparison, in a study where individuals were randomised to sleep in rooms that were either completely dark or had an overhead light on, those who slept with the light on spent less time in both deep sleep and REM sleep and had higher heart rates and worse insulin sensitivity the next day, suggesting that light at night and its effect on sleep quality can add a type of stress.[84]

Temperature

As melatonin increases and we get ready for bed, our body temperature drops. The body needs this drop in temperature to trigger sleep. Have you ever felt really sleepy after a hot bath? That's because of the drop in body temperature after you get out of the water. A hot bath or shower is even something you can use to help accelerate a decrease in temperature and trigger the onset of sleep in the evening. It also helps to keep the bedroom on the cool side—no more than 70 degrees, if not closer to 65. In a recent study where participants were confined for ten days in a simulated heat wave (96 degrees in the day, 79 degrees at night), core body temperature was higher during early sleep, and the warmer people were, the shorter their sleep.[85] There will be some personal preference involved, and maybe some compromise between the people sleeping in the bed or house (says the guy whose wife accuses him of freezing her to death with the house at a *lovely* 62 degrees at night), but feeling cool when you head to bed is about right. Cooling mattresses and mattress toppers are all options if you still get hot overnight. Funnily enough, wearing socks in bed has also been found to help people fall asleep by helping them to regulate temperature.[86]

Food and Drink Timing

Though food should be considered within the context of your overall needs (see chapter 7), changing the timing of food around bedtime can help with sleep. For instance, if you are very active and need a lot of calories, having a small amount to eat before bed can improve sleep by making sure you're not hungry, which can impair sleep. On the other hand, for some people, having a large meal close to bed (within approximately two hours of sleep) can make sleep less restful. After we eat, our body temperature increases as we digest, which may prevent the natural tendency of body temperature to decrease with sleep. Eating a large meal before bed can also trigger acid reflux in some people. If you often wake up during the night to pee, avoid drinking a lot right before bed. If not, having some kind of warm (caffeine-free) beverage can help with relaxation as part of an evening routine.

Air Quality

When we breathe, we take in oxygen and release carbon dioxide. If we're sleeping in a small, enclosed space, especially if there are multiple bodies in the room, this carbon dioxide accumulates and can reach levels where it starts to impair sleep quality and makes us feel sleepier and more sluggish the next day.[87] Opening a window or having the door open so air can circulate to the rest of the home can help with this, and can also help to regulate temperature in the room.

Noise

People respond very differently to noise when they sleep.[88] For some, noise from the street, neighbours, or planes or trains passing by can disturb them during the night and worsen sleep quality. Others adapt to it and can sleep through anything. Ask anybody who lives in New York City or central London whether the street noise affects them, and for most people it doesn't. This is because we get better at filtering out these sounds if they are relatively constant or happen at a predictable frequency. However, for people who do have trouble sleeping due to noise, using a low-level white-noise machine or app can help.[89]

Caffeine

Everybody's favourite stimulant is double-edged. It can give us a boost in mood and improve cognitive function when we're sleep-deprived, but it can also decrease both sleep time and sleep quality. Deep sleep seems to be particularly negatively affected by caffeine.[90] Because of the time it takes to be metabolised, it's best to have your last significant dose of caffeine around nine hours before bed, though drinks with less caffeine such as tea can usually be consumed in the afternoon, as long as you're not having trouble hitting your sleep goals.[91] As an example of this, a recent study looked at the timing of coffee intake and risk of death. They found that coffee consumed in the morning was associated with a lower risk of death, but coffee later in the day was not. All-day coffee drinking wasn't *harmful*, but those who are drinking coffee in the evening are probably also sleeping less well, which might offset some of the potential benefits of coffee (like polyphenol antioxidants).[92]

Relax
This probably goes without saying, but relaxation is a critical part of getting into the right frame of mind to initiate sleep. Many of the tools mentioned in chapter 9 can help here. This includes writing out thoughts or to-do lists before bed, as well as breathing exercises. A breathing pattern that involves a long exhale, like the physiological sigh, can help decrease the time it takes to go to sleep by promoting relaxation. In a group of people with insomnia, doing the 3:7 breathing exercise from chapter 11 significantly decreased the time it took them to fall asleep. Guided meditations such as yoga nidra can also help to improve sleep, as can avoiding screen-based or other activities that are especially stimulating in the hour or so before bed, like video games and intense exercise.[93]

Track (Maybe)
Depending on whether you find the information useful, sleep trackers can be a helpful tool to understand trends as well as to get a picture of your sleep opportunity and regularity. While most current sleep trackers built into rings, watches, mattresses, or wrist straps aren't good enough to tell you a lot about your sleep stages (like the balance of deep sleep and REM), they do a reasonable job of telling you when you were in bed and when you were asleep.[94] They can also help you identify factors that cause large changes to your sleep, such as caffeine, exercise, or alcohol. When used properly, many people—but not all—can find insights from sleep trackers to be helpful. Others can find the data distracting or stressful as they worry about perfecting their sleep, sometimes even resulting in a condition called "orthosomnia"—an obsessive focus on sleep and sleep data from trackers and wearables.[95] So sleep trackers are an option but certainly not essential and not for everybody. Their usefulness will probably also improve over time as technology advances.

Breathe

Health issues like obstructive sleep apnea and upper airway resistance syndrome, which cause people to struggle to continue breathing properly during the night, are another common cause of impaired sleep quality. Sleep apnea may occur in more than 30 percent of the population and is more common in men and in those with evidence of excess energy availability. Due to impaired sleep quality, sleep apnea is associated with impaired cognitive function on a day-to-day basis and higher dementia risk.[96] Luckily, this risk can be reduced with treatments like CPAP as well as better positioning during sleep. If you snore a lot, or if it feels like your sleep is rarely refreshing and you don't know why, it might be worth speaking to your doctor to see if there is anything you need to pay attention to.

Build a Routine

The best way to build sleep regularity and support sleep quality and quantity using the parametres and ideas above is to develop a routine. When creating a routine around sleep opportunity and regularity, it is practical to think about when you need to wake up. For most people, this is fairly consistent because of when we need to work, and having a consistent wake-up time every day (even on weekends) can help set you up for good sleep the following night. Bright light early in the day can also help to set your circadian rhythm and improve sleep that night.[97]

Because most people don't sleep from the minute they get into bed until the minute their alarm clock goes off, subtract thirty minutes to an hour from your sleep opportunity (time between going to bed and getting up) to estimate the amount of time you spend actually sleeping. If the number you get is less than seven hours and you're regularly waking up not feeling fully refreshed or are sleepy during the day, it's likely that you need more sleep opportunity.

The next step is to use the above ideas, or a small subset depending on what you need, to build a routine. Remember to be kind to yourself rather than expecting to be able to sleep eight hours every night right away. Start by trying to get in bed fifteen minutes earlier than usual every (or most) nights and increasing that over time if you're able. In a recent study of more than three thousand participants in the Adolescent Brain Cognitive Development study, going to bed earlier and sleeping longer was consistently associated with better cognitive function.[98] Though it might seem silly, many people like having an alarm for bedtime, just like they have an alarm for waking up. This stops you from having to think about going to bed and makes it easier to develop a routine.

An example is the routine we have in our house. We know we will wake up around 6 A.M. because that's when the dogs decide it's their breakfast time. Knowing that I would like to aim for around eight hours of sleep, I try to be in bed around 9 P.M. Before that, we turn the lights down and my wife enjoys a cup of herbal tea. In bed I read a physical book so that I'm not staring at a screen. We use a low-level white-noise machine to minimise noise disturbances, because we keep the window open for cooling and airflow. My wife often reads longer than I do, so I use a sleep mask. And on the rare occasions when I can't sleep, I usually do some slow-paced breathing or transcendental meditation until I drift off again. The goal of this or any routine is just to help build a slow period of winding down before bed to maximise the likelihood of sleeping well, even when we're busy and have a lot to think about.

Get Help If You Need It

Unsurprisingly, not all sleep issues can be fixed with a cool, dark room and a nice cup of tea. If that's the case for you, one first step that can be beneficial is cognitive behavioural therapy for insomnia (CBT-I), which involves improving some aspects of sleep hygiene—using tools that include some of the other techniques in this chapter—as well as reframing the way you think about sleep. One core component of CBT-I is making sure that you associate your bed with sleep. This means avoiding other non-sleep activities (except maybe one) while you're in bed—especially those that are arousing for other reasons, such as work. When you can't sleep, CBT-I methods often suggest getting out of bed until you feel sleepy again; otherwise, you might start to think of your bed as a place where you *can't* sleep. Studies have shown that CBTI-I improves multiple aspects of sleep in people with insomnia, and it is even available via apps.[99] But if you still struggle with insomnia despite all your efforts, you should always aim to consult with your doctor. Importantly, biological sleep-regulation systems are normally intact in people with insomnia—it's just a case of retraining your body to feel relaxed, comfortable, and safe enough to drift off.[100]

Finally, it's also important to remember that sleep need is driven by demand and stimulus. Exercise during the day increases sleep drive and tends to improve sleep quality that evening.[101] Because of the accumulation of metabolites like adenosine as a result of cognitive activity, we see more sleep pressure and sleep activity in areas of the brain that received a lot of stimulus during the day. So, in addition to starting the process of plasticity and repair, activating a specific area of the brain—for instance, by taking on a new challenge or making complex decisions—

results in more accumulation of the chemicals that drive sleep. This, in turn, means that increased cognitive stimulus can help to initiate and support sleep.

One fascinating—though admittedly small—study looked at the effects of online cognitive training on sleep in adults in their sixties and seventies. Half the group was randomly assigned to the intervention group, doing cognitive training for twenty to thirty minutes three times per week. The others were in a control group that did simpler computer-based tasks that involved reading and drawing for the same amount of time. The cognitive training group significantly improved on several measures of sleep quality after eight weeks, including how quickly they fell asleep each night as well as the total hours they slept. These improvements were associated with better memory and an increased ability to avoid distractions.[102] By comparison, sleep quality and cognitive function in the control group didn't really change. In this way, cognitive and physical stimulus, sleep need, glymphatic function, and the processes of adaptation that occur during sleep all seem to be intertwined. If you want to sleep well, you need to stimulate your brain, and if you want your brain to work well, you need sleep after you stimulate it so that it can adapt, reset, and be ready to do it all again the next day.

In summary, sleep is a highly evolutionarily preserved and highly coordinated activity that is essential to brain health. It allows for the processing, interpreting, and integrating of all the stimuli we've experienced during our waking hours. One might even argue that stimulus is only important because our sleep allows us to benefit from those new inputs afterwards. The whole system is governed by a set circadian rhythm determined by sleep quantity, quality, and regularity, which align synergistically to create a balance of NREM and REM sleep. This all comes together to optimise connections in the brain. Add on the waste removal provided by the glymphatic system, and you can clearly see that sleep is a critical daily reset that clears the decks, allowing your brain to function at its optimal level the next day—helping you to stay sharp, build headroom, and lower your long-term dementia risk.

CHAPTER 13
SEX, DRUGS, AND ENVIRONMENTAL TOLL

I mentioned in part 1 that it's common to find long, evidence-based lists of risk factors for dementia that can become daunting checklists to address. But if we think about the topics covered in part 2 so far—movement, nourishment, cognitive stimulation, human connection, and adequate recovery and sleep—we've hit the areas that are likely to have the biggest overall impact on headroom and long-term dementia risk for all of us. These factors are the primary determinants of human brain health, relevant to everybody, and should form the core of any plan to future-proof your brain.

In Professor Livingston's *Lancet* Commission report on dementia prevention, of the 45 percent of dementia that they felt was preventable (probably a conservative estimate), at least three-quarters of the risk factors were related to complications of excess energy availability and lack of physical activity such as obesity and high blood pressure, social isolation, low education, and sensory loss. Similarly, a massive overview of 182 meta-analyses found nearly twenty modifiable and overlapping risk factors that increased the risk of three big age-related brain disorders—stroke, late-life depression, and dementia. The most protective factors were cognitive activity followed by physical activity (did somebody say *stimulus*?). The biggest risk factors were variables that we know are intimately linked to excess energy availability and being sedentary: high blood pressure, poor kidney function (most commonly due to type 2 diabetes), and high blood sugar. Stress and sleep disturbances were also high up on the list of major risk factors for all three major brain disorders. Therefore, by tackling the big topics we've already covered, you will automatically be addressing the biggest modifiable risk factors that lead to poor brain health.[1]

That doesn't mean that there aren't other important factors to consider. Most of these additional factors, however, can be understood in terms of how they influence either our engagement with stimulus or how our physiology responds to and supports adaptation and recovery.

FIRE AND FERMENTATION

There are two common major determinants of cognitive health that we still have to cover—smoking and alcohol. The *Lancet* Commission included smoking and excessive alcohol use as two of the ten risk factors that contribute to significant dementia risk in midlife. The large analysis examining risk factors for stroke, dementia, and depression estimated that smoking increased the risk of dementia by around the same amount as having poor sleep, high blood pressure, or type 2 diabetes. However, the relationship between alcohol and dementia in this study was more ... complicated. Let's start there, acknowledging that most people who ask my opinion on alcohol usually do so in order to find a way to justify their own intake, whether that's none at all or a tipple every day.

There are two main schools of thought on alcohol, both of which have some scientific evidence to support them. One says that a little is good, but lots is bad. The other says that consuming *any* alcohol at all is fraught with peril. The differences in approach are largely due to discrepancies in how the data are collected and analysed, plus a little bit of personal ideology in the interpretation. Of course, everybody agrees that excessive drinking is bad. Alcohol is addictive, impairs sleep, and at high enough doses acts as a neurotoxin by increasing oxidative stress.[2] Studies consistently show that those who regularly consume more than two drinks per day have an increased risk of cognitive decline, stroke, heart disease, several cancers, and overall death.[3] But what about more moderate consumption?

For a long time, it was thought that small regular doses of alcohol—that nightly glass of red wine—had several health-promoting benefits, particularly in terms of reducing the risk of heart disease.[4] There are some interesting reasons that this might be the case. For instance, red wine can be high in the kinds of polyphenols that benefit cardiovascular function (though I would argue that some dark chocolate and a nice bowl of berries would be better). There's also some evidence from animal studies that small doses of alcohol trigger hormesis, the "what doesn't kill you makes you stronger" idea we met in chapter 11—providing a small biochemical challenge that can boost function, including our capacity to tolerate oxidative stress.[5] Along these lines, several large population studies and meta-analyses suggested that those who drank moderately—up to one or two alcoholic drinks per day—had a lower overall risk of death compared to those who completely abstained.[6] But more recent studies in humans have suggested that the real answer may be even more nuanced.

It seems that a big part of the "benefit" of moderate alcohol consumption in earlier studies was driven by the study design and the participants themselves. On average, moderate drinkers are healthier than abstainers or heavy drinkers. They eat better, exercise more, and are less likely to smoke. When this is taken into account, the supposed benefit of moderate alcohol consumption decreases.[7] Then there's the fact that the definition of a nondrinker can be a bit murky. For example, some studies include *previous* drinkers in their nondrinking group. As people who have stopped drinking entirely may have a prior history of heavy drinking that will affect their future health, this could make the abstainer group have worse health on average than they might otherwise. And while small amounts of alcohol (less than one drink per day on average) do still seem to be associated with a slightly lower risk of heart attacks, this is balanced out by a slightly increased risk of stroke and several cancers. As a result, the best studies suggest that moderate alcohol intake has a minimal net effect on long-term health, either positive or negative.[8]

The picture is similar when it comes to alcohol and the brain. Early meta-analyses suggested that those who averaged around three or four U.S. standard drinks per week might have a lower risk of dementia,[9] though these studies were probably confounded by some of the same issues mentioned above. Other studies found no overall benefit of low or occasional alcohol intakes on either cognitive function or cognitive decline (but also no evidence of harm), mainly because the data were all over the place.[10] Then three large studies from the UK Biobank found that those who averaged two or more UK units of alcohol per day had smaller brains, showing decreases in both grey matter and white matter. And, notably, as alcohol consumption increased, brain volume decreased further and dementia risk increased.[11] For those who are counting, it's worth bearing in mind that one UK unit (eight grams of ethanol) is about half a U.S. standard drink (fourteen grams of ethanol—a twelve-ounce beer or a five-ounce glass of wine).

The upshot is this: while studies suggest that daily alcohol consumption—especially if averaging more than one drink a day—is associated with smaller brain volumes and a higher risk of dementia, there's no strong evidence that we need to listen to the (often quite puritanical) calls to completely abstain. While there's probably little overall *benefit*, one or two drinks once or twice a week probably won't negatively affect brain health or cognitive function. As a result, a drink now and again can absolutely be part of a brain-healthy lifestyle if you so choose. This is the approach I take myself. My wife and I rarely drink at home, but I will partake in a nice cocktail on date nights. And it's this kind of context that can make a big difference. If you *are* going to drink, savor something you really enjoy while having a nourishing meal or spending quality time with loved ones or friends.

MAKING A HABIT LESS OF A HABIT

There are behaviours we sometimes fall into even though we know they might not be supporting our larger goals around (brain) health. Reaching for a beer or glass of wine at the end of the day is a very common example. For others it might be a pint of ice cream or skipping the gym in favour of a night on the sofa. Of course, none of these things are a problem if they happen once in a while. But if you find yourself falling back on these habits on a daily basis, it's probably worth considering your actions a little more deeply.

Rangan Chatterjee is a close friend of mine who has decades of experience as a physician and health educator. He has also written multiple successful books about behaviour change and why we develop the patterns of behaviour that we do. When he works with patients trying to break a habit, like drinking multiple glasses of wine every night, he uses the 3-F framework—*feel*, *feed*, and *find*. When an urge arises—such as reaching for the wine bottle—Rangan recommends that people ask themselves three basic questions:

- What am I feeling?
- How does this habit feed the feeling I'm having?
- Can I find an alternative for when I feel this way?

The idea isn't to immediately stop the behaviour but instead gain some self-awareness about why it is happening. Over time, this understanding can help to shape our actions. As he says, "Understanding why you have a behaviour immediately changes your relationship with it."

Feel

Ask yourself, "What am I feeling?" Is it hunger? Or stress? Have you been on Zoom calls all day and just need a moment to yourself with a nice glass of wine? Asking this question immediately adds a pause between thought and action, which gives us a moment to think about what's *really* going on and what might be triggering our behaviour. Rangan says that, of all the three questions, this one is the most important.

Feed

Then ask yourself, "How does this habit feed the feeling I'm having?" Does it make you feel less stressed for a short time? Does it make you feel like you've regained some control over your day? Often, we fall into less-than-ideal habits when we feel stressed or depleted. We gravitate toward them because we know they are a surefire way to feel a little better in the moment, even though it's not what we want long term. But knowing how the habit feeds your feelings can help you answer the final question so you can get what you need in a different way.

Find

Ask yourself, "Can I find an alternative for when I feel this way?" For some people, it's the ritual—that moment when you pour yourself a drink and can finally sit down and relax in the evening. But does that beverage need to be wine or spirits? There are many non-alcoholic options that can provide the same ritual, complete with the nice glass, the fizz, and the taste. Or maybe you could substitute with an entirely new ritual to help you relax—a bath or a nice walk outdoors to release tension. Whatever gets you that break from the workday and vital time to yourself. If the feeling driving the habit is loneliness, you could phone a loved one or make plans to hang out with a friend. Knowing what you're feeling can help you identify a number of ways to feel better without resorting to one particular habit.

Restructure the Environment

Most habits occur in cycles that involve some sort of trigger, a comforting ritual, and a reward that results from executing the habit. That's why one

> of the most important parts of reshaping a habit is changing the environment by either removing your triggers or making the ritual less automatic. For example, if there are bottles of wine within easy reach in the kitchen, alcohol will likely be in your line of sight while you are preparing dinner. That makes it much easier to trigger the ritual. The easiest way to address a particular trigger, whether it's wine or ice cream, is to not have it available in the house. Yet, even adding some friction can be enough to help you reshape your habit. For example, Rangan once told me a story of a patient of his who didn't want to completely ban alcohol from the house. Instead, he started storing it in a shed in the garden. He could still have a glass of wine or beer every once in a while, but the added friction meant he wasn't reaching for it every night.

In contrast to alcohol, explaining the relationship between smoking and the brain is fairly straightforward. Smoking can negatively impact most of the organs in the body, thanks to increased inflammation and oxidative stress,[12] and as a result smokers tend to have smaller and older-looking brains. Therefore, it's not very controversial to say that there's no amount of smoking that's beneficial regardless of the health outcome you happen to be looking at, including cognitive decline and dementia. One meta-analysis of nearly one million people found that current smokers have a significantly increased risk of all types of dementia, including Alzheimer's disease. Strikingly, the analysis they used found that the effect was linear—the more cigarettes smoked per day, the higher the risk. However, *former* smokers were not at increased risk compared to those who had never smoked.[13] Although these researchers didn't look at how long you had to abstain from smoking to decrease your dementia risk, we know the risk of related diseases like heart disease and stroke is halved within a few years—and gone entirely within ten to twenty years of quitting.[14]

Once you get beyond tobacco products, the research on nicotine gets more nuanced. When administered as a patch or gum to nonsmokers (usually at a dose of one to four milligrams), nicotine improves some aspects of cognitive function, including focus and working memory.[15] This is because nicotine binds to and triggers acetylcholine receptors in the brain. Acetylcholine is a neurotransmitter that plays a critical role in arousal, sustained attention, and motivation. Some of the most commonly used drugs to treat the symptoms of Alzheimer's disease—cholinesterase inhibitors—work in a similar manner by preventing acetylcholine from being broken down, increasing the acetylcholine signal that assists cognitive functions like initiating the processes of storing a memory (also called memory encoding). Of course, none of this means that nicotine should be something we regularly turn to for a cognitive boost. Nicotine delivery methods that don't involve tobacco or inhalation are clearly much less problematic from a health standpoint, but nicotine is still neurotoxic at high doses and highly addictive. It can also result in dependence, tolerance (where you need more to get the same effect), and withdrawal.[16]

These latter points are particularly important when it comes to vapes and e-cigarettes, which have made it much easier to consume large doses of nicotine. The health risks of these products are still debated, largely because they haven't been around long enough for us to gather the necessary long-term data. Some people suggest that they probably carry lower health risks compared to cigarettes, but depending on the quality of the product, the level of regulation, and additives like solvents and flavourings, it's likely that e-cigarettes and vapes can still be detrimental to your overall health.[17] Though it's too soon for there to be high-quality data available on dementia risk, some very preliminary research suggests that e-cigarette use may be associated with lower cognitive function, especially in adolescents.[18]

MATTERS OF THE HEART

Another critical factor—just as important as smoking and alcohol in terms of cognitive decline and dementia—is cardiovascular disease. Several large population studies show that risk factors for heart disease—for instance, smoking, high cholesterol, and high blood pressure—also increase the risk of dementia and the rate of cognitive decline, while therapies that decrease heart disease risk tend to be associated with decreased dementia risk.[19] As mentioned in part 1, the cells of your brain sit inside a network of hundreds of miles of blood vessels that support the function of the whole organ. Healthy blood vessels are essential so that you can respond to stimulus and deliver the oxygen and nutrients that activated brain networks need to function. And as we saw in the previous chapter, pulses of blood flow in healthy blood vessels also help drive the glymphatic system, clearing debris and resetting the brain while you sleep.

As we get older—particularly if we're sedentary or experience chronic excess energy availability, high allostatic load, or inadequate sleep—the function of our blood vessels declines. They become stiffer and develop atherosclerosis, and the cells that line the vessels stop responding to changes in blood-flow demand. This latter change is known as *endothelial dysfunction*. As a result, the body's normal processes of stimulus and recovery become impaired. Though we've seen that the brain can still respond and adapt to stimulus at any age, if we want to maximise our capacity to build and maintain headroom for as long as possible, it will always be important to pay special attention to our cardiovascular health.

The critical importance of the role a healthy vascular system plays in maintaining long-term brain health is underpinned by the fact that almost all the major lifestyle factors we have discussed so far affect both heart disease risk *and* dementia risk. Even though there are technically multiple subtypes of dementia, the vast majority of cases include some aspect of vascular disease. That's one reason I often talk about dementia more broadly rather than delving down into specific subtypes (the other reason is that dementia is typically a clinical diagnosis based on symptoms, and it can sometimes be hard to diagnose exact types).[20] Vascular disease is implicated in the two most common forms of dementia—Alzheimer's disease and vascular dementia—that account for up to 90 percent of dementia cases.[21] This can be due to either small clots causing very tiny strokes that you don't notice in the moment but that slowly add up over time or a more chronic decrease in blood flow to the brain that increases inflammation, oxidative stress, and impaired neuronal and glymphatic function.[22] These effects likely explain the findings from a recent study from the Chicago Health and Ageing Project where those who had better cardiovascular health had lower blood levels of a neurofilament light chain (NfL), a biomarker tied to neuronal injury, which is associated with both cognitive decline and future dementia risk when elevated.[23]

In addition to the broader need to supply blood to the brain, variations in blood supply might explain why certain brain regions are more susceptible to damage in Alzheimer's disease. Consider the hippocampus. Using high-powered MRI scans, a team at the University of Washington recently measured both blood flow and tissue properties of different parts of the brain, including the hippocampus. What they found was, of all the structures they studied, the hippocampus had the richest blood supply, with its physical function intimately tied to the amount of flow through the blood vessels. As a result, they hypothesised that when blood flow is impaired, the hippocampus would be particularly susceptible to impairment—as is seen in Alzheimer's disease—because a good blood supply is critical to its function.[24]

The relationship between cardiovascular health and dementia risk can also start early in life. In an analysis of nearly 2,000,000 people in South Korea, the components of metabolic syndrome—waist circumference greater than or equal to 35.5 inches in men or 31.5 inches in women, high blood pressure (above 130/85 mmHg), fasting blood sugar greater than or equal to 100 mg/dL, triglycerides greater than or equal to 150 mg/dL, and HDL cholesterol above 40 mg/dL in men or 50 mg/dL in women—were all associated with an increased risk of being diagnosed with Alzheimer's and vascular dementia before sixty-five years of age.[25] When looking at the size of the risk associated with each component of metabolic syndrome, high blood sugar and high blood pressure were consistently associated with the highest increase in risk. A similar analysis in more than 350,000 people using data from the UK Biobank also found that heart disease was one of the greatest risk factors for young-onset dementia.[26]

The good news is, this risk is modifiable. There are a number of ways to improve cardiovascular health, most of which we have covered already. For example, physical activity improves blood pressure and blood sugar control. It also directly improves the function of the blood vessels by working the whole cardiovascular system. You might even recall a study mentioned in chapter 7 in which older adults saw significant improvements in blood pressure by just standing up more frequently. Many stress-management techniques, such as meditation and improved sleep, can also improve blood pressure. And, as many of the risk factors for heart disease are related to excess energy availability, improving diet quality (increasing nutrient density and decreasing calorie density) can significantly reduce cardiovascular disease risk.

While all of us can have a significant impact on our cardiovascular health and dementia risk through lifestyle changes—and this is where our focus should always be—we also have to acknowledge that sometimes medications may be necessary as well. For example, one of the reasons that GLP-1 receptor agonists such as semaglutide (Ozempic, Rybelsus, Wegovy) and tirzepatide (Zepbound, Mounjaro) are thought to be promising for the prevention of dementia is that they can offer dramatic improvements in blood sugar, blood pressure, and heart disease risk.[27] If you are considering starting one of these drugs (or even making a significant lifestyle change) to help you lose weight, not only should you have a full discussion with your doctor about the risks and benefits, but this is also a critical time to start resistance training and hitting your protein goals to help you maintain as much muscle (and bone) mass as possible.[28]

Two other categories of drugs that can help support cardiovascular health if needed are those that control blood pressure (antihypertensives) and cholesterol (particularly statins). There are differing degrees of evidence that one or both are beneficial for decreasing dementia risk. In part 1, we discussed the fact that the risk of being diagnosed with dementia at any given age has recently decreased, with experts hypothesising that this may be due to a population-level focus on treating and preventing heart disease. Drugs for high blood pressure and cholesterol, in combination with increased physical activity, improved diet, and smoking cessation, have played an important role in that approach.

The evidence for reducing dementia risk with medications that help manage blood pressure is particularly robust. In general, once your blood pressure is considered high (above 130/80 mmHg), your dementia risk continues to increase as your blood pressure does.[29] Meta-analyses of randomised controlled trials—one of which included nearly one hundred thousand people from twelve different trials—have found that treatment with antihypertensives in people with high blood pressure decreases the later risk of both cognitive impairment and dementia. When data from individual patients was available from these trials, the average reduction in blood pressure associated with this benefit was 10 mmHg for systolic blood pressure (the top number) and 4 mmHg for diastolic blood pressure (bottom number).[30] The goal isn't necessarily to get your blood pressure as low as possible, and your doctor may have specific targets based on your age and other risk factors, but even small improvements can lead to notable reductions in dementia risk.

Outside of medications, the intake of sodium and potassium can be critical for helping to control blood pressure. In general, the medical field has focused on reducing sodium—primarily from salt—to improve blood pressure, but increasing potassium intake is just as important.[31] Several trials and meta-analyses show that reducing sodium intake significantly improves blood pressure, especially in those with hypertension.[32] Similarly, increasing potassium intake or swapping regular salt for a low-sodium substitute that includes potassium (like Lo Salt or Lite Salt) significantly improves blood pressure.[33] However, the greatest impact will probably come from shifting your overall dietary pattern. In the United States and Europe, most sodium intake comes from foods that already contain it, not from the salt we add ourselves during cooking.[34] In general, processed convenience foods tend to have a higher amount of salt and low potassium, which is often lost during processing. Foods high in potassium include many of the nutrient-rich foods discussed in chapter 8—fruit, lentils, beans, vegetables, potatoes, milk and yoghurt, and fresh meat and fish. Therefore, by moving toward a more nutrient-dense dietary pattern that relies less on processed high-sodium foods and makes you less likely to eat above your needs (excess energy availability is also a major risk factor for high blood pressure), you can automatically decrease salt intake while increasing potassium and improving energy balance.

Shifting your dietary pattern can also help boost the intake of nitrate from vegetables like beets and leafy greens. This nitrate is converted to nitric oxide (NO) in the body, which is critical for dilating blood vessels and keeping them functional, including those in the brain. By increasing NO production and blood vessel function, consuming nitrate-rich vegetables can also help to improve blood pressure as well as exercise performance.[35]

In addition to blood pressure, when it comes to determining your heart disease risk, physicians tend to look at LDL cholesterol (LDL-C—sometimes referred to as "bad" cholesterol, though that's an inaccurate term because LDL-C does have its uses). LDL-C is an approximate marker for the level of apolipoprotein B (ApoB) containing lipid particles, which play a role in the accumulation of atherosclerotic plaque in blood vessels—not just in the heart but also in the brain.[36] Your diet, genetics, and overall health all influence your LDL-C levels. For instance, insulin resistance can decrease the number of receptors available to take up LDL-C particles from the blood, increasing their likelihood of being left behind in a blood vessel.[37] When you improve your metabolic health through diet or exercise, cholesterol levels often improve as a result.[38] Dietary fat can also increase LDL-C levels, though it is more complicated than just whether or not you are consuming too much saturated fat. For example, one meta-analysis of randomised controlled trials showed that butter, in particular, increases LDL-C more than most other fats—even other sources of saturated fat like beef fat and coconut oil.[39] By comparison, intake of unsaturated fats like those from olive oil and nuts and seeds are associated with lower LDL-C and heart disease risk.[40] As with everything, though, overall dietary pattern is most important, and I absolutely enjoy having some butter in my diet occasionally. But knowing these relationships can help you decide where you might need to make changes based on your own risk. Increased fibre intake also decreases uptake of cholesterol and related compounds from the gut and has been shown to decrease levels of LDL-C and ApoB, which is one reason fibre has been consistently associated with lower heart disease risk.[41]

Though there are multiple ways to treat high cholesterol, statin medications are by far the most common. Statins decrease the production of cholesterol while increasing the uptake of LDL particles from circulation, decreasing the risk of cardiovascular events like heart attacks as a result. However, in the few randomised controlled trials of statins that have looked at cognitive outcomes, no consistent benefits have been found.[42] Much larger studies have looked at big population datasets (often including millions of people) and found that those with high cholesterol who were prescribed statins had a decreased risk of dementia, particularly Alzheimer's disease.[43] Though we might initially expect statins to have a bigger effect on vascular dementia, this finding isn't necessarily surprising. Firstly, Alzheimer's disease is more common than pure vascular dementia, so it may be easier to see an effect there. Secondly, statins can also decrease inflammation, which we know plays an important role in the development of both heart disease and Alzheimer's disease.[44]

It's worth mentioning, however, that, as there is no strong evidence of benefit (or harm) from statins on cognitive function and dementia risk from clinical trials, current medical guidelines do not recommend them specifically for the prevention of dementia.[45] At least two ongoing randomised trials—STAREE and PREVENTABLE—are specifically looking at statins and whether they help to decrease dementia risk. Their results will provide some clarity in the coming years.[46] In the meantime, it is still worth assessing your cardiovascular risk with your doctor as part of a long-term brain health plan. In a study of more than 450,000 people from the UK Biobank, ApoB was more strongly tied to dementia risk than LDL-C was, with an increased likelihood of dementia in those with an ApoB above 118 mg/dL.[47] This is in the range that would likely result in treatment for those at higher risk for heart disease.[48]

On the whole, converging evidence suggests that your cardiovascular disease risk and your dementia risk go hand in hand. If your risk for heart attack or stroke is high or remains high after trying to address it with exercise, diet, or stress reduction, your plan for future-proofing your brain should include a discussion with your doctor about medications that may help improve both your heart health and your brain health.

THE OTHER SIDE OF MEDICATIONS

While medications can play an important role in supporting various aspects of health related to longer-term risk of cognitive decline and dementia, there is also evidence that your brain may benefit from stopping, avoiding, or monitoring side effects of certain drugs.

Antihypertensives

Sometimes the dose or type of blood pressure medication can make blood pressure too low, increasing the risk of dizziness and falls. Falls can cause head trauma (a risk factor for dementia in its own right) or injuries that put you out of action for long periods of time (decreasing opportunities for stimulus). People who experience symptoms of low blood pressure when taking these medications should discuss alternative strategies with their doctor. Big swings in blood pressure have also been shown to increase the risk of dementia,[49] so the ideal approach is one that helps to prevent prolonged high blood pressure without overcorrecting.

Statins

Some people experience muscle pains (myopathy) when taking statins, which may prevent them from participating in exercise or other physical activities. One potential reason is that statins decrease the production of coenzyme Q10 (CoQ10), which is important for mitochondrial function. While there is little overall evidence that statins impair cognitive function, their impact on CoQ10 may be why a small number of people report fatigue or brain fog when taking a prescribed statin.[50] Supplementing with CoQ10 (100–600 mg/dL) can help with fatigue and muscle symptoms caused by statins,[51] but alternative types of lipid-lowering medications might be a better option if you are experiencing these side effects. (If you notice your cognitive function changing after starting *any* medication, it's time to get in touch with your doctor.)

Metformin

Metformin is a drug used to manage blood glucose in individuals diagnosed with type 2 diabetes. In general, this medication is very safe and works well. It is even being studied in large trials as an anti-aging drug for those without diabetes (though I wouldn't recommend using it for that purpose until those trials are completed). In those with diabetes, there's some evidence that metformin use is associated with a decrease in dementia risk.[52] The reason I mention it here, though, is that metformin can also cause a B12 deficiency, which we know is linked to an increased risk of dementia.[53] If taking metformin long term, be sure to have your B12 levels checked regularly, and consider a B12 supplement if needed.

Proton Pump Inhibitors (PPIs)

Along the same lines as metformin, drugs that decrease stomach acid to treat acid reflux such as the PPIs omeprazole and esomeprazole (Prilosec and Nexium) may alter the absorption of certain nutrients such as magnesium and B12.[54] Some studies have suggested that PPIs are associated with an increased risk of dementia,[55] though other studies have not found an effect.[56] While the jury is still out, if you're unable to manage reflux symptoms without PPIs, it may be particularly important to focus on your diet's nutrient density and to consider checking B12 levels.

MIND THE BEERS

As we get older, there are certain medications that may provide more harm than benefit, including an increased risk of cognitive issues. These medications are assessed using the Beers Criteria (named after geriatrician Mark Beers rather than the world's most popular hoppy beverage).[57] While you don't have to completely avoid all these medications, their use should be carefully considered in adults over sixty-five, especially in those already experiencing some cognitive or physical decline.

First-Generation Antihistamines
Antihistamines that make you drowsy, like chlorpheniramine and diphenhydramine—often found in the evening versions of flu medications or sleep aids—inhibit acetylcholine signaling and can increase the risk of confusion and falls, as well as dementia, if used for extended periods.

Antipsychotics
First-generation (typical) and second-generation (atypical) drugs like haloperidol, quetiapine, risperidone, and olanzapine can accelerate cognitive decline in individuals already diagnosed with dementia.

Benzodiazepines
These drugs are used for a variety of conditions including anxiety, insomnia, and seizures. The Beers Criteria suggest that all benzodiazepines increase the risk of cognitive impairment in older adults.

SEX AND THE BRAIN

Any discussion of brain health would be incomplete without acknowledging that men and women can experience a number of neurological conditions—including dementia—very differently. While the risk of vascular dementia is similar in men and women, around two-thirds of Alzheimer's disease patients are women. Once Alzheimer's disease is diagnosed, its progression in women also tends to be faster. As a result, the global burden of dementia is much greater in women.[58] While men are more likely to experience strokes, Parkinson's and motor neuron diseases, and brain cancers, women experience a greater burden of other neurological conditions such as depression, multiple sclerosis, and headache disorders like migraines.[59] Ultimately, the core steps for building headroom and preventing cognitive decline are the same for everyone, but it is important to understand some of the biological differences between males and females, and where further research is needed. That can also help guide personal decision-making in the quest for better brain health.

Historically, there have been a lot of missteps (and that's putting it nicely) with respect to understanding how biological sex affects health outcomes, particularly when it comes to the brain. Though things have improved over the last decade, neuroscience has consistently been one of the worst offenders. Studies either focused only on males or didn't bother to explore whether sex impacted brain function or outcomes.[60] Part of this stemmed from an assumption that hormonal fluctuations during the menstrual cycle in humans (or equivalent oestrous cycle in rodents) would introduce too much variability into the data. So, rather than being curious about the impacts of hormones on the brain, scientists tended to exclude females entirely. However, when my wife and I wrote a large review paper covering the ways that physiology and the environment can impact development and treatment of neurological disorders, all the evidence we found suggested that, in both humans and animals, data from males and females is similarly variable.[61] This variability is also important because there is a huge amount of critical information hidden inside our differences.

Luckily, the past few years have seen a surge of interest in the female brain, with 2025 hopefully being a significant turning point. Special features on sex and the brain, and women's health in general, were published by top scientific journal groups like *Nature* and *Science*,[62] and the Wellcome Leap foundation launched a $50 million initiative called Cutting Alzheimer's Risk through Endocrinology (CARE), focused specifically on the burden of dementia in women. These efforts joined other large initiatives like the Ageing Adult Brain Connectome (AABC) project funded by the National Institutes of Health, which will examine the effects of stress, allostatic load, inflammation, lifestyle behaviours, and menopause on the trajectory of cognitive function in adults.

CARE is led by Lisa Mosconi, a neuroscientist who has pioneered studies looking at how women's brains change during perimenopause and the menopausal transition. While the long-term goal of CARE is to dramatically reduce the risk of dementia in women by better understanding the effects of hormones on the brain, work by Mosconi and others suggests that there's a lot that can be done right now, even while additional research is ongoing.

There are many reasons that men's and women's brains might be more susceptible to different neurological conditions and then experience those conditions differently once they occur. Some of this stems from differences in the genes expressed by the X and Y chromosomes.[63] For example, even when brain cells or tissue are studied in isolation—removing the influence of other organs and hormones—those taken from males and females respond differently to injury. Male cells from many species show lower antioxidant capacity, making them more susceptible to oxidative stress and certain aspects of aging. However, the greater expression of certain genes on the X chromosome in women—many of them related to the brain, including some that regulate white matter structure and protein handling—might increase the susceptibility of the female brain to the kinds of changes that happen in Alzheimer's disease.[64]

Of course, we are not isolated cells in dishes, and hormones do have a major impact on long-term brain health (though whether and how we might intervene is still being figured out). While it was once thought that the increased prevalence of Alzheimer's disease in women was simply because they lived longer, this doesn't make sense based on the data. Lifespan differs from country to country but, on average, women only live four to six years longer than men. This is not enough of a difference to explain the added cognitive decline and dementia risk that appears to slowly accumulate over multiple decades in women. It's this lengthy timeline that has resulted in a lot of focus on perimenopause and the menopausal transition as the time during which the risk of dementia diverges between the sexes.

One of the important recent shifts in focus when it comes to sex and the brain is the increasing realization that "sex" hormones do much more than simply regulate reproduction. Oestrogen is important for regulating body composition, and it provides support for neuronal function in the brain in all humans, regardless of sex.[65] In women, oestrogen is also responsible for regulating multiple aspects of brain metabolism like glucose uptake. As women enter perimenopause (usually some time in their forties, though it can occur earlier), oestrogen levels start to decline, resulting in irregular periods as well as a number of other symptoms that can last for several years. Many of these symptoms have a neurological component, including hot flashes, mood changes, and insomnia.[66] Some women also experience changes in cognitive function, with decreased verbal memory (recall and processing of written or spoken information) being the most common.[67]

When Dr. Mosconi scanned the brains of women at high risk for Alzheimer's disease, she discovered that glucose metabolism in certain areas of the brain decreased from premenopause to perimenopause, and then again in menopause. This led to the idea that decreasing oestrogen levels were resulting in decreased glucose uptake into the brain (though others have pointed out that ageing may play a role in addition to these transitional hormonal changes).[68] In another, similar study, Mosconi found that oestrogen receptors in the brain *increased* during perimenopause, suggesting that the brain was trying to make the most of the declining oestrogen levels.[69] In areas like the hippocampus, higher oestrogen-receptor levels were associated with lower scores on memory tests. The research team interpreted this as the hippocampi feeling like they weren't getting enough oestrogen to function optimally and therefore increasing oestrogen receptors in order to get as much oestrogen signal as possible.

The correlation between hormonal changes during perimenopause and changes in brain metabolism during that period logically raises the question of whether hormone treatments (menopausal hormone therapy, MHT) might be beneficial for the brain. In many ways, the current state of the evidence is similar to that for statins: some promise from big population datasets, but less support from clinical trials. After a lot of initial promise for MHT, the Women's Health Initiative Memory Study (WHIMS), published in 2003, found that MHT in women over sixty-five increased the risk of dementia and cognitive decline.[70] This resulted in a dramatic decrease in interest in and research on MHT and cognitive function, though many of the results from WHIMS could potentially be explained by the fact that the trial started treatment late (more than a decade after the average age of menopause) and used conjugated equine oestrogens (a group of oestrogen compounds extracted from the urine of pregnant mares) rather than more recent versions of oestrogen that mimic what humans produce.

Several randomised trials have tested MHT in younger women, with no clear effect seen on cognitive function (though treatment groups were often quite small and some of the same comments about the form of oestrogen used could still apply).[71] As a result, MHT is not recommended for dementia prevention based on current treatment guidelines.[72] However, it would also be fair to say that a large trial adequately addressing timing and type of MHT—as well as exploring who might benefit from it most—has not happened yet, which is why initiatives like CARE are so important. In the meantime, large meta-analyses of population data by Lisa Mosconi's group have suggested that early initiation of oestrogen-only MHT may reduce the risk of dementia and improve global cognitive function in women who have experienced surgical menopause after a hysterectomy that included removal of the ovaries.[73] Due to the sudden loss of hormones in these patients, MHT until the age of normal menopause is often suggested both for symptom control and to decrease the risk of cardiovascular disease, osteoporosis, and dementia.[74]

By comparison, the evidence for MHT in women who go through the full menopausal transition remains mixed. In population studies, early initiation of combined oestrogen and progesterone (necessary to prevent an increased risk of endometrial cancer in those taking oestrogen) may be associated with a lower risk of dementia, but in a meta-analysis, the effect was not statistically significant.[75]

Some important answers might lie in the fact that oestrogen seems to be only indirectly related to cognitive function during perimenopause. All women who live long enough will go through menopause, but not all of them experience cognitive decline or dementia. As a result, it's clear that hormonal changes do not automatically increase dementia risk, and some evidence suggests that cognitive changes are potentially secondary to other symptoms. For instance, women who have more hot flashes are more likely to experience cognitive symptoms, with changes in temperature and metabolism thought to potentially alter the connectivity or function of regions of the brain like the hippocampus.[76] In a small study that used a nerve block (injecting an anesthetic into some nerves in the neck) to control hot flashes—a treatment that has nothing to do with hormone levels—cognitive function improved in the treatment group but not the placebo group. In addition, those who experienced greater symptom relief saw greater cognitive improvements.[77]

Another symptom of perimenopause that could influence cognitive function is insomnia, which we know affects cognitive function no matter what the cause. Mood changes and changes in sexual function may also contribute to cognitive symptoms, and these can often be addressed with MHT. It's the specific symptoms of menopause, then, that will best guide the use of MHT, and this is what is recommended by treatment guidelines.[78] While the direct hormonal effects of MHT on the brain are still being investigated, appropriate treatment of symptoms affecting a woman's quality of life would be expected to have a knock-on effect, helping those women better maintain headroom and cognitive function throughout and after the menopausal transition.

It's also worth noting that perimenopause appears to be a time when the effects of other risk factors for dementia might be amplified. The glucose-metabolism changes seen during perimenopause mirror those seen with metabolic disease (and ageing in general). So, if individuals are already experiencing issues with excess energy availability, it is likely to be exacerbated by perimenopause. For example, the Study of Women's Health across the Nation (SWAN) followed more than two thousand women for over seventeen years and found that those who had metabolic syndrome during the menopausal transition years experienced an accelerated decrease in cognitive processing speed (though not in memory).[79]

Many of the factors covered in the preceding chapters may also impact symptoms during menopause. Being sedentary or having lower levels of physical activity during menopause is associated with more severe symptoms, and multiple meta-analyses of randomised trials show that physical-activity interventions improve hot flashes, as well as depression and anxiety symptoms.[80] Both physical activity and relaxation techniques involving mindfulness or slow-paced breathing can also improve insomnia symptoms during (peri)menopause.[81] Diet quality and nutrient status can also play an important role. For instance, symptoms like fatigue and changes in cognitive function in perimenopause are commonly related to iron deficiency.[82] Iron-deficiency anaemia (haemoglobin below 12 g/dL in women or below 13 g/dL in men) is also associated with an increased risk of dementia.[83] On the other hand, if haemoglobin is high (more than 15 g/dL in women or 17 g/dL in men), one of the most common causes is obstructive sleep apnea, which has also been linked with higher dementia risk, as mentioned in the previous chapter.[84]

Finally, it's worth reiterating that studies suggest cognitive changes or other symptoms during the menopausal transition are temporary— it is a transition rather than a permanent state. As an example of this, data from the SWAN study suggested that cognitive functions that worsened during perimenopause bounced back to previous levels after menopause.[85] Longitudinal studies of women from midlife to late life also suggest mood will improve as they move from their mid-fifties into their sixties and seventies.[86] And other studies that ask women about their menopause experiences often find that they report positive aspects of this important life transition, including feelings of personal growth and an ability to focus on themselves.[87] Cognitive flexibility (the capacity to switch between tasks or adopt alternative viewpoints) and crystallised intelligence peak in midlife, and well-being increases steadily for both sexes as they enter their sixties and seventies.[88] This is thought to be a combined effect of increasing wisdom, as well as a greater likelihood of focusing on the positive, rather than negative experiences and memories, as we approach our golden years.

Overall, the data seem to suggest that the strategies you can use to build headroom and support cognitive function will also make it easier to navigate the menopausal transition. However, if you have symptoms that decrease quality of life or prevent you from being able to implement those brain-supporting strategies, personalised application of MHT can be an important part of the bigger picture of long-term well-being, physical health, and brain health. As the field advances in the coming years, future research will no doubt also improve the tailoring of route, dose, and timing of MHT to the individual risks, needs, and lifestyle of each patient.[89]

HORMONES AND THE MALE BRAIN

Testosterone plays a greater role for men than for women in some aspects of brain metabolism, including neurotransmission and the regulation of glucose uptake.[90] Interestingly, in certain areas of the male brain, testosterone is important because the brain converts that testosterone into oestrogen that modulates the function of neurotransmitters like serotonin (involved in mood, sleep, and memory). In large population studies, low testosterone levels in males have been associated with an increased risk of both dementia and depression.[91] As you age, it's also important to have adequate testosterone to maintain muscle mass and strength. Yet, in spite of the societal assumption that high testosterone is required for maximum manliness, testosterone replacement therapy is not exactly a cure-all. As you might expect, studies so far suggest that the full picture is nuanced.

Though testosterone levels do decrease with age, some of the most prominent decreases in testosterone levels are more related to core health and lifestyle factors—metabolic disease, diet, poor sleep, and being sedentary.[92] Perhaps, then, it's not a surprise that studies of testosterone supplementation have found inconsistent effects on cognitive function, with no clear evidence of benefit.[93] This may be because many men stop using testosterone therapies within twelve months of starting,[94] or because the symptoms the individual is experiencing are more related to other factors or health problems that testosterone supplementation does not have the power to fix.

That said, there are some smaller studies that suggest, in men with low testosterone and cognitive complaints, testosterone therapy can improve cognitive function.[95] For men experiencing low testosterone and depression, low libido, or erectile dysfunction, replacement can also improve these symptoms as well as quality of life overall.[96] So, as with MHT in women, hormone therapies in men should be guided by symptoms as well as the bigger picture of other risk factors. If you are experiencing a recent decrease in testosterone levels along with other symptoms, talk to your doctor about replacement—but don't forget that your focus should always remain on addressing core lifestyle factors that are also likely to be driving those changes.

FINDING THE FINAL PIECES

One of the most important things you can do as a scientist is to go out into the real world so others can kick the tyres on your thoughts and ideas to help you refine, improve, or sometimes completely reject them. While I have a lot of varied experience working with healthy individuals to improve cognitive function and have done my time studying interventions in the lab, I have to admit that my experience working with patients who already suffer from significant cognitive decline and dementia only makes up a short chapter of my early medical career. And while there's a lot that a professional scientist can glean from the published literature, it's also important to consider on-the-ground experience from physicians who are seeing these patients, like Deborah Gordon.

Deborah and I first met at a conference more than a decade ago when we talked about how multimodal lifestyle interventions might significantly impact cognitive decline and dementia. This was supported by some promising early work by Dale Bredesen, who at the time had just published data from ten patients for whom a comprehensive and highly personalised set of lifestyle interventions appeared to reverse some aspects of cognitive decline.[97] Having started out his academic life as a highly acclaimed neuroscientist specialising in the search for drug targets to treat Alzheimer's disease, Dale later realised that holistic lifestyle- and metabolism-based approaches were more likely to be successful.[98] Some small trials using Dr. Bredesen's approaches suggest improvements can be seen even in those who are already experiencing some cognitive decline.[99] Deborah Gordon was one of the doctors who helped run those pilot trials.

Deborah is a primary care physician in Oregon who specialises in the promotion of cognitive health in her patients, most of whom are older adults. Every day she sees how risk factors and lifestyle choices contribute to long-term cognitive function. As a result of this as well as her formidable medical training, Deborah makes sure to walk the walk. In her mid-seventies, she is a competitive rower, lifts weights, and gets critical nutrients, as part of a whole-foods diet, from her own vegetable garden as well as the chickens and livestock she keeps. I recently asked her about common clusters of risk variables she sees in her patients, which I thought would help flesh out an overall approach to sustaining long-term cognitive health and function for all of us.

Though I'm obviously biased, I was not surprised when Deborah quickly mentioned the impact of retirement. Even in people who are otherwise active and in good health, she told me, she's seen several patients whose function declined almost as soon as they lost the cognitive stimulation and social connection received through work. (This is one reason she plans to keep working into her eighties.) But while we've already discussed the critical importance of ongoing stimulus for maintaining long-term cognitive function, Deborah's statement also cemented the idea that we need to do whatever we can to minimise the risk of experiencing long periods of reduced cognitive activity.

In chapter 9, I mentioned the Adult Changes in Thought study, where periods of significant illness were associated with drops in cognitive function. Similar results were seen in the Rush Memory and Ageing Project.[100] Though there's a lot that somebody can do to regain function after illnesses—by applying the ideas in this book, for instance—a practical approach to future-proofing your brain would be to minimise the likelihood of major illness. Part of this we've covered by addressing risk factors for major health events like heart attacks, but prevention of falls and infections is also critical.

A common problem Deborah sees across many of her patients is frailty. Frailty has some specific diagnostic criteria—unintentional weight loss, slow walking speed, low grip strength, physical exhaustion, and low physical activity. It also usually comes with increases in inflammation (measured by CRP levels on a blood test).[101] Having at least one symptom of frailty makes you *prefrail*, but checking three or more of these boxes merits an official diagnosis of frailty.[102] However, each of these characteristics occurs on a spectrum, and it's important to recognise that loss of muscle and strength is important even if your body weight stays the same. For example, sarcopenic obesity (low muscle mass in the setting of a higher BMI) is increasingly common in older adults due to decreases in physical activity as well as a general decline in overall population health. Sarcopenic obesity is also associated with an increased risk of cognitive decline and dementia.[103]

As discussed in chapter 7, the structure and function of the brain and body—and their decline over time—are intimately connected. Frailty increases the risk of falls, which can result in brain trauma as well as long periods of being bedbound thanks to broken bones—especially broken hips. There are also multiple other ways that frailty can create a vicious cycle for the brain. Having more muscle and moving it more frequently helps to regulate blood sugar and prevent insulin resistance, but the opposite also holds true. Not only can loss of muscle increase the risk of insulin resistance, but insulin resistance due to excess energy availability can negatively affect muscle mass and strength.[104] This is probably why a recent meta-analysis found that resistance training was the best exercise for improving overall cognitive function in older adults.[105] The combination of being sedentary and having low muscle mass (sarcopenia) can also increase inflammation, which is one of the key links between ageing and cognitive decline.[106]

Chronic inflammation appears to impair cognitive function through a number of mechanisms. In the short term, inflammation is incredibly important because it drives healing and repair. Just like the stress response, inflammation is needed to keep us healthy and able to respond to challenges like infection or injury. Think about the last time you had a cut on some part of your body, or you twisted your ankle. You'll have seen the four cardinal signs of inflammation—heat, pain, redness, and swelling. In medical school you learn these in Latin, mainly because it's more fun to say *calor, dolor, rubor,* and *tumor.* You can even add a fifth sign, *fluor,* which means "secretion." Yummy. When you see these signs, you know your immune system is creating inflammation to hasten the repair process. This happens in a similar way in your brain when it's injured or exposed to environmental elements that might cause damage.[107]

Inflammation, however, becomes a problem when the immune system does not switch it off, or we continue to be exposed to whatever caused the inflammation in the first place. This kind of chronic inflammation might originate within the brain itself (for instance, after a head injury) or elsewhere in the body (such as inflammatory signaling molecules that get released from sedentary or sarcopenic muscles). Even if they're made elsewhere in the body, many of the inflammation messengers (called cytokines) released by the immune system can cross into the brain, affecting its function. As a result, elevated cytokines are often seen in the brains of people suffering from depression or dementia and other neurodegenerative conditions such as Parkinson's disease.[108]

Inflammation can clearly affect our mood and the way we think. Just remember how well your brain worked the last time you had the flu. You probably felt fairly fatigued and maybe even a bit depressed. You also probably struggled to think straight and later found it difficult to remember some of the conversations and interactions you had, or what Netflix shows you watched while hiding under a blanket on the sofa waiting for the misery to pass. All these experiences are direct results of inflammation and its effect on the brain.

Long-term chronic inflammation can have similar effects on mood and cognitive function, though maybe not in such an obvious and dramatic manner. As mentioned in part 1, inflammation in the brain seems to increase well before we see other changes associated with dementia. In particular, this inflammation can directly impact not only the function of neurons but also microglia, changing their ability to support the generation and maintenance of synapses that are critical to learning and neuroplasticity.[109] As a result, a chronic pro-inflammatory state of microglia is implicated in almost every neurological, psychiatric, or neurodegenerative condition.

The chronic inflammation and insulin resistance seen in those with sarcopenia is thought to directly impact the brain, providing the link between frailty and dementia.[110] But, in addition to preventing falls, tackling frailty fits into a bigger picture of promoting overall well-being. This is because the immune system changes in those who are frail can make them more susceptible to infections like the flu and pneumonia. Maintaining physical strength can therefore help support the brain from a variety of angles, including decreasing the risk of major illness—which helps to protect you from further cognitive decline.[111]

ANTI-FRAILTY TOOL KIT

Though some of my advice on preventing or treating frailty is, by now, hopefully self-explanatory (lift some weights and then chase them down with a protein-rich dinner), there are some other things you can do if you are already experiencing a decrease in physical function.

Jump

When Deborah first introduces her patients to resistance exercise, she has them start with jumping. As people lose their muscle and strength with age, the first thing to go are the "fast-twitch" muscle fibres. This is the type of muscle responsible for our maximal strength and power. Fast-twitch fibres are also the part of the muscle we use to catch ourselves when we stumble, allowing us to quickly put a foot or hand out to steady ourselves. The loss of fast-twitch muscle is a major reason our risk of falling increases as we age. By directly stimulating fast-twitch muscle fibres, even relatively small amounts of jumping, bouncing, or hopping can have a big effect on muscle size and strength, as well as bone health.[112] For example, one study had women in their sixties jump from side to side over a box for three to four sets of fifteen to twenty seconds, twice per week. This resulted in significant improvements in both leg strength and function.[113] If you do the maths, this is less than five minutes of jumping *per week*. A similar study had men in their sixties and seventies hop on one leg at a time for five sets of ten repetitions every day for six months, which improved both muscle mass and strength.[114] Jumping is an intervention that requires an almost unbelievably small amount of effort to see some benefits—and it also requires nothing more than a bit of space. Feel free to use bands or straps or even the side of a door or wall to help stabilise you while you jump. Taking five minutes to do around fifty jumps or hops as part of another workout, or just to break up your sitting time, is another great way to start working toward improving your strength.

Blood-Flow Restriction

Thought to have been developed by Yoshiaki Sato in the 1960s, blood-flow restriction (BFR, also known by Sato's term, *Kaatsu*) training is a way of triggering improvements in muscle and bone without heavy weights. Cuffs are placed around the top of the arms and/or legs at a pressure of around 30 to 50 percent above systolic blood pressure.[115] This restricts blood flow returning from the limbs without preventing the blood getting into them. As a result, the muscles have to work harder, triggering improvements in muscle and strength while using higher repetitions of very low weight. Though it sounds daunting, this type of training has been extensively used in those who are frail, elderly, or undergoing rehabilitation.[116] Formal guidelines recommend checking with your doctor first, but as long as it is done according to the normal procedures, BFR is incredibly safe.[117] Though it does not always produce the same improvements in strength and bone mass that heavier resistance training does, BFR is an excellent option when you don't have access to a gym, or if you're frail, recovering from an injury, or new to training.[118] Whenever I travel, I keep a set of BFR cuffs and some resistance bands in my bag so I can get in a good resistance training session no matter where I am. I gave Deborah her first set of BFR cuffs several years ago, and now she's using BFR regularly with her patients. The best cuffs include a hand pump that allows you to measure the pressure and keep it consistent. They also provide general pressure guidelines for those who are just starting out. You can get BFR cuffs easily by searching online, but the ones I use are from a company called B Strong. (I have no affiliation with them, but they support a number of military, academic, and professional sports groups.) Once you get your cuffs, inflate them and perform three to five sets of twenty to thirty repetitions of your given exercise (squats, lunges, bicep curls, push-ups, etc.). Rest for thirty to sixty seconds between each set and don't deflate the cuffs until all your sets are done. This should take about five minutes. You'll get your heart rate up and feel the burn in a short period of time, getting gains without having to lift heavy.

Protein Hacks

Deborah's older and more frail patients often don't eat enough food, which can make it even more of a struggle to get enough protein. Inadequate protein intake is implicated in sarcopenia, metabolic disease, and frailty. This is why one of the diagnostic criteria for frailty is weight loss, which can be offset by consciously increasing protein and calorie intake. For example, in a recent randomised trial in individuals with type 2 diabetes and evidence of sarcopenia, higher protein intake (0.55–0.7 grams per pound per day, as recommended in chapter 8) resulted in improvements in strength and function compared to a control group eating to standard protein guidelines (0.35–0.45 grams per pound per day), who *lost* muscle and strength over twelve weeks.[119] Though Deborah focuses on increasing nutrient density overall by improving the quality of the diet her patients eat, she'll recommend protein bars or protein powders if needed to make sure her patients are taking in enough protein to support muscle mass, strength, and all the jumping they've started to do . . .

Vitamins and Omega-3 Fats

One nutrient that seems to synergise with exercise to help manage sarcopenia is long-chain omega-3 fats like the EPA and DHA found in seafood. Meta-analyses show that omega-3 supplementation improves muscle mass and function in the setting of sarcopenia, potentially by decreasing inflammation.[120] Consuming at least three or four servings of fish per week, or supplementing with 2–4 grams of omega-3 fats per day, provides the intake generally shown to be beneficial in clinical trials for sarcopenia.

When working to improve muscle and bone health in the setting of sarcopenia and frailty, fat-soluble vitamins can be critical as well. Several studies suggest that vitamin D deficiencies increase the risk of sarcopenia, though vitamin D supplementation alone will probably not be enough to change muscle mass or strength.[121] Vitamin K2 can also play a role in improving bone health in those who are older or frail, with benefit seen at doses of at least 1 mg a day (as MK-4 or MK-7), but usually more like 40–50 mg a day.[122] Food sources of K2 include natto and other fermented foods like sauerkraut, eel, cheese, liver, and chicken. Adequate magnesium intake is important too (see chapter 8), with magnesium, calcium, vitamins D and K2, protein, and physical activity all required to provide the necessary components for improving bone health.[123]

INFECTION, IMMUNITY, AND COGNITIVE DECLINE

As we've seen, significant illness can have a major impact on the trajectories of cognitive function. In addition to focusing on interventions that keep her patients physically robust, Deborah recommends other interventions that can prevent illnesses, such as vaccinations. Flu and pneumonia are common causes of illness as people get older, so vaccination can help prevent you from being out of action for several weeks—and therefore help you avoid periods of extended loss of stimulus and function. One particularly interesting example that may provide dementia-prevention benefits beyond just a reduction in illness is the shingles vaccine.

Shingles (herpes zoster) is caused by reactivation of the chickenpox virus, which can lie dormant for decades in the spinal nerves of people who were previously infected.[124] When immune function drops—during periods of extended stress, for example—the virus can pop back up and cause a painful rash in the area of skin associated with the nerve where the virus was hiding.[125] Though the rash usually resolves in a few weeks, some people end up with significant pain in that area for months or years. Since immune system function decreases with aging, shingles is more common in older adults, which is why a shingles vaccination is now recommended for anyone over the age of fifty.

A fascinating recent study looked at the effect of the shingles vaccine on dementia risk.[126] On September 1, 2013, the National Health Service (NHS) in Wales rolled out a shingles vaccine programme, but only for those who were seventy-one years old. If you were born before September 1, 1933, your chance of getting the vaccine was essentially zero percent, but almost 50 percent of the people born the following year got the vaccine. This kind of study is about as close as you can get to a randomised trial without actually doing a controlled study, because you wouldn't expect many other things to change so immediately that they would significantly affect the results.

What the researchers found was that there was a sudden decrease in shingles diagnoses (as you'd expect) in those eligible for the vaccine. There was also a sudden drop in future dementia diagnoses. Not much else seemed to change—healthcare utilization was about the same, and other vaccinations (flu and pneumonia) stayed at similar levels too. Additional analyses suggested that part of the benefit probably came from preventing or minimising reactivations of the virus, but it wasn't enough to fully explain the effect. The authors suggested that there might be a broader benefit of the vaccine for inflammation and the immune system. The same team used a similar approach to study data from when the shingles vaccine was implemented in Australia in 2016 and found the same association with lower dementia rates.[127]

At this point we can't definitively say that the shingles vaccine helps to prevent dementia. Both studies also only looked at one specific type of shingles vaccine—a disabled version of the live virus called Zostavax—that is no longer widely used. However, these studies provide fascinating insight into the fact that infection and inflammation may be contributing to dementia in ways that we don't expect. As an example, another virus implicated in dementia risk is herpes simplex virus 1 (HSV-1), the virus that causes cold sores. Though the connection hasn't been proven, studies have found HSV-1 DNA inside amyloid plaques,[128] and the authors of the shingles studies suggested that the immune response to the shingles vaccine might also be suppressing other viruses like HSV-1.

While we wait for more definitive studies, I think current data gives us something to apply practically as we look for ways to future-proof our brains. We know that it's impossible to completely avoid viral infections, and it could be counterproductive to try. Being exposed to common viral infections is an important part of building a healthy immune system. We also know from chapter 10 that if we completely isolate ourselves from other humans, we can put ourselves at risk of other issues with both our physical and mental health. At the same time, as we get older, we are increasingly susceptible to viral infections that have the potential to knock us back for long periods, or worse. A lot of this risk can be mitigated by doing the things we know build headroom to maintain better physical health, but an increasing body of evidence suggests that it would also be prudent to take advantage of vaccinations and early treatments for viral infections like flu and shingles to minimise the time spent out of action.[129] The less time you spend being sick, the more time you can spend building and taking advantage of your remarkable brain.

FROM THE MOUTH TO THE BRAIN

Viruses aren't the only microbes we need to consider when thinking about factors that can cause chronic inflammation and influence long-term cognitive function. Though an exhaustive list of all the microbes that colonise our bodies would be rather overwhelming—and we're still just starting to plumb those depths from a scientific perspective—the bacteria that colonise our mouths and guts can play a large role in brain health. This is why another one of Deborah's top tips for her patients is to floss every day.

Now, don't get me wrong: the irony of a Brit writing about the importance of dental health is not lost on me. I have one crown in my mouth from back when I was a medical student, and the first time my dentist in Seattle saw it, he immediately said, "You *definitely* didn't get that done in the U.S." This particular piece of dental work is still going strong after two decades, though, so I guess I (and he) can't complain. I do, however, see my dentist much more regularly now than I did in the past, largely because of the ever-increasing evidence linking the mouth to brain health.

The most impactful story I've heard on this topic isn't *directly* related to dementia risk, but it definitely could be. In part 1, I mentioned the work my lab does looking at preterm birth. In those born preterm, once they reach adulthood, there's evidence that they're at an increased risk of many of the diseases of aging, including dementia.[130] One of the triggers for preterm birth is elevated levels of inflammation in the mother, including from infections.

One of my friends and close collaborators at the University of Washington is Greg Valentine, who does a lot of his research in Malawi, a country in southeastern Africa. Malawi has the highest rates of preterm births in the world,[131] and most pregnant women in Malawi show evidence of gum disease. Periodontal disease, as it is more formally known, can start as inflammation of the gums (gingivitis) that can eventually affect the underlying ligaments and bone (periodontitis). Periodontal disease is caused by an imbalance of the microbiome in the mouth, which leads to the overgrowth of certain bacterial species like *Porphyromonas gingivalis*. This imbalance of bacteria can cause systemic inflammation and provide a route for bacteria in the mouth to enter the body. Several studies have found bacteria originating from the mouth in the placenta after pregnancy. Having travelled to the placenta through the blood, these mouth bacteria are then implicated in some cases of preterm birth.[132]

As part of a large international team, Greg helped lead a trial in Malawi in which more than ten thousand women were randomised to a control group that received oral-health education or one that was given xylitol gum to chew twice per day during pregnancy. Xylitol is a sugar alcohol that inhibits the growth of *P. gingivalis* and can improve oral health as a result.[133] In the xylitol group of this trial, there was a significant reduction in preterm births, as well as the number of babies born very small (three pounds or less).[134] This is pretty much the first time that any intervention—especially one as simple as this—has been found to improve preterm birth on this kind of scale. Though he's planning bigger trials to include a placebo chewing gum and cognitive assessments in the babies, Greg's work to date clearly shows how our mouths can affect our whole bodies.

There is also evidence that gum disease may play a more direct role in cognitive decline and dementia risk. More than twenty years ago, *P. gingivalis* was found in arterial atherosclerotic plaques known to cause heart attacks and strokes.[135] And since then, researchers have collected reasonably strong evidence to suggest that poor oral health plays a direct role in the risk of heart disease—either because of bacteria invading the arteries after they enter the bloodstream or through an increase in chronic inflammation.[136] More recently, *P. gingivalis* has also been found inside amyloid plaques in the brains of individuals with Alzheimer's disease.[137] As amyloid can have antimicrobial effects,[138] it's believed that one reason for it to accumulate in the brain is as an immune response to the presence of bacteria and viruses that are causing local inflammation. In line with this, though the results of individuals studies are inconsistent, meta-analyses suggest that those who have periodontal disease are at an increased risk of cognitive decline and dementia, while treatment of gum disease is associated with decreased risk.[139] Periodontal disease is also associated with other issues related to the brain that are often linked to increases in inflammation, such as depression and fibromyalgia.[140]

One recent study of more than six thousand adults using data from the NHANES database in the United States tried to find a more direct link between oral health and dementia risk.[141] They found that those with worse oral health were more likely to be diagnosed with Alzheimer's later in life. The study also measured the amounts of antibodies against oral bacteria like *P. gingivalis* circulating in the bloodstream. Higher levels of antibodies that fight bacteria from the mouth were associated with an increased risk of Alzheimer's disease, suggesting that those with an invasion or infection by those bacteria were more likely to experience cognitive decline.

Just as we might think about minimising significant periods of illness as a part of future-proofing the brain (even if some of the evidence is circumstantial), staying on top of oral hygiene likely has both direct and indirect benefits to brain health—and it is easy to do and low risk. So, if you don't already, brush your teeth every day (ideally, at least two minutes twice a day) and find a way to clear out stuff that accumulates between your teeth and near your gums (floss, water flossers, or interdental toothbrushes). See your dentist or dental hygienist at least a couple of times a year and treat any periodontal disease promptly. In the case of periodontitis specifically, you could also consider chewing xylitol gums (two or three grams of xylitol, two or three times per day), like in Greg's trials, or using a xylitol mouthwash. These can balance your oral microbiome without negatively affecting it in other ways.[142]

THE OUTSIDE THAT'S ON THE INSIDE

As another part of the body teeming with microbes that can affect our health, the gut has recently received a lot of attention for its influence on the brain.[143] The gut has always fascinated me, as it is essentially a continuation of the skin (meaning that the contents of your gut are technically outside your body) that is highly specialised for absorbing nutrients yet also has to act as a barrier to control what gets in.

Just like the brain, the gut is incredibly good at adapting to the environment. This is one reason that humans can thrive on such a wide variety of diets, with many different sources of nutrients. While we're often told that one particular dietary approach is "best" for the gut, most of the evidence suggests this isn't true. Some colleagues and I recently published a paper summarising the literature showing how metabolically flexible the gut can be.[144] While it's traditionally thought that the gut primarily runs on the by-products of gut bugs metabolising fibre (which generates butyrate that our gut cells use for energy), the human gut also seems to work just fine in scenarios where the majority of calories come from protein or fat. This doesn't mean that fibre isn't important—just that the gut is a lot more robust and adaptable than we're often told it is.

When it comes to the brain in particular, there are a lot of factors that make the gut worthy of consideration. The gut and the brain are in direct, bidirectional communication (known as the gut-brain axis), and changes in gut function and the gut microbiome are implicated in a number of neurological disorders, including Alzheimer's disease and dementia.[145] The problem is what to do with this information. Though there are several large studies tying different bacterial species to cognitive decline and dementia,[146] there's little evidence to suggest that we should be trying to directly manipulate our gut bugs in order to future-proof our brains.

One of the problems is that, despite the huge depth and detail of data that scientists have collected about the gut microbiome, the tools we use to collect that information are quite blunt. This means that we don't really know what's going on in there, let alone what we should do about it. For example, if you were inclined to send off some poop for testing to determine what bugs are in it, the most common technique used is called *16S sequencing*. 16S sequencing isn't particularly accurate beyond the genus level. In nonscientist speak, that means the method can tell you that an animal is a dog but can't determine whether the dog is a wild coyote or labradoodle.

More sophisticated tools are increasingly being used, but even these only go one more level down to species. So they could tell you the animal is, in fact, a domestic dog, but not whether it's a Chihuahua or a boxer. And even if it *could* tell you a Chihuahua was residing in your bowels, the problem is that these tests don't have the ability to tell you what that dog (or bug) is actually doing in there—which is what we really care about. Is this a friendly lap Chihuahua that just likes to snuggle or is it possessed by a doggie demon that makes it determined to remove all your fingers at the knuckle? With most commercial gut tests today, it's impossible to know.

Another problem is that our guts are incredibly variable. Two healthy people standing next to each other might only have about one-third of their microbiome in common, and we have no idea whose remaining two-thirds is "better."[147] In reality, I think the most evidence-based statement you can make is that the microbiome *you* want is the one that *you* have when *you're* healthy. This is why many experts in the field have promoted a focus on the idea that changes in the gut microbiome are largely influenced by the health of the host.[148]

This is great news because we already know how to improve the health of the host. You may also know what I'm going to say next: the best and most evidence-based ways for improving gut health or gut symptoms include physical activity, decreasing stress, and improving sleep and diet quality.[149] Even companies that give you personalised diet advice based on your gut microbiome are really just finding ways to give you sensible advice that is largely geared around improving your diet quality (decreasing calorie density and increasing fibre and nutrient density).[150] In fact, studies that employ gut-microbiome-based personalised interventions have often found that the results aren't different from standard dietary advice and support, and results are usually driven by how well people adhere to improving their diet.[151]

If you do want to make a dietary change to support your gut, incorporating some fermented foods would be a great start. A small but well-done trial recently looked at the effects of fermented foods like fermented dairy (e.g., kefir, yoghurt, and cheese), fermented vegetables (e.g., sauerkraut and kimchi), and fermented nonalcoholic drinks (e.g., kombucha) on gut health. They found that fermented foods increased the diversity of the gut microbiome (usually a good thing) and decreased several markers of inflammation.[152] For now, at least, providing a variety of bacteria in the diet with fermented foods—building on a whole foods–based diet that will automatically provide the variety of polyphenols and fibre that have consistently been associated with improved cognitive function and overall (gut) health[153]—is probably better than using probiotic supplements, which often don't work as well as promised unless you're able to find the exact source and strain used in a particular study.

Overall, the best way to keep the gut-brain connection in fine working order is by using the strategies for future-proofing your brain that you already know about—because they also have the power to support the health of your body more broadly. In many ways, that's not surprising. The brain, the gut, and the rest of the body are all part of the same system. The same core factors can improve gut health and, through the gut, continue to enhance headroom and support cognitive function.

IT CAN BE A LITTLE TOXIC OUT THERE

It often feels like our world is becoming increasingly toxic—especially as we read headlines about pollutants in the air we breathe and the food we eat. As a result, it can be tricky to judge how much we need to worry about toxins. There's certainly evidence that the environment can play a role in our risk for cognitive decline and dementia, but some simple steps are probably enough to manage most of that without having to be too paranoid about everything we breathe and put in our mouths.

Air Pollution

Several recent studies have found that air pollution, including from roads, local industrial activity, or wildfires, can increase the risk of dementia.[154] Globally, poor air quality both indoors and outdoors has been ranked as the second-highest cause of death, just below high blood pressure and just above smoking.[155] Inhaling tiny particles (including microplastics), nitrogen oxides, and ozone that are released into the air can trigger inflammation and oxidative stress, as well as physiological stress and increased allostatic load.[156] While it can be impossible to escape the air around you without completely and permanently relocating, a measured approach would include wearing a mask when you're outside on very smoky days—for instance, during wildfire season (an N95 mask will filter out the 2.5 micron particles thought to be particularly problematic). But it's also important to recognise that the air inside can often be several times worse than the air out of doors.[157] So it might be worth considering an air purifier in spaces where you spend a lot of time, which in a recent randomised trial improved blood pressure in people with hypertension.[158] Though there is wide variety in these devices, with some being able to filter more than others, if you live in an area with a lot of air pollution, anything is probably better than nothing. And once you have it installed, you can forget about it. A recent study from the University of Washington also found that the effect of air pollution on dementia risk was attenuated in those who had good B vitamin intake, potentially because B vitamins counteract the increase in homocysteine that can result from air pollution exposure.[159] This wasn't a randomised trial, but it's another good reason to focus on getting enough B vitamins in your diet.

Water Quality

Though the municipal water supply is very safe, depending on the region and your local plumbing, there are several possible contaminants that can potentially affect your health. It would be difficult to cover an exhaustive list, but lead and polyfluoroalkyl substances (PFAS, or "forever chemicals") are two good examples. Lead exposure is associated with an increased risk of dementia, and though exposure has decreased with the banning of lead in petrol, there are still millions of lead pipes that supply water in certain areas of the United States.[160] The risk from PFAS has only been appreciated more recently, but early evidence suggests you can commonly find them in food packaging, nonstick cookware (especially if old or damaged), and drinking water. These forever chemicals can accumulate in the brain, potentially increasing your risk of metabolic disease and dementia.[161] Though not everybody needs it, and it's usually fairly easy to check your local water quality online first, a simple approach would be to start using a water filter. This could be either a jug that you can place in the fridge or something that filters water that flows through the water dispenser or out of your sink tap. As with air filters, there are many different options on the market, but even the basic versions can remove the majority of heavy metals and PFAS in the water, which can add up to a lot of benefit over time.

Microplastics

Microplastics are tiny particles shed from plastic containers, tubes, and pipes and can end up in what we eat and drink. Recent studies on microplastics have received a lot of attention—especially those that have found microplastics throughout the body, including in blood vessels and the brain.[162] One study even suggested that microplastic levels were much higher in the brains of people who had dementia than those who didn't.[163] However, we don't yet know if microplastics play a role in the development of dementia. For instance, the vascular disease that is common in dementia—resulting in slow or inadequate blood flow to the brain—probably makes it more likely that any microplastics in the blood will eventually lodge themselves in the brain. So microplastic accumulation in the brain may well be a consequence, rather than a cause, of dementia. With that said, even if the estimates of microplastic exposure are exaggerated,[164] this is not a problem we should ignore entirely. Other components of plastics, such as bisphenols and phthalates, have been linked to neurodevelopmental disorders in children and heart disease in adults.[165] We can dramatically reduce exposure to (micro)plastics by drinking (filtered) tap water instead of plastic bottled water, using wooden or metal cooking and eating utensils, storing and microwaving food in glass containers, and increasing intake of fresh foods that have not been stored in plastic. While many microplastics are probably eliminated by the body, one very interesting scientific paper suggested that anthocyanins from fruits and vegetables might help counteract some of the negative effects of plastics on health.[166] Another study in mice found that β-glucan—a fibre found in oats and mushrooms that can also help to reduce LDL-C and ApoB—might decrease absorption of PFAS.[167] Though this work was done in animal and test tube studies, and there are currently no trials in humans yet, if the recommendation is simply to eat more fibre and berries, I'm OK with it.

NAVIGATING AN UNFORGIVING WORLD

Having thought a lot about the *internal* environment—blood vessels, the mouth, and the gut—we should also think about some additional ways that the external environment can affect our brain health. This includes the influence of society and our place within it. In addition to the differences by sex, the burden of cognitive decline and dementia disproportionately affects those from more disadvantaged backgrounds. And just like with sex, we're talking about *average* effects across entire populations rather than any single person's experience. But societal effects have been observed to influence dementia risk in multiple large studies, and these make particular sense in light of what we know about the brain from chapters 9 ("Stimulate") and 10 ("Connect").

Though the biological effects of sex no doubt play a large role in the differences in dementia burden in men and women, many have argued for a societal role as well. For example, we know that education is a critical factor in building early headroom and decreasing long-term dementia risk, but at a global level educational opportunities are not always equal for men and women. This seems to explain some of the differences in dementia risk by sex.[168] Similarly, we know that varied, complex, and engaging work can provide an important lifelong cognitive stimulus, and occupational opportunities can also vary by sex. Across the globe, women have historically been disproportionately excluded from higher-paying and more complex jobs, as well as jobs with significant leadership responsibilities that, one could argue, would provide higher levels of stimulus.[169] In the United States, the workforce as a whole was male dominated until the second half of the twentieth century, with women generally expected to take on the majority of caregiving responsibilities in a family.[170] This prevented many women from entering the workforce entirely or hindered their opportunities for advancement at work.

An example of how sex differences in work might play out at the societal level comes from the Seattle Longitudinal Study discussed in chapter 9. When looking at the types of cognitive environments associated with higher likelihood of cognitive decline, one that was highlighted was the role of "homemaker"—which, in this study from the 1950s to 1970s, was a category made up of almost exclusively women.[171] Being a homemaker was associated with more time spent alone and a higher level of disengagement. Even now, women still bear a greater burden of caregiving for both young and old family members, which is also thought to contribute to a higher overall burden of allostatic load.[172] This is, of course, not meant to be a commentary on anyone who performs this kind of job. After all, these roles can look very different from person to person and, depending on the situation, can be very rewarding and involve a lot of cognitive stimuli and social activity. But the results from the Seattle Longitudinal Study do support the idea that traditional societal roles may have resulted in different levels of cognitive stimulus, contributing to the sex differences in dementia risk we see today.

Another critical factor related to sex that potentially explains other disparities in dementia risk is societal support and belonging. I've focused on differences in dementia based on biological sex because that's where we have the best data, but we know the picture is much more complicated than whether somebody has two X chromosomes, especially when it comes to the world that people experience and the ways that world can affect their health. In chapter 10 we saw how social stress can come from many different places, but regardless of its source, it can drive a fundamental shift in our physiology and biology. That shift has the power to impact our long-term health by increasing allostatic load, triggering chronic stress responses and increased inflammation.

Any time somebody feels disconnected from, or unsupported by, the society around them for any reason, their fundamental need for connection and belonging can be disrupted and result in additional social stress. This is incredibly hard to study and measure, but reasons people might experience some kind of social stress that could reasonably be expected to affect their later dementia risk include their sex, race, sexual orientation, and gender identity.[173] Reasons for experiencing a disconnection from society can also come in many forms, from how somebody is treated on a day-to-day basis by others to differences in access to educational or occupational opportunities—or even healthcare—based on their demographic or financial background. Most importantly, it doesn't matter whether we agree that discrimination against a given person—or a hardship experienced by a person—truly exists or not, because the physiological responses to social stress and their downstream effect on health are driven entirely by the experience and feelings of that individual.

As we zoom out again, there are some clearer—though equally hard to solve—reasons that we see differences in dementia risk based on an individual's background. A recent study in the United States using data from more than fifteen thousand people in the Atherosclerosis Risk in Communities (ARIC) study found that dementia burden was greater in Black individuals.[174] By comparison, in the UK, data from nearly one million people showed that the burden of dementia risk factors is greatest in those of South Asian ancestry.[175] In both cases, at least part of this was thought to be due to differences in access to education and healthcare. These factors are often outside of the individual's control due to barriers like a lack of financial resources or speaking a different language. If you can't afford a university degree, or if you struggle to get your high blood pressure treated by a doctor, you have fewer opportunities to improve your headroom and support brain health than you might otherwise have.

As an example of this, the impact of the socioeconomic environment on dementia risk was examined in the Chicago Health and Ageing Project. They found Black participants had more than twice the Alzheimer's disease risk seen in white participants. But this difference seemed to be driven by average differences in socioeconomic status based on the Social Vulnerability Index, which measures factors including education, income, and housing and household structure. When comparing individuals of different skin colours with the same socioeconomic background, dementia risk was not affected by race.[176]

In addition to education and healthcare access, your socioeconomic status can change a variety of factors we know are important for brain health. This includes the type of food you can afford, your access to nature and the quality of the air you breathe, the time and equipment available for exercise, and how safe you feel in your environment. It can also affect the type of work you do, with many lower-paying jobs including shift work, which can influence health by interfering with circadian rhythms.[177] These reasons, as well as many more, might explain why socioeconomic status is such an important determinant of how fast we age as well as our risk of dementia, regardless of other factors like our individual genetics.[178]

Unfortunately, I don't have any good answers for how to solve these broad and complex issues, but I think it's important to know that they exist and can have a real impact on somebody's long-term brain health through no fault of their own. If we're truly going to decrease dementia burden at the population level, societal changes will be needed to support underserved populations who have higher baseline dementia risk as well as less time and fewer financial resources to access education, healthcare, and other tools to support overall health—including brain health. Only we ourselves can know how much any of this might relate to us individually, and how that might impact our ability to build and maintain headroom. But I think an important take-home message (again) is that small changes can have a big impact, no matter who we are or where we come from. And above everything else, I think there is one fundamental approach to leveraging the rules of the brain game that could make at least a small difference when it comes to the importance of a supportive social environment: be kind to others.

As this second part of the book draws to a close, let's take stock of what we've covered so far. We know from part 1 that the brain is more than the sum of its parts and is perhaps too complex to ever fully understand. But, critically, if we step outside of the traditional reductionist approaches to neuroscience, we can have a huge impact on our cognitive function by leveraging our lifestyle and the environment. The strategy is to build headroom—creating physical and functional buffers in our skulls through appropriate stimulus and adaptation. In part 2, we covered the main tactics, tools, and important risk factors that influence headroom. And now that we have those pieces, in part 3, I will present a model of the brain that puts all these pieces of the puzzle together and show you how to leverage what we've learned to support and build cognitive function today, as well as for decades to come.

HOW DO I KNOW IT'S WORKING?

While it can sometimes be important to get hard numbers—tracking your sleep as part of your recovery strategy, examining the nutrient markers mentioned in chapter 8, or identifying and treating metabolic disease or heart disease risk—it is equally important to track, or at least think about, how you *feel*. If we consider that the brain is constantly surveying its environment, filtering an incredible amount of information through all its inputs and outputs, then our mood is arguably a metric that summarises the current state of our brains. Remember my definition of brain health from part 1—*a healthy brain is one that performs the functions you want, at the time you want it to perform them*. If this statement resonates with you and you feel good overall—alert, focused, sociable, and generally like yourself—chances are that things upstairs are in reasonable shape. If you don't feel this way, tracking how you feel over time can help you determine whether something is working as you start to apply changes in your daily life to improve your brain health.

Believe it or not, tracking how you feel is incredibly popular with coaches and athletes, because it can make a strong impact on performance. In fact, mood disturbances and fatigue are much more consistently associated with overtraining (or under-recovery) than most blood tests.[179] Therefore, asking an athlete how they feel is often used to help determine whether they are experiencing low energy availability or are at an increased risk of injury.[180] For the brain, the equivalent of overtraining might be something like "brain fog," or subjective cognitive decline.

Brain fog is often reported by patients with chronic pain and chronic inflammatory conditions, after traumatic brain injury or viral infections, or by women during their menopausal transition. Subjective cognitive decline has a more formal definition and is now considered to be part of the first symptomatic stage of Alzheimer's disease. While this makes it sound fairly concerning, adding subjective changes to a formal dementia diagnostic framework is helpful because that means people are more likely to take it seriously. Though they're not *technically* the same thing, brain fog and subjective cognitive decline have a lot of similarities. Symptoms of both include difficulties with concentration, memory, planning, decision-making, and language, and can also include fatigue, anxiety, depression, and sleep disturbances.[181]

When you're experiencing subjective cognitive decline or brain fog, you'll usually get normal scores on a cognitive function test, so the only people who can really tell that something is different are you and maybe the people who live with you. Historically, this meant that it was difficult for neurologists or other physicians to act upon these early cognitive changes. Now, at least, with expanded guidelines and increased interest in brain fog after the Covid-19 pandemic, people are paying more attention.[182]

You might also notice that many of the symptoms of brain fog and subjective cognitive decline overlap with the symptoms of allostatic overload and burnout mentioned in chapter 12. Though I'm sure there will be a lot more effort to dissect the different patterns of symptoms and their causes across these conditions, for our purposes here, I'm not sure that's necessary. Just know that there are a number of subtle (or not-so-subtle) symptoms we might experience before you can see changes on a cognitive test. And while subjective cognitive decline is associated with an increased risk of dementia later in life, that should be a call to action rather than a source of worry. All the cognitive changes associated with brain fog, allostatic overload, and subjective cognitive decline appear to be reversible.[183]

It's clear that when the brain isn't getting everything it needs, symptoms like brain fog and subjective cognitive decline start to show up. This might be due to lack of stimulus, such as the cognitive changes seen when we're socially isolated. It could be due to being overly sedentary or deficient in nutrients like iron or vitamin D. Or it could be due to inadequate sleep or a high level of chronic stress. Many of the conditions associated with brain fog also include an element of chronic inflammation. But just as each case of Alzheimer's is slightly different based on the individual's genetics, exposures, and lifestyle, we will each experience slightly different symptoms when our brains are struggling.

If you're experiencing any cognitive changes, there are a few things to take away from all this. The first is that your symptoms *matter*. In the process of trying (and generally failing) to apply the reductionist model to cognitive function and the experience of the individual, we've often ignored these subjective changes because they're very hard to quantify, leading people to assume that there's nothing specifically "wrong." Of course, there are common and addressable causes of cognitive changes—like thyroid disorders and nutrient deficiencies—so it's always worth speaking to your doctor and addressing anything that comes up. But beyond that, I think it's worth acknowledging that a lot of the time our brains do a good job integrating our experiences, so any cognitive symptoms you might be experiencing are the equivalent of your car turning on the check-engine light.

So, in addition to measuring important risk markers for general health and cognitive decline, take some time to introspect. Think about how things are going for you and your brain. This will give you another way to track changes as you work to build additional headroom. If you start to feel better, chances are you're moving in the right direction.

PART THREE

A Brain for Today and the Future

CHAPTER 14
THE 3-S MODEL OF BRAIN HEALTH

As I'm sure you can tell by now, I'm fascinated by the history of physiology and neuroscience as well as the wide range of biological, psychological, and societal factors that contribute to brain health. However, as we think about the huge range of factors that can affect long-term cognitive function, it's easy to feel overwhelmed and unsure of where to begin in order to start future-proofing your own brain. In this chapter I'll outline my personal framework for building and maintaining a healthy brain and explain the science behind it. When thinking about what's happening in the brain as we build and take advantage of our headroom, it quickly becomes clear that small changes can have a big impact. More importantly, it's fairly easy to adopt activities that can influence multiple aspects of brain health at the same time.

Though it wasn't what I had initially imagined when I started my career in medicine, a lot of my time in medical school was spent learning how to solve problems. This started with the way our group tutorial sessions were structured in the first year. I should mention first that my path through medical school—doing it as a graduate degree—is relatively unusual in the UK. Though it's becoming more common to do graduate-entry medicine (as we call it), British medical students typically start straight out of secondary school, becoming qualified doctors five or six years later. When I started medical school, however, the graduate-entry path was still fairly new, and there was a lot of flexibility in how the first year was structured before students joined those on the typical medical degree course for the final three years.

The standout feature of my first year of medical school was the regular sessions where we were tasked with diagnosing various weird and wonderful conditions simply by asking the right questions. Everybody would sit in a big circle facing our less-than-expressive course director as he told us about a patient who had come in with a specific symptom. From there we would take a medical history and ask for the results of some basic tests in order to come up with a diagnosis. As we moved through the process, we would see there were often multiple issues to consider—for example, a patient with symptoms of a vitamin B12 deficiency caused by a medication given for acid reflux that wasn't actually acid reflux but was instead a more complex issue with the gut.

While these sessions could be quite frustrating (and could make us feel a bit stupid), everyone I trained with remembers these discussions very fondly. This is because they taught us to think about a medical problem at multiple levels. Rather than simply learning how to recite lists of biochemical pathways and medical diagnoses (which happens during a lot of medical training), the goal was to instead approach the problem logically—understanding what information we needed and how to get it while filtering out red herrings purposefully thrown in to distract us. We learned to take all these pieces of a puzzle and put them together into a bigger picture.

A couple years later, I had the opportunity to apply this type of problem-solving to a less fictional scenario. Sometime around my final year of medical school, my stepbrother—who is about the same age as I am—was diagnosed with multiple sclerosis (MS). MS is an autoimmune neurodegenerative disease where the body's immune system attacks myelin—that fatty sheath that surrounds neurons in the white matter and helps them transmit signals quickly. There is no cure for MS, and it can be difficult to control, even with the latest therapies designed to block the immune response that breaks down myelin. While these drugs can be very helpful for slowing the disease and have continued to improve over time, they can also have severe (though thankfully rare) side effects.

Shortly after my stepbrother's diagnosis, we embarked on a family project led by my then stepfather (a professor of chemical engineering) to try to understand all the possible factors that might contribute to the development and progression of MS. As you would expect, much of the research on MS has focused on treatments for the disease once it is established. Therefore, even though I had studied MS in medical school, the risk factors and environmental components that might make someone more susceptible to MS were fairly unfamiliar to me. In order to better understand the disease, we went to the scientific literature and read everything we could find on the subject. The goal was to assume nothing and then incorporate all related data into a bigger model of the disease. This involved reading well over a thousand research papers on genetics, sun exposure, diet and nutrient status, infections, stress, and other environmental factors that might contribute to the risk and progression of MS.

As part of this process, I learned the basics of systems dynamics—an approach commonly used in engineering fields to model and understand the behaviour of complex systems by describing how individual components interact and influence one another. One of the main outputs of a systems dynamics analysis is something called a *causal loop diagram*. In these diagrams, all the nodes are variables, and arrows between nodes depict how the variables in the system affect one another in feedback loops (figure 1). These diagrams can be incredibly helpful for figuring out common pathways, or understanding how the parts of a system might interact with one another.

When thinking about new or complex topics, or when I'm just wanting to have some casual fun, I often start by drawing out causal loop diagrams. My wife, Elizabeth, who is also a professor of chemical engineering and therefore much more experienced with these techniques than I am, often says that there's a secret engineer inside me just trying to get out. According to her that's a good thing. In fact, it might even have helped to convince her that I was a viable long-term prospect.

When we first met, I was a PhD student in Norway and she was doing her postdoctoral research at Johns Hopkins in Baltimore. For more than two years our relationship consisted mainly of long emails and video calls, but one summer she was able to visit me for nearly a full month. One of my most vivid memories of that time is working together on a large systems dynamics model of metabolic disease. We sat around a table in my tiny studio flat in Oslo, and I called out nodes and their relationships while she built an ever-increasing causal loop diagram to try to explain the interactions between different factors. (If you were ever curious about the weird mating habits of academics, look no further.)

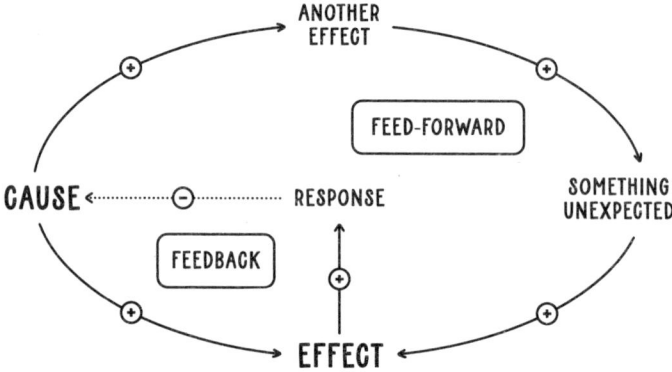

FIGURE 1. An example causal loop diagram. Usually, we think about cause and effect, but in biology the effect normally generates a response that feeds back and decreases the initial cause. At the same time, the cause rarely has just one effect—it might change some other part of our biology in a way that does something else entirely or it might further modify the initial effect through a feedback loop. Solid lines indicate positive effects (one variable increases the other). Dotted lines indicate negative feedback (one variable decreases the other).

In figure 2 you can see a version of a causal loop diagram I made for a biohacking conference a decade ago on the benefits of having a dog, slightly altered here to focus on the brain. I'll admit to being a little biased about the advantages of dog ownership—you'll often find my two boxers, Morgan and Bowen, curled up on the sofa next to me. Of course, you don't have to get a dog to have a healthy brain, and hopefully it goes without saying that you should get a dog because you love dogs rather than as a way to boost your own health. But either way, dogs provide a perfect example of how multiple aspects of health interact and can be shifted by a single new variable.

Starting on the left of the dog model, one of the first things you'll notice is that you have to take your dog for walks. Walking does a whole host of things for the brain, as we know from chapter 7. There are direct improvements to vascular health, blood sugar regulation, and inflammation. Movement can also help us sleep. All these factors support cognitive function. Walking can also boost creative thinking,[1] helping you solve problems you might be facing, which decreases stress and improves well-being.

If you're walking your dog outdoors, then you're more likely to be

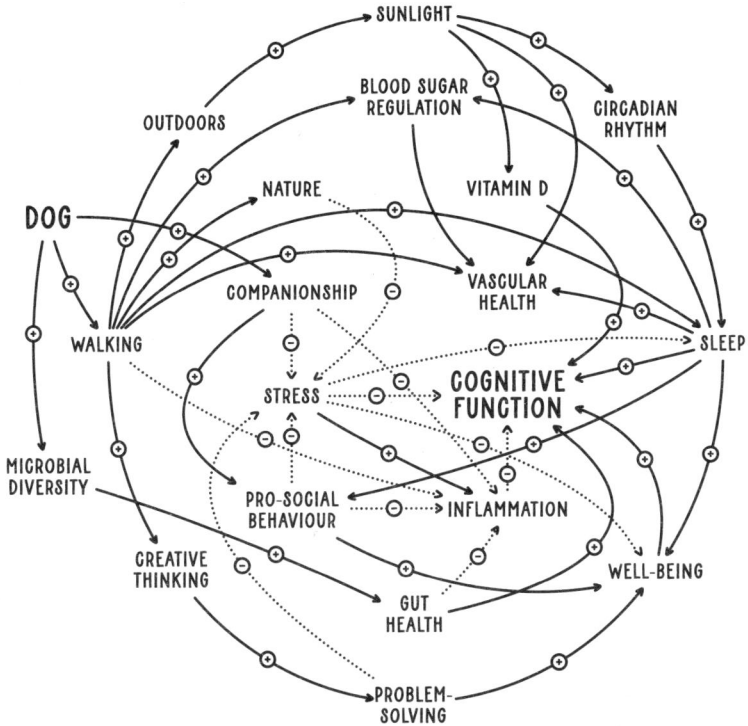

FIGURE 2. How dogs can improve your cognitive function—a causal loop diagram. Solid lines indicate positive effects (one variable increases the other). Dotted lines indicate negative feedback (one variable decreases the other). See text for full description of the model.

spending time in view of nature or at least a tree or two, which can decrease stress. If you're lucky enough to be somewhere with some sun, you may get the added benefit of increasing your vitamin D level. The action of (moderate amounts of) sunlight on the skin has some other surprising health benefits, like increasing production of nitric oxide—a signaling molecule that's important for regulating blood pressure as well as being responsible for directing blood flow changes in the brain as it responds to cognitive tasks and stimuli. As a result, moderate sun exposure can improve blood pressure and potentially decrease the risk of cardiovascular disease.[2] And even if the sun isn't shining, as long as it's light outside during your morning dog walk, that light will help to sync your circadian rhythm, which can also help to improve sleep.

We also know from chapter 10 that dogs (and pets in general) provide companionship and opportunities for prosocial behaviour that can decrease stress and improve overall well-being. People who walk their dogs outside are also more likely to meet other dog-loving humans, which can provide more opportunities for social connection. Though it's admittedly a bit speculative at this point, as our pets expose us to a wide variety of microbes that help to shape our microbiomes, the increased diversity may even support overall health through modulation of the gut microbiota.

You'll see that even in complex models like this one there are some core common features where brain-boosting factors coalesce. For example, many of the paths in the figure act through decreased stress and inflammation, which can then help to reduce the risk of cognitive decline. There are also quite a few paths that result in improved cardiovascular health and sleep. So, while the mechanisms are varied, they often come together in common pathways that help to build headroom. And though we can't (and I would argue we shouldn't) isolate all the individual effects that dogs can have on our brains, even using this theoretical example we can see why evidence shows that dog ownership is associated with a lower risk of cognitive decline and dementia.[3]

As you can see, causal loop diagrams can get very large, even when you are working from a simple starting point. The final versions of the MS causal loop diagrams included several hundred nodes with thousands of connecting arrows, describing the many, many relationships observed in the network. But the benefit of this kind of approach is that you can distill common nodes or areas—like sleep or stress in the dog model—to identify potential intervention points.

Though I can't say that my family's deep dive *solved* MS, for the first time I could begin to see how we might develop a model to explain how a huge range of interacting fixed (e.g., genetics) and modifiable (e.g., lifestyle) factors could come together to influence brain health and function. For my stepbrother, it also allowed him to better understand his condition and come up with approaches to his diet, physical activity, and stress management that have helped to support his energy levels and well-being for fifteen years and counting.

A few years ago, I again found myself thinking about systems dynamics as I tried to better understand how to manage all the variables involved in brain health across the lifespan. From everything we've covered so far, it's clear that there is an incredibly long list of factors with the power to affect our brain health, including sleep, nutrition, cognitive stimulation, stress, and physical activity. And there are still more items to add to that list, as we saw in the last chapter. But one thing that I'm certain of: if we are to successfully leverage these factors to future-proof our brains, we need to stop thinking of these items as a *list*.

AN UNLIMITED CORNUCOPIA OF COGNITIVE FUTURES

As you know by now, there are a vast number of ways that we each can influence our brain health and cognitive function, both today and for decades to come. But when we consider how just a single, simplified model shows that one intervention (getting a dog) can impact multiple pathways related to brain health, it becomes clear that we have to think about the brain, the body, and the environment as one intimately connected network full of feedback loops rather than a list of individual variables.

The dynamic system that influences the function of our brains is one reason I am so hopeful about the potential to dramatically decrease dementia risk at both the individual and population levels. There are so many places where we can start to intervene, and each of those interventions can have knock-on effects across the whole system. This is also why I think current estimates for the proportion of dementia that may be preventable—such as the 45 percent estimated by the *Lancet* Commission—might be too low.

The *Lancet* Commission estimates are based on traditional reductionist approaches, where scientists try to statistically isolate the effect of each individual risk factor. But when you take that approach, you can dilute the impact that a certain factor has on the whole picture of dementia risk. Take, for example, the estimates in their 2024 report—7 percent of dementia due to hearing loss, 3 percent due to depression, 2 percent from diabetes, 2 percent from smoking, 2 percent from high blood pressure, and 2 percent from vision loss. Looking at smoking in particular, we know that smoking increases the risk of all of the other factors I just listed. People who smoke are more likely to get type 2 diabetes and have high blood pressure, and they're at higher risk of presbycusis (age-related hearing loss) and cataracts. There are also bidirectional links between smoking and depression. So, while listing the relative contributions of individual factors to dementia risk can make it easier to get a message across, it ignores how interconnected all these variables really are. If you currently smoke and decide to quit, you will see the *whole* dementia-risk network shift in your favour.

As a result of interactions like these, a huge number of possibilities open up for each of us as we seek to lower our dementia risk. And importantly, our cognitive function does not have one direct predetermined path that we're destined to follow. Rather than following a single path of cognitive function over time—like the lines shown in the figures in part 1—we each have a wide band of potential cognitive function that we are able to achieve or experience depending on how we live our lives (figure 3). This means there are an infinite number of cognitive trajectories that each person could travel along depending on how they choose to stimulate their brain and the ways that their environment and lifestyle contribute to ongoing brain adaptation and function. It also means that there isn't any one way you *have* to live in order to build and maintain your brain health.

Figure 3 is adapted from a paper by Christopher Hertzog, a psychologist and former student of Warner Schaie, who founded the Seattle Longitudinal Study (SLS) mentioned in chapter 9. Simply reading Hertzog's paper, which clocks in at nearly fifty thousand words, could be considered a cognitive stimulus in its own right. But it also perfectly captures the wide range of outcomes we might experience as we create an environment in which our brains can thrive—an environment in which we're able to keep learning and taking on new challenges, can put our skills to use while connecting with others, and are able to support our brains with our other lifestyle choices like a healthy diet and regular physical activity.

Thanks to the SLS, we can be reassured that our brains are surprisingly robust, because all our varied stimuli and supportive lifestyle factors help build critical redundancies into the system. Even if we lose a night of sleep or miss a few workouts, our investment in building headroom means we will continue to have the capability to work at a high level, bringing in additional cognitive resources when necessary. And, though some decline in certain functions with age is probably going to happen to all of us eventually, our brains are capable of increasing func-

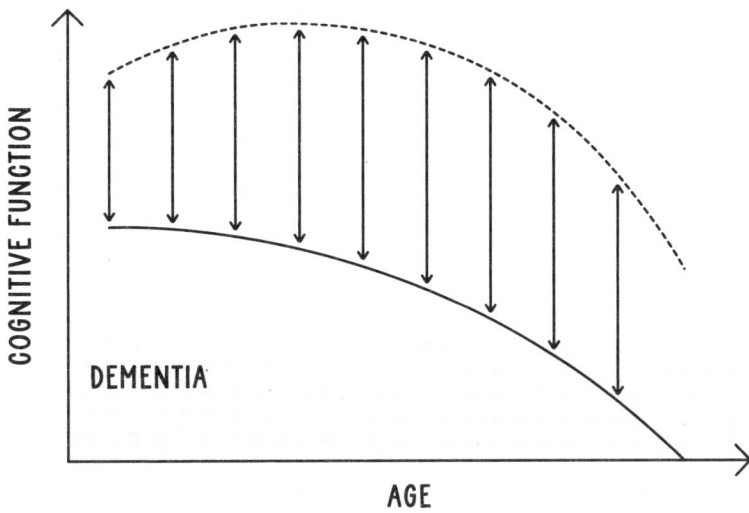

FIGURE 3. Depiction of the band of potential cognitive function that we each have across our lifespan, with age along the bottom (x-axis) and cognitive function along the side (y-axis). Though some decline with age is inevitable if we live long enough, no matter where or when you start, the arrows show that you can increase cognitive function at any time based on how you use your brain and support it with lifestyle factors such as exercise and nutrition. The grey area represents a level where function is low enough that an individual is not able to function as they need, such as in dementia. Each of us has a different graph, but depending on how we navigate it, dementia does not have to be inevitable. Adapted from Hertzog et al., *Psychological Science in the Public Interest* 2008.

tion at any point in life, as long as the right stimulus is provided. This means that, for each of us, there will always be multiple scenarios that will allow us to stay toward the top of our band of potential function, minimising decline over time no matter where we might start.

With that said, we still need to bridge the infinite complexity of the human brain to an actionable framework to build our *own* unique path to a future-proofed brain. If you recall the radio example in part 1, our brains are a collection of billions of infinitely tunable components that interact with one another. Each factor has its own set of causal loop diagrams just like the one for dog ownership earlier. And all those individual diagrams must be combined to develop one big model to explain how everything might fit and work together.

BUILDING A MODEL OF THE BRAIN

The first thing that any model of the brain should be able to account for is that each of us has a unique brain, with our own trajectory of cognitive function and risk of cognitive decline and dementia. Though dementia has a formal definition (a decline in cognitive function severe enough to interfere with daily life and independence), patients all have very different experiences. Each case is particular in its own way, suggesting that each individual's personal set of lifestyle factors, environmental exposures, and genetics will interact in distinctive ways to influence long-term brain function.

This huge variability can even be seen when you look at brain tissue under a microscope. A recent study by the group who performed the Rush Memory and Ageing Project in Chicago (which was used to construct the MIND diet discussed in chapter 8) looked at the brains of more than a thousand older adults after they had died. Pretty much all of them had pathology—accumulations of proteins like amyloid and tau or evidence of blood vessel disease or other injuries—regardless of whether or not they had dementia. Those who had more pathology had worse cognitive function on average, but the researchers found more than 230 different combinations of pathology.[4] This means that in a group of more than a thousand people, one brain might only look similar to one or two others. And that's before we even take into the account the fact that most cognitive function is completely unrelated to how that brain looks under a microscope.

All this variability means that any version of a systems model of the brain has to account for multiple moving parts. Yet it also has to be simple enough to identify the actions to take in order to improve brain health. So, in my model of brain health, I focus on areas that are potentially modifiable—those we are likely able to change—while factors like genetics are given a bit of a back-seat role. Though genetics do play a role in determining our cognitive function and dementia risk, we can't change them. Most importantly, as of right now, there's almost no evidence to suggest our individual genes mean we need to take different actions to support brain health.

As an example of how genetics might contribute to dementia risk but don't necessarily change the actions we need to take to build headroom, let's look at the ApoE4 gene. Apolipoprotein E (ApoE for short) plays a role in how we metabolise fat and move it around the body, including in the brain. We each have two copies of the ApoE gene, and for most of us, each gene can take one of three forms—ApoE2, ApoE3, or ApoE4. ApoE3 is the most common (nearly 80 percent of all ApoE copies), and ApoE2 is the rarest. Evolutionarily, ApoE4 is the oldest form of ApoE, and it seems to be associated with certain benefits, such as improved infant survival early in life.[5] However, later in life, ApoE4 may accelerate some of the effects of aging. Those with at least one copy of ApoE4 also tend to have higher cholesterol levels and a higher risk of heart disease.[6] In the brain, the main producers of ApoE are glial cells, where ApoE4 can cause impaired cholesterol handling, increase inflammation caused by microglia and other immune cells, and contribute to astrocytes becoming dysfunctional as we get older.[7] As a result, those who have one or two copies of ApoE4 tend to have a higher risk of developing Alzheimer's disease, and ApoE4 is considered the most common genetic risk factor for dementia and earlier death.

However, the relationship between ApoE4 and dementia is fairly complicated. The effect of ApoE4 varies depending on your ancestry, and there are several populations where ApoE4 is not associated with a higher risk of dementia. This includes the Bolivian Tsimané, the Yoruba population in Nigeria, and certain groups of Indigenous Northern Americans.[8] Similarly, ApoE4 does not appear to affect longevity in people of Italian descent living in Italy, but does have a negative effect in people of a similar ancestry living in the United States.[9] Therefore, the environment likely plays a large role in the effect of ApoE4 on long-term health.

A large study in Finland found that ApoE4 doesn't change which lifestyle factors are associated with dementia risk. Instead, having one or two copies of ApoE4 *amplifies* the risk of dementia associated with factors such as excessive alcohol intake or physical inactivity.[10] Studies have also found that, though everybody benefits from lifestyle changes regardless of their ApoE genes, those who have at least one copy of ApoE4 often get *more* benefit from physical activity, social engagement, adherence to a Mediterranean-style diet, and treatment of high blood pressure—offsetting their otherwise increased risk of dementia.[11] And similarly, though the data don't come from randomised trials, there is some evidence that those with at least one copy of ApoE4 might be more likely to benefit from statins and omega-3s, and that preventing worsening risk of heart disease over time can also mitigate some of the increased risk of dementia in ApoE4 carriers.[12]

As ApoE4 is the most evolutionarily ancient version of ApoE, it may be that those who carry a copy of ApoE4 experience more mismatch in the modern environment when it comes to common dementia risk factors like being sedentary or socially isolated, or the effect of lifestyle on heart disease.[13] However, as there are potential benefits to all of these interventions and lifestyle factors regardless of genetics, they will still be important to consider even if you don't have a copy of ApoE4. What this means is that knowing whether you have a copy of ApoE4 might change how serious you are about making lifestyle changes to support your brain health and decrease your risk of dementia, but it doesn't really change what you need to do in order to achieve that.

CAN YOU TEST FOR DEMENTIA RISK?

For many of us, having some hard data on our individual dementia risk could be helpful, especially as we try to decide what we might need or what to do in order to decrease that risk. But how might you get such a number? There are dementia-risk calculators out there, but most of them just cover the basics. Your risk is higher if you have a family history of dementia, a lower level of education, or are a woman. Your risk also—obviously—increases with age. Beyond that, with the exception of cognitive stimulus, all the risk factors for dementia are almost identical to those for heart disease, metabolic disease, and many cancers. So far, unfortunately, there's no medical test that accurately predicts dementia, though a lot of work has been done in the area of brain-health biomarkers in recent years, and this area will continue to see improvements.

Blood Tests

Many of the blood tests currently in development for Alzheimer's disease, as you might expect, focus on amyloid and tau. This includes measuring the levels of different forms of amyloid (e.g., Aβ40 and Aβ42) and phosphorylated tau (e.g., pTau181, pTau217, and pTau231) in the blood. Other markers might include levels of proteins associated with injury to neurons (neurofilament light chain, NfL) or astrocytes (glial fibrillary acidic protein, GFAP). The problem is that—at least for right now—what these markers can actually tell us is quite nuanced. Blood tests for amyloid and tau, for example, do increase more rapidly—on average—in those who end up with dementia, and they are quite good at determining who has a lot of amyloid or tau in the brain. As a result, blood tests that examine the levels of certain forms of amyloid and tau were cleared for clinical use by the FDA in 2025.[14] However, we already know that the amount of these proteins in your brain is only part of your cognitive function and dementia risk, a lot of which is also determined by other things like lifestyle factors related to cognitive resilience and reserve (headroom).

A recent study looked at amyloid, tau, NfL, and GFAP markers in more than two thousand Swedish people who were followed for approximately ten years.[15] Having low levels of these markers was associated with a very low risk of dementia, though 5 percent of participants with low marker levels still developed the disease. But even the best combination of these markers could only find a cutoff where 43 percent of people would be diagnosed with dementia. This is definitely much better than not having *any* information, but even those who had high levels of these markers still had a more than 50 percent chance of *not* developing the disease over the period of the study.

One reason for the imperfect degree of accuracy may be that these measures are firmly rooted in the amyloid cascade hypothesis. As we already discussed, this hypothesis only partly explains why some people get Alzheimer's disease and others don't. Without a more holistic group of markers that covers the wide range of pathways and risk factors that can affect dementia risk, we're probably always going to have problems predicting who will or won't get dementia. And while it is possible that these tests and the associated medications developed to target amyloid and tau will have broad utility one day, no one really knows exactly what to do with a patient who has high levels of amyloid or tau in their blood when they don't have any current cognitive issues.[16] So, for now, at least, these markers probably require expert or specialist interpretation and management.

In the coming years, though, we will hopefully have a better ability to map these brain markers to specific risk factors and interventions. Early work by neurologists Richard Isaacson and Kellyann Niotis at the Institute for Neurodegenerative Diseases in Florida found that personalised approaches to dementia prevention—including both medications and lifestyle changes—decreased levels of amyloid and tau markers in the blood in those attending an Alzheimer's disease clinic.[17] Similarly, a study of nearly ten thousand adults in Germany found that NfL and GFAP increased with age, but NfL tended to be higher in men while GFAP was higher in women.[18] Work like this opens the door for exploring specific disease processes based on each individual patient, with the goal of tying them back to targeted interventions, but a lot of work needs to be done before this is possible outside of the research setting or specialist centres.

Genetic Tests

Beyond ApoE4, polygenic risk scores have been developed to amalgamate small effects across hundreds or thousands of genes to help determine dementia risk. Some studies suggest that polygenic risk scores can improve the prediction of dementia when added to ApoE genotype.[19] However, polygenic risk scores are also notoriously unreliable. If they're developed in one population or group of people, they don't do well in another group of people.[20] And if you have a high polygenic risk score, what should you do with that information? Studies show that a healthier overall lifestyle is associated with a lower risk of dementia, regardless of your polygenic risk score.[21] So, just like with ApoE4, the information wouldn't really change what you need to do to lower your dementia risk.

Family History

One of the most common questions I'm asked is, "Will I get dementia because my mum (or dad, grandparent, or sibling) did?" Genetics will absolutely play a role, but one main reason that dementia runs in families has nothing to do with genetics: the environment and lifestyle you share with other family members can contribute to your dementia risk beyond your DNA. For example, one study of nearly ninety thousand people in the Netherlands found that those with a family history of dementia were also more likely to smoke as well as have risk factors for—or evidence of—heart disease and metabolic disease.[22] While these diseases also have a genetic component, they are largely modifiable through lifestyle. Similarly, though it hasn't been published in a peer-reviewed journal yet, a study using data from more than three hundred thousand people in the UK Biobank found that lifestyle changed the relationship between family history of dementia and an individual's dementia risk. In those with a family history of dementia, their risk was dramatically reduced if they followed a healthy dietary pattern, met government physical activity guidelines, slept at least six hours a night, and didn't smoke or drink excessive amounts of alcohol.[23] So, if you have a family member who suffered from dementia, think about any shared lifestyle risk factors you might have with them. This is a great starting point for building new habits.

While diagnostic and genetic tests for dementia risk can be helpful to some people as a motivating factor,[24] right now there isn't much evidence that the results of these tests should influence your approach to future-proofing your brain. The utility of these tests may well change in the com-

> ing years, but for now, the best way to lower your dementia risk is to focus on big-impact areas like diet, exercise, or other things we discussed in part 2. Start with areas where you're confident you can make some positive changes and stick with them for the long haul.

As we saw in parts 1 and 2, potentially modifiable lifestyle and environmental factors may account for the majority of dementia risk. When you add in the data from the different ApoE4 studies, there's no question that these same modifiable lifestyle factors should make up the core of any model of brain health. These are the activities that will increase our brain's ability to function over time by building headroom, no matter who we are.

The same lifestyle factors that contribute to headroom seem to define what some people call *superagers*—people whose cognitive function remains stable from their fifties well into their eighties. Compared to others who experience age-related cognitive decline, superagers have better physical function (strength and fitness) and physical health (are less likely to have high blood pressure, diabetes, or prediabetes), sleep better, and are more likely to engage in cognitively stimulating activities and be socially connected.[25] And despite their name, these individuals do not necessarily have to be super rare or undertake superhuman efforts to achieve their cognitive longevity. In fact, Warner Schaie's work in the Seattle Longitudinal Study suggests that most of us are capable of becoming superagers, as long as the right variables are in place.

While a core set of lifestyle components seems to consistently be associated with improved cognitive function and headroom, there are many different ways to navigate those components. There's no one-size-fits-all approach to brain health. Think about the people you know who have remained sharp into their golden years. Though you might see some commonalities, they probably differed significantly in terms of education level, type of job, hobbies, physical activity, and diet. Therefore, any model for brain function should be able to explain how an almost infinite number of lifestyles and life trajectories can all support long-term brain health.

The fact that there are so many different combinations of lifestyles and activities that seem to support long-term cognitive health suggests that dementia prevention may be less about specific actions and more about common mechanisms that support the brain.[26] For example, we know that high-intensity physical activity is really important for brain health, but exactly *how* you accomplish it matters much less. Similarly, there are core nutrients the brain needs (e.g., B vitamins and omega-3 fatty acids), but as long as you get enough of them their source matters much less. Based on shared mechanisms that seem to explain the majority of what we know about long-term cognitive function, three key areas stand out:

1. Stimulus—cognitive demand or challenge through social or mental activities
2. Supply—the energy, oxygen, and important nutrients that allow us to respond to stimuli
3. Support—the processes of neuroplasticity, maintenance, and repair that occur during rest and sleep

The stimulus, supply, and support that your brain experiences will directly influence its structure and function. It is important to note that structure and function are also tightly linked—to improve function in the long term you need improvements in brain structure, and together these provide greater capacity in the system. That extra capacity is your headroom. This whole process can also support a big virtuous cycle: if you improve function, you're able to expose yourself to a wider range of stimuli. By exposing yourself to more stimuli, you improve function even further. Just like lifting weights—the stronger you get, the more you can lift, and the more you can lift, the stronger you get. Repeat.

For all the reasons we discussed in chapter 9, my model of brain health focuses on how we use our brains, because stimulus drives how our brains function. This is true in terms of both our unique skills and more universal brain functions like memory, information processing, and decision-making—during development and as we get older. These cognitive processes involve multiple regions and coordinated networks of cells in the brain. The connections within those networks are cemented and then refined over time based on how they are used.

But brain health needs more than just stimuli. Areas of the brain that are activated by a given stimulus require resources in order to respond.

This includes a constant and adaptable supply of oxygen, energy, and nutrients delivered through the bloodstream, which requires a healthy heart and vascular system. We also need good energy regulation and physical health, avoiding states of excess energy availability and insulin resistance. Oxygen and energy sources like glucose, delivered by the bloodstream to our brains, combine in the mitochondria to produce ATP, the main energy currency for our cells. Mitochondria require the nutrients discussed in chapter 8 in order to function optimally, and these nutrients are also critical to the growth and maintenance of cells and connections in the brain. So, taken together, the health of our blood supply, energy supply, and nutrient supply all underpin the response to brain stimulation.

Finally, to physically change the brain—and even just to maintain it over time—we need support, which encompasses the adaptation and repair processes that drive new connections while strengthening old ones and performing maintenance on our cells. The most important support process of all is sleep, which is when memories are stored and cells are repaired. But, as discussed in chapter 12, we can activate similar restoration and replenishment processes by allowing ourselves adequate breaks around cognitively challenging or stressful stimuli.

Support and recovery processes can be further augmented by hormones (like testosterone or oestrogen), or trophic factors like BDNF and IGF-1 that are produced during exercise. Recovery can be impaired by unresolved stress (high allostatic load) or a variety of other exposures that affect the function of our cells by increasing inflammation or oxidative stress, such as excessive alcohol intake, smoking, or the various environmental factors discussed in chapter 13.

The three main nodes of the model—stimulus, supply, and support—are intimately connected. When we challenge our brains, the parts of the brain that we're using increase their blood supply to obtain more oxygen and nutrients through neurovascular coupling. And as the cells in the brain are challenged, they initiate the processes that will result in repair and adaptation during sleep and rest. Many of the activities that drive stimulus, supply, and support also overlap. For instance, exercise can directly stimulate the brain, but it also improves heart health, which improves the supply of oxygen and nutrients to the brain. Exercise can also improve sleep as well as triggering the production of supportive trophic factors like BDNF that help strengthen the function of parts of the brain that have recently been stimulated.

By altering the inputs of stimulus, supply, and support, the net result is changes in brain structure and improvements in brain function that influence our ability to focus and perform. As those outcomes improve, our long-term risk of dementia decreases. Thinking about all the ways stimulus, supply, and support interact, you can also see why you can't treat dementia risk factors as one long checklist. Instead, we should think about brain function in terms of a systems model of interconnected common pathways. A slightly simplified overview of this systems approach, which I call the 3-S model for *stimulus, supply,* and *support* (essentially, a causal loop diagram in slightly sexier clothing), is shown in figure 4.

Understanding this figure, and thinking about how it might apply to you, is probably the second most important part of this book. I almost said it was the *most* important, but I still think the most important part of this book is the message that your brain is incredibly adaptable and that you have a huge amount of control over your cognitive destiny. By applying the right stimulus, you have the power to change your brain at any age. How you go about achieving this change can be explained by the 3-S model.

THE 3-S MODEL IN PRACTICE

The interconnected nature of stimulus, support, and supply helps to explain at least some of the variability we see in individuals with dementia. It also explains why sometimes the benefit of one thing requires something else, or the negative effect of one risk factor can be offset by another. The fact that we're unable to fully understand how the brain works through the reductionist scientific approach is at least partly due to these different interactions and synergies that come together to create the final output of cognition.

In one person, a single major issue in one variable might be enough to dramatically increase the risk of cognitive decline. But, in those who have good long-term cognitive function—like superagers—it's likely that lots of small effects across the entire model come together to produce what seem to be age-defying brains. Knowing this allows us to

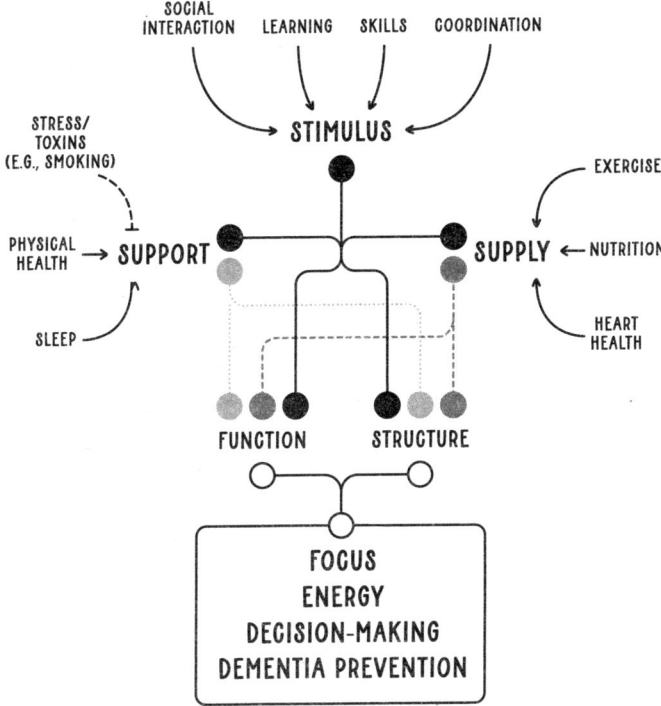

FIGURE 4. The 3-S model of brain function. Critical components of brain health are depicted as an interacting network, like train lines. The solid "stimulus" line is where the journey starts, connecting to all the other stations. Stimulus results in greater supply of blood and nutrients to an area of the brain as well as driving adaptation and repair processes and sleep the following night. Feeding into the stimulus station are factors that can beneficially challenge our brains like skill learning and social interaction. The dashed "supply" and dotted "support" lines then come in and support the "demand" line to change brain structure and function. Inputs to the supply station include heart health and exercise, with the support station having inputs like sleep but also physical health (e.g., levels of inflammation or blood sugar) and other exposures like smoking that can impair the ability of the brain to respond to increased demand. The outputs of this network are improved brain structure and function, which together result in a brain that has better focus and performance as well as a lower risk of dementia.

identify the big-ticket items that are most likely to be beneficial for us individually. It also allows us to see incremental improvements when we make smaller tweaks.

One of the most widely studied lifestyle-factor interactions when it comes to the brain is the relationship between sleep and exercise. Several large population studies suggest that the increased risk of dementia and early death associated with inadequate sleep is reduced in those who are physically active.[27] When scientists explored data from four hundred thousand people in the UK Biobank, they discovered that those who slept an average amount (around seven hours per night) had not only the lowest risk of dementia but also the largest brains. However, in those who slept for six hours or less per night, the increased risk of dementia they experienced seemed to be offset by doing just a moderate amount of physical activity. And the amount of physical activity required was relatively low—the equivalent of doing at least fifteen to twenty minutes of brisk walking, or seven minutes of intense exercise or sports, per day.

Sleep and exercise interact in a number of other ways that benefit our brains in both the short and long term. Exercise can improve alertness, mood, and cognitive function when we haven't slept as well as we'd have liked. In several studies, a twenty-to-thirty-minute aerobic exercise session of moderate intensity (such as a brisk walk or a light jog) improves almost every aspect of cognitive function. It also boosts mood, and that's regardless of how well somebody has slept. Some of those benefits, however, may be greater in those who slept less well. This includes minimising increases in stress hormones and inflammation that occur with long-term sleep loss.[28] High-intensity interval/sprint sessions can also help offset some of the negative metabolic effects of poor sleep, like increased blood sugar.[29]

This doesn't necessarily mean you have to hit the sprints if you didn't get a good night's rest—it just shows that multiple types of exercise can be beneficial even after you slept badly, which helps to explain the interaction we see between sleep and exercise in dementia risk. As sleep loss can affect our overall motivation to exercise, any movement you do after a night of poor sleep is likely to be beneficial, so just stick with your regular workout plan (if you have one) or pick something that you enjoy and are willing and able to do.

In addition to overcoming some of the negative effects of sleep loss, exercise also helps improve sleep quality. One recent study of exercise trials demonstrated that all types of physical activity—even those of low-intensity—were effective for improving sleep in all populations studied.[30] In general, exercise helps people fall asleep faster and increases deep sleep by supporting circadian rhythm and melatonin production.

It also improves the internal temperature regulation critical for falling asleep and adds to the drive for sleep caused by stimulating the brain.[31] With that said, some studies do suggest that intense exercise within an hour or so of going to bed might make it harder to fall asleep at night and decrease the amount of REM sleep we get. While lighter exercise in the evening is fine, high-intensity exercise can delay melatonin release and increase arousal afterwards.[32] Therefore, keeping intense sessions to the morning or afternoon is likely to be most beneficial for sleep. But, assuming you're not doing sprints in your pyjamas, sleep and exercise tend to work together to support the cognitive function we have the next day—and the headroom we build for the future.[33]

Though the research is still relatively new, exercise also seems to offset some of the effects of social isolation and loneliness that are seen in the brain. During the Covid-19 lockdowns, several studies found that mental health declined as people felt increasingly alone. However, this effect was lower in those who were physically active.[34] Physical fitness is associated with lower inflammatory responses to mental stress,[35] and studies in the lab simulating the effects of isolation during space missions show that exercise can counteract its negative effects on sleep, stress, and cognitive function.[36] These studies show that exercise somehow makes us feel less lonely, even when we're isolated—and, luckily, we can benefit from this information in multiple ways. For example, for those of us remaining on earth, group exercise classes are a great way to decrease loneliness—through the direct beneficial effects of exercise as well as the opportunity to create supportive relationships with the people sweating alongside us.[37]

If we look at the 3-S model, complex relationships like those seen between physical activity, sleep, and social isolation all start to make a bit more sense. While social connection and sleep may primarily act on different nodes (stimulus and support, respectively), social isolation and feelings of loneliness can increase stress and inflammatory responses that impair our sleep and overall ability to support adaptation processes. Similarly, long-term sleep restriction can increase both inflammation and stress, which is part of the reason that sleep is critical to long-term cognitive function. Though we shouldn't rely on exercise as a way to ignore sleep or relationships, it seems that it can make up for some of the cognitive stimulus we lose in the absence of social interaction. This is because physical activity has the power to decrease stress and inflammation while improving sleep—targeting common mechanisms that underpin brain health. This knowledge gives us some flexibility as we start to think about how to adopt more brain-healthy activities, because the data suggest that we don't have to be perfect in every area of our lives, at all times. Just having a few core components in place (such as a regular basic exercise routine) helps to cover multiple bases at once, which is particularly useful during those times when we're spread thin.

There are also several other interesting interactions with sleep that can potentially be explained by the 3-S model. For example, in older adults with normal cognitive function, greater engagement in cognitively stimulating activities like reading books or newspapers, writing letters, and playing games may counteract the negative effects of poor deep sleep on executive function and memory.[38] This again suggests that brain stimulation is the main driver of cognitive function, even if we are struggling with aspects of supply and support.

While this is encouraging, it doesn't necessarily mean that going for a jog and doing the crossword is a replacement for a good night's rest. Sleep is still critical to adaptation and recovery, and prolonged periods of short sleep affect a range of cognitive functions as well as increasing inflammation, blood sugar, and blood pressure.[39] As we saw in chapter 12, sleep is also important for supporting other lifestyle changes. For example, when we don't sleep enough, it impacts our satiety and stress hormones. That can make us hungrier while also making it more likely that we'll choose calorie-dense and hyperpalatable foods. In a study of adults with obesity who slept 6 hours per night on average, a simple intervention that increased sleep opportunity—aiming for 8.5 hours in bed each night—increased sleep by at least an hour and decreased the amount people ate. These results were likely caused by decreased hunger signaling and an increase in the release of satiety hormones.[40] So even though we may be able to offset some of the negative aspects of poor sleep, we should still aim to sleep enough so that we wake up refreshed every day. Just as stimulus is critical for determining brain function, sleep will remain a core requirement to keep your brain healthy as you age.

BRAIN BENEFITS EVEN IN UNEXPECTED PLACES

In early 2024, a journalist asked me to comment on a study that had just been published exploring the relationship between phosphodiesterase 5 (PDE5) inhibitors and dementia risk. These drugs help to dilate blood vessels and were initially developed as a treatment for angina.[41] Though the first breakthrough drug of this type—sildenafil—was a failure for treating heart disease, a common side effect seen in the initial trials breathed new life into a drug that soon became world-famous for helping men achieve and maintain erections. Yes, that drug is Viagra. Simon Campbell, one of the scientists who developed the little blue pill, even received a knighthood from the queen of England for his "services to chemistry."[42]

Using data from a large health database in the UK including over 250,000 men, researchers from University College London looked at the risk of Alzheimer's disease in men prescribed drugs for erectile dysfunction that act on the PDE5 pathway, like Viagra and Cialis. Surprisingly, they found that being prescribed one of these drugs was associated with a lower risk of dementia, especially for those who were getting regular prescriptions.[43] The effect seemed to be strongest in those who took Viagra, which was the most common drug of this type used by the men in the study. This study, which resulted in some rather cheeky headlines, wasn't even the first time the relationship between Viagra and dementia had been described—a previous study of more than seven million people in U.S. insurance databases found something similar in 2021.[44]

It is typical, when we think about drugs and brain health, to consider the *mechanism*—the direct effects that Viagra might have on the brain that could produce this result. That's what the journalist asked me about. Though these studies were not randomised controlled trials, and we have to be cautious about interpreting population data like this, there are several things that could be going on. Viagra could be increasing blood flow to the brain, which we know is critical for *supply*. It is also being explored as treatment for many brain injuries, because—in animal models, at least—sildenafil can increase neurogenesis and decrease inflammation, providing *support* for critical adaptation processes in the nervous system.[45]

But what is most interesting to me about this finding, which has generally been left unsaid, is that you usually go to your doctor for a Viagra prescription because there's a *stimulus* you want to respond to. If you think about a group of men with erectile dysfunction, those who seek solutions are more likely to be in relationships, as well as being willing to discuss their bedroom issues with a physician. This means they have not only more social connection in their lives but more social support. Depending on how you do it, sexual activity can also count as physical activity—so a regular Viagra prescription probably comes with a little more movement on the side too.

Therefore, while many excited men have probably thought an erectile dysfunction drug might provide a new way to prevent dementia, it's more likely that those prescribed Viagra have found a way to hit all the nodes of the 3-S model at once. Assuming this is a real finding, it's the combined stimulus, supply, and support that goes with a Viagra prescription that are likely producing the outsized brain benefits. These *other* reasons are also why we don't all suddenly need to queue up for a Viagra prescription to help future-proof the brain—the magic is probably in the synergistic effects in those who need it.

THE FUTURE OF TRACKING AND TREATMENT

One way that I think we will soon be able to benefit from advancements in technology is by using it to help us implement activities that support brain health. As wearables, trackers, and health data collection become more accurate and commonplace, they will also become better at sharing meaningful personalised recommendations. At some point, we will have collected enough data from enough people about their lifestyle, health, exposures, and dementia risk that we will be able to determine the best levers for a specific individual to pull. Even better, these models won't necessarily require that we understand the neuroscience in a reductionist way, because the decisions will be based on how certain inputs influence the outputs that we care about—in this case, cognitive function.

One advance I'm quite excited about is digital twins.[46] Imagine a scenario where, if you choose to, all your health and lifestyle information is tracked and entered into a database, creating a "twin" of your data online. Using all the information collected about how lifestyle and the environment affect cognitive function, this can then be mapped on to your "twin" to help you decide which interventions are likely to have the biggest impact on your own dementia risk. Though there will be some noise and error in these models, as there always is with statistics, access to your digital twin can help you predict what would happen if you changed your diet, or sleep, or exercise in a certain way. These technologies have remarkable potential to guide our decisions regarding where to start our journey of building headroom.

I also look forward to improvements in how cognitive function is measured and tracked. The current methods can be expensive, hard to access, or just too rudimentary to really capture the full spectrum of human abilities. Cognitive tests also commonly suffer from learning effects, which means that you'll get a better score on the test the second time you take it, even if your brain hasn't really changed that much. Some of these problems are being solved with new tests that will hopefully be incorporated into easily accessible technology so we can keep an eye on our cognitive function over time—as well as track the effects of the activities we use to build headroom. Similarly, it's getting easier to measure activity in the brain using electrodes built into headphones or stickers placed around the head, which can quantify and track focus, attention, processing speed, and cognitive load, as well as future dementia risk.[47]

It's also likely that some of these assessments will become built into the devices we use every day.[48] For instance, you can track elements of cognition by the way people type on their phone,[49] and you can assess stress or depression levels based on changes in somebody's voice.[50] These are all technologies that are likely to become commonplace at some point. In the future, I can certainly imagine using them to receive feedback on how we're doing. (Though hopefully we will also be able to opt out if we want to!)

With that said, we will need to remain aware that technologies that track our sleep, exercise, and blood test results can easily become the goal themselves rather than being what we *really* want them to be—tools to achieve the bigger goal of long-term brain health. If you get to the point that you're stressed about what your sleep tracker or glucose monitor tells you, or if you become so focused on the perfect exercise regimen or recovery score from your wearable that it's stopping you from getting out into the world and enjoying the brain you're building, these technologies may be more hindrance than help. But if you can use the data to help you implement the 3-S model—and still do the hard work yourself—these tools will hopefully be able to show you where to begin and how to track your progress over time.

While health tracking apps and tools will probably be best suited to helping with the *supply* and *support* arms of the 3-S model, there will soon likely be many more technological advancements that may help directly apply stimulus to the brain. In chapter 9 we touched on the fact that more advanced virtual reality (VR) solutions are likely to overtake app or web-browser-based technologies for cognitive training because of their immersive multisensory inputs. They provide an environment that takes advantage of how the human brain normally receives complex information in the world. I expect similar enhancements in assistive technologies and brain-computer interfaces to help restore lost elements of function, whether that involves physical movement, speech and other forms of communication, or senses like sight, touch, and hearing. While these technologies are nascent, they could one day help us maintain stimulus as well as connection to the outside world in a way that supports an individual's brain after a function or input is lost.

In a final look at future developments in brain health, we turn now to the various new therapies coming down the pipeline with the promise of either treating or preventing cognitive decline and dementia. This includes both drugs that target certain mechanisms—tau and amyloid, but hopefully also the other cells that contribute to brain health: the glia. Some of these new therapies may also include neurotrophic peptides, hormones, or stem cells or their components. I certainly hope that some of these therapies will be successful. But regardless of any new interventions on the horizon, I remain confident the 3-S model will still have a role to play. If a therapy puts the brakes on a process that's impairing brain health—like inflammation or the accumulation of brain pathology—the best way to regain or improve brain function with treatment will still be to stimulate the brain, supply the necessary nutrients, and support adaptation and recovery.

MULTIPRONGED APPROACHES TO DEMENTIA PREVENTION

The nodes in the 3-S model give us a strong jumping-off point to understand how the balance of lifestyle and environmental factors might explain differing trajectories of cognitive function. They can also help us choose interventions based on our own needs. Importantly, the nature of the 3-S model predicts that multiple smaller changes across the network can have significant impact, since they will interact and synergise with one another. At this point there are countless examples of supplements and drugs that, as single interventions, had underwhelming effects on long-term dementia prevention. Ultimately, pulling just one biochemical lever in a complex system and expecting a large-scale impact is unrealistic. Each of us has a different balance of risk factors and different needs that are unlikely to be addressed by a medication that targets a single biochemical pathway.

On the other hand, once you start looking for the ways that lifestyle factors overlap through common mechanisms, you'll see that the scientific literature is full of interesting interactions between variables that combine to affect brain health. For example, one study in older Japanese adults found that greater cognitive engagement (regularly reading newspapers and magazines or using computers and game consoles) and higher intake of the omega-3 fat DHA were both associated with small (but not significant) improvements in the risk of cognitive decline. The risk was only significantly decreased in the study participants who had higher cognitive engagement *and* ate more omega-3s—better stimulus plus improved supply and support.[51] Another Japanese study found a similar relationship between open-skill exercise and omega-3s, with the combination of both associated with having larger brain volumes (more stimulus and supply leading to more headroom).

Risk factors can also interact. For instance, in one study, the effect of poor sleep (impaired support) on brain structure and function appeared to be particularly exacerbated in the setting of high blood pressure (impaired supply).[52] In practical terms, you're much more likely to move the needle by identifying what's most important for you (say, getting more exercise if you already sleep well) but also by making several smaller lifestyle changes that play off one another. The small beneficial effects of a slightly better diet, slightly more exercise, slightly more sleep, and slightly better stress management can work together to have a large effect on overall brain health.

There are now several trials that show the benefit of this kind of multipronged approach. The first is the Finnish FINGER trial, which we discussed in part 1, where a combination of four interventions—diet, exercise, cognitive training, and cardiovascular risk monitoring—significantly improved cognitive function over two years in older adults. This finding has now been reproduced in multiple trials in multiple countries around the world.[53] The best example is POINTER (Protect Brain Health Through Lifestyle Intervention to Reduce Risk) a recent

U.S. trial that replicated FINGER in adults ages sixty to seventy-nine at risk of cognitive decline and dementia. The intervention group received a training programme that included resistance, aerobic, and balance training in a social setting, followed the MIND diet (including a monthly budget to buy blueberries), were cognitively challenged using BrainHQ (mentioned in chapter 10) for fifteen to twenty minutes three times per week, and received health coaching to track and improve their cardiovascular risk.

Compared to an active control group who received advice to change the same areas of lifestyle in a self-guided manner, the intervention group saw significant improvements in overall cognitive function, especially executive function and processing speed. The benefits of the intervention were the same regardless of the individual's ApoE4 genotype or sex. Notably, both groups improved over the two-year study, suggesting that engaging with lifestyle changes in a self-guided manner was also beneficial for the control group.

The Maintain Your Brain study—a similar trial to FINGER and POINTER but much larger and conducted entirely online—shows that similar improvements are possible when lifestyle changes are personalised based on individual need. Maintain Your Brain included more than six thousand people aged fifty-five years or older who had dementia risk factors but no evidence of cognitive decline. The intervention group identified one or more of four areas where they were at increased risk for dementia—diet, physical activity, cognitive activity, and depression or anxiety—and received personalised recommendations based on their unique risk factors. Over three years, those who received personalised dementia prevention advice saw significant improvements in cognitive function compared to a control group.[54] These types of personalised multidomain interventions may be particularly important for closing the sex gap in dementia risk. Even though it benefitted both males and females, Maintain Your Brain found a greater improvement in cognitive function in females.

To give you an idea of the simple but impactful interventions from FINGER and Maintain Your Brain, summaries are shown in the table on the next page:

INTERVENTION	FINGER	MAINTAIN YOUR BRAIN
Exercise	Aerobic: 2–5 moderate-intensity sessions of 30–60 minutes/week. Resistance: 1–3 sessions (2–3 sets of 8–20 repetitions for 8–10 exercises) of 30–60 minutes/week.	300 minutes of moderate-to-vigourous aerobic exercise/week. Resistance training 3 times/week. Balance training every day.
Nutrition	Focus on whole foods while limiting sugar and alcohol. Vitamin D and fish oil supplementation if not getting them from the diet.	Mediterranean dietary pattern focused on increasing intake of whole foods. Counseled against excess alcohol.
Cognitive stimulus	10–15 minutes of online brain-training programme 3 times/week. Social interaction through group meetings as part of the interventions.	45 minutes of online brain training 3 times/week for 10 weeks, then once per month.
Cardiovascular risk monitoring	Regular assessment of blood pressure, blood sugar, and cholesterol. Medication was prescribed if needed by the patient's doctor.	N/A
Peace of mind	N/A	Online cognitive behavioural therapy (CBT) using a digital mental health programme over 10 weeks.

In addition to these two large studies, smaller trials suggest that a similar approach may be helpful in those who are older or who are already experiencing some degree of early dementia. The Systematic Multi-Domain Alzheimer Risk Reduction Trial (SMARRT) randomised participants seventy years or older to create personalised goals around ten targets. Each participant worked with a health coach to address areas where they had the biggest issues or were most interested in making changes. These goals included controlling blood pressure or diabetes, aiming for at least eight thousand steps per day, increasing cognitive stimulation and social engagement, cognitive behavioural therapy for depression symptoms or insomnia, reducing smoking, and eating a MIND-style diet focused on whole foods. Over two years, the intervention group decreased their Alzheimer's disease risk and improved their cognitive function more than a control group.[55]

More promising data for those who are already seeing some cognitive decline comes from a small (fifty people) trial that implemented twenty weeks of changes to diet (a plant-based whole-foods diet plus multiple supplements, including omega-3s, magnesium, vitamin B12, a multivitamin, and a probiotic), exercise (thirty minutes of walking per day and resistance training three times per week), stress management (yoga and breathing exercises), and social support (online and in-person groups) significantly improved cognitive function and slowed decline in individuals who were diagnosed with mild cognitive impairment.[56] A South Korean trial that implemented the same strategies as FINGER in individuals with mild cognitive impairment also saw improvements in cognitive function after just six months.[57]

Across all these studies, it's clear that when identifying and addressing the big-ticket lifestyle items covered in part 2, we can see improvements in cognitive function across a wide range of ages and levels of risk. The interventions can be relatively simple and tailored to the individual, which makes complete sense when you think about how these different components might interact as part of the 3-S model. The combination of stimulus, supply, and support can provide outsized benefits that reductionist approaches have failed to provide so far. And what's even better is that there are many activities that can result in improvement in multiple areas at the same time, whether you are looking at exercise, sleep, or dietary changes. With these individualised approaches, each of us can start to plot our own path to increased headroom and a future-proofed brain.

WHERE SHOULD I START?

I vividly remember the first time I arrived at a Formula 1 race to support some drivers and their coaches. I had been contacted a year earlier by Dr. Luke Bennett, who at the time was the medical and sports performance director for a company called Hintsa Performance—the company through which I do my work in motorsports. Luke had heard me speak on a podcast and, perhaps recognising a fellow sports-and-performance nerd, sent me what ended up being a fairly life-changing email. After several months getting to know Luke and the rest of the Hintsa team, I joined the company as a scientific advisor. The first time my skills were really put to the test was at the U.S. Grand Prix in Austin, Texas.

I have been a huge fan of Formula 1 racing for most of my life—ever since my early teenage years, when I spent a summer watching it religiously with my aunt and uncle. So, as you might imagine, I spent a lot of time preparing before this trip. I came armed with every tip, trick, and scientific paper I could think of, and all that information was locked and ready for me to dispense at high speed to any unsuspecting driver or coach who might ask me a question. I probably had a list of a hundred things that I felt could help to improve a driver's health, well-being, and performance.

Up to this point, I had done most of my work as a coach in solo or small-team endurance sports, where I was usually one of only a few advisors working with an athlete. This made it fairly easy to help those athletes implement several different ideas at the same time. But in Formula 1, even though I was an invited expert, I was one of dozens of people trying to give the drivers advice. And that's before you remember that they must also consult with huge teams of people involved with the car, the tactics, and the logistics of the sport (while taking part in an intense number of additional media commitments). These athletes are constantly on the road, often finding themselves in multiple countries and time zones in a single week. Beyond the physical demands of racing, the cognitive and allostatic loads really add up across their season.

It's all well and good to show up with a long list of tools and recommendations, but much harder to decide which to implement when time and cognitive resources are already stretched to their limit. I remember a coach saying during that trip to Austin, "We have the ability to maybe try *one* thing. What should it be?" This is a question I have heard hundreds of times in the years since. In fact, somebody asked me very recently whether they should focus on their diet *or* exercise in order to support their brain health and performance. Clearly, the evidence shows that *both* are important, and that's what I would have said ten years ago. But when you only have the capacity to do *one* thing, focusing on two makes it likely that zero will happen.

This is where the rules of the brain game and the 3-S model start to come into their own. Regardless of where you start, we have consistent evidence that *everything counts*. Rather than trying to hit optimal goals for exercise, sleep, or protein intake, pick one of those areas where you're motivated to make some progress. Then decide to make *one* consistent change that will move you in that direction.

The interconnected nature of the factors that influence health means that when you change one thing, you're not really changing *one* thing. At the beginning of chapter 13, I mentioned a huge meta-analysis investigating common lifestyle risk factors for dementia, stroke, and depression. Sanjula Singh, the neurologist at Harvard who led the study, recommends that people focus on one risk factor at a time rather than the more than twenty her study identified. Because "if you're starting to work on one of them, very often you're actually improving multiple at the same time."

When you increase physical activity, you're automatically decreasing sedentary time. You are also improving other risk factors like blood pressure, blood sugar, and sleep. Some evidence even suggests that starting a new exercise regimen could shift food preferences toward a healthier dietary pattern.[58] Similarly, improving sleep or finding more time for brain recovery decreases cognitive load and improves mood, making it more likely that we will engage in other health-promoting behaviours. This is why we can think about brain health as a network—any one change can make big shifts across the entire system that synergise and help build greater headroom.

As you think about where to start in your quest to build headroom, there are a few different ways you could do it. For all the reasons we've already discussed, the most important place to start is with something that you can define in a concrete way, are interested in doing, think you might enjoy, and are at least reasonably confident you can achieve. It can also be useful to think about where you might get the biggest bang for your buck. If you have a busy and demanding job (plenty of stimulus), maybe the best place to focus is on finding some time to exercise, sleep a bit more, or spend time with your friends or family (more supply or support). If you don't feel cognitively rewarded at work or are at or near retirement (lower stimulus), consider starting a new hobby, joining a class, or volunteering. If you feel like you are always pressed for time, you could start by picking something you can set and forget, like a water filter or air purifier—or adding a high-quality multivitamin (or tin of sardines) to your breakfast. Ask yourself what you think you can consistently do that will have a big payoff. And then, once that habit is firmly in place, you can think about the next thing.

Beyond all that, if you *really* want to know where to start, the most important thing for your long-term cognitive function is to make sure that you do, in fact, start.

A BEGINNER'S GUIDE TO THE 3-S MODEL

The nature of the 3-S model suggests that there are certain activities that will have an outsized effect on brain health and function because they act on multiple nodes of the network at once. If you're thinking of starting with just one new thing to break into the brain game (and the thought of adopting a dog or getting a Viagra prescription doesn't quite tickle your fancy), any of the activities below would be an excellent option.

Group or Coordinative Physical Activity

As discussed in chapter 7, there's something special about exercise that involves complex coordinative movements. They're a stimulus, improve supply through cardiovascular health, and help support the brain through better sleep and decreased stress and inflammation. Add in a social component and you're hitting all three nodes of the 3-S model in multiple ways. Think dancing, doubles pickleball (or any team ball sport), yoga and Pilates, or martial arts (ideally varieties that don't involve getting hit in the head).

Outdoor Volunteering

Parks, gardens, and farms are always looking for volunteers to help maintain trails, plant trees, remove invasive species, and grow and harvest vegetables. This provides all the social benefits of volunteering, in combination with time spent outdoors in nature and physical activity (all three S's in one go). If there aren't good volunteering opportunities near you, then almost any outdoor physical activity can still hit multiple nodes in the 3-S model at once.

Classes and Time with Friends

Any kind of quality social connection—especially in person—with loved ones provides a beneficial cognitive stimulus. It can also improve multiple aspects of support by decreasing stress and inflammation responses associated with high allostatic load. So how about hosting a dinner party with family or friends each week? Alternatively, take up a group class related to a skill like a musical instrument or language. Though they might not start out as your friends, the people you take classes with will provide much-needed social connection alongside the cognitive stimulation.

Sardines

OK, hear me out. Small fish like sardines, mackerel, and herring are nutritional powerhouses. They also tend to be lower in contaminants while being excellent sources of protein, omega-3 fats, vitamin D, most B vitamins, and several minerals such as copper and selenium, and creatine. We know from chapter 8 that B vitamins and omega-3 fats synergise when it comes to brain health, so why not get both at the same time? In fact, a recent study found that having low omega-3s and vitamin D plus high homocysteine (which increases when people are low in B vitamins) was associated with a more than four-fold increase in dementia risk. Sardines could be the perfect antidote![59] The B vitamins might even help minimise the impact of local air pollution.[60] And if you buy the sardines that have skin and bones (which you can't tell when you eat them, I promise), you'll get in some extra collagen and calcium too.

Sleep

Technically sleep only belongs to one arm of the 3-S model (support), but from chapter 12, we know that sleep facilitates everything else. When we sleep well, we're more sociable, less stressed, more likely to engage in cognitively challenging tasks, and more likely to exercise. Physical health factors like blood pressure and blood sugar also improve, and we're less likely to fall back into old habits that we're trying to change. If you need something to grease the wheels of the 3-S model, sleep is an incredible place to start. Even just starting with an additional fifteen to thirty minutes of sleep opportunity each day can make a big difference in helping you get the rest your brain needs.

CHAPTER 15
FUTURE-PROOFING YOUR BRAIN

Now that we understand the core principles and common mechanisms involved with future-proofing our brains, it's time for the rubber to meet the road. Broadly speaking, the activities with the power to build headroom can occur in two windows: today and the future. But as they both rely on the same underlying physiological and cognitive processes, these windows of time aren't mutually exclusive. In fact, they're mutually *inclusive*. By working in one, you're inherently working in the other.

When people think about dementia prevention or future-proofing their brains, often they think about what they need to do when they're sixty years old. This means that any action is put off until some unknown time in the future. Or, perhaps just as frequently, people assume that there's nothing they can do to prevent dementia, so they avoid action entirely. This is despite the fact that we know that the trajectory of cognitive decline begins, and remains modifiable, right from the start of life. You can see this in the influence that parental education has on babies born preterm, and then again in the slowed decline in superagers who engage in activities that stimulate, supply, and support their brains. We also know that the brain changes associated with later dementia risk, such as changes in the volume and structure of the brain as well as accumulation of pathology, can begin decades before a diagnosis is made. Just like you (hopefully) wouldn't wait until you're seventy to start an exercise routine, the time to start future-proofing your brain is right now.

This is particularly important when we think about the fact that, as mentioned in part 1, our brains seem to be struggling no matter who we are or how old we are. This includes many adolescents, a group experiencing an increasing prevalence of mental health struggles, and the more than 10 percent of adults over forty-five who report some element of diminished cognitive function—and did so even *before* the Covid-19 pandemic.[1] Because of this, it can be easy to feel stuck. We are stressed, distracted, overwhelmed, and believe there isn't anything we can do for our brains *right now*. Or maybe being stressed, distracted, and overwhelmed prevents us from being able to fully engage in the activities that can help us build headroom in the first place.

Having gotten to this point in the book, we see that multiple scenarios are possible. Maybe you've realised that you're already doing a lot for your brain and that the constant urge to do *more* can be counterproductive. Maybe you've seen that everything counts and have started small—partaking in some exercise snacks, a bit more broccoli, and a slightly earlier bedtime—knowing from the 3-S model that these changes can synergise to have outsized benefits for your brain. Or maybe the thought of doing *anything* still feels overwhelming considering everything else you have to accomplish in a day.

Regardless of the starting point, and even after starting the process of building long-term headroom, there are a few more ideas that can benefit any of us when it comes to thinking about cognitive function *today*. And, perhaps unsurprisingly, a lot of it comes down to how we're using our brains. We've talked about the problems with social media, and about the importance of truly challenging ourselves cognitively in order to build capacity—better function, bigger brains, and more headroom. But all this has to occur in the context of the modern work environment, which in many ways can make it harder to engage in challenging and meaningful activities—either by fracturing our attention or by leaving us so cognitively fatigued that even the *idea* of lifting weights or attending a French class at the end of the day becomes too much to consider.

When we already feel like we have too much on our plate, the thought of adding even more to support a long-term dementia-prevention plan may seem unrealistic. And let's face it: humans suck at doing the things they know they should be doing when the payoff might not come for years or even decades. This is especially the case when you are working to make something (dementia) *not* happen. So, one important way to get started with building a future-proof brain is to start incorporating the underlying principles in ways that can provide immediate feedback.

As our jobs provide some of the most consistent cognitive stimulus (or stimuli) that most of us will experience across decades of our lives, this is a place where we can achieve some immediate wins, given that applying the 3-S model can improve how we feel and perform each day. By tweaking our approach to work—or, in fact, any number of tasks that we might have to get done in a given day—we can feel more productive while also feeling less drained. But that doesn't mean work has to be the centre of your life. Even if your occupation isn't your passion, focusing on how to apply the tools and ideas we've discussed in and around your workday can ensure that you come away from work with more energy for all the other things you want to do with your brain.

Of course, the amazing diversity of human brains (as well as all the varied professions in the world) means that there are an infinite number of objectives any one of us might want to achieve on a given day. We also don't know what the work environment is going to look like several years from now (though deadlines, long to-do lists, and endless messages and emails are unlikely to go anywhere). As a result, we need a range of approaches to support cognitive performance now *and* in the future, no matter what tasks are in front of us. We also need frameworks rather than strict rules, because each of us will differ slightly in the practices we might benefit from. With all that said, there are some common basics we can apply to help us make the most of our brains' capacity.

Once again, this concept has a lot of overlap with how you would work to improve athletic performance. Athletes obviously rely on a wide range of approaches to meet the demands of their specific sport. But, to achieve the gains they seek, they also consistently attend to similar areas around training and recovery, whether they are trying to row faster or lift heavier. When it comes to future-proofing the brain, think of yourself as a cognitive athlete and your brain as a muscle you need to stimulate. Applying some athletic principles to the way we use our brains at work every day can have a big impact on both short- and long-term brain health.

GETTING IN GEAR

Hintsa Performance was founded by Finnish orthopedic surgeon and Olympic team physician Aki Hintsa, who in the 1990s worked with legendary marathon runner Haile Gebrselassie and two-time Formula 1 world champion Mika Häkkinen.[2] Three decades later, Hintsa has supported multiple world champions in Formula 1 as well as several other sports. A core extension of my and Hintsa's work with Formula 1 drivers is taking what we know about the principles of elite athletic performance and showing how they can be used by anyone who wants to feel and perform better both physically and cognitively. One of the first people I worked with at Hintsa was James Hewitt, a former professional cyclist who now specialises in supporting cognitive athletes—knowledge workers who pay the bills using their brain power. One of the most impactful concepts I learned from James, taken from *Exponential,* a book he wrote with Aki Hintsa, is the idea of cognitive gears.

Across a typical day or week, we use our brains for a wide variety of tasks that require different levels of focus and engagement. Each of these tasks therefore requires a different set of cognitive resources. The particular resources we engage for a specific task then dictate the downstream adaptations or physiological responses. A good workday or workweek, just like a good training programme, should include a balance of activities—with different intensities that drive different adaptations while providing enough time for recovery. And though we don't always have control over what we do or when, in situations where we do have some control over our schedule, it can help to map certain activities to certain times of day or blocks of work in order to get the most out of them.

If we're thinking about how to structure a day so we can perform all the tasks we need to in a way that supports focus while minimising avoidable allostatic load, James's idea of cognitive gears helps. It involves categorising the tasks we need to accomplish based on their mental requirements. Just as movement has different levels of intensity—low, moderate, and vigourous—so does cognitive activity. In James's model, there are three gears of cognitive work: high, middle, and low.

High gear is like a sprint workout or heavy gym session. It requires all your focus and attention, and minimal distractions. In short, it's the time during your workday when actual *work* is done. Think problem-solving, crisis management, strategic planning, writing, research, and learning. All of these are best accomplished when they have our full attention.

Low gear is more like walking. This keeps the wheels turning and can be restful and restorative, but it doesn't really push the boundaries of our fitness. Low-gear cognitive activity includes reading for pleasure, social interaction, creative thinking, and maybe even some of the rote activities discussed in chapter 12 (simple games, reading the news, or light social media use), when we're engaged but not overly challenged or stressed. Low gear is where we should spend a lot of our time—recovering from high-gear work but also exploring the ideas and connections we can make when we're not overloaded or singularly focused on one particular task.

Where we *actually* spend most of our time, thanks to the demands of the modern work environment, is in middle gear. Because some of this is self-inflicted, restructuring our middle-gear work is where we can make some of the biggest gains in terms of how we use our brains during the day. Middle gear is like running. You can keep going for longer than you can sprint, but if you were to try running all day every day, those miles would add up, resulting in a lot of fatigue and frustration. The middle-gear category includes meetings, administrative work, and dealing with emails or messages on business-collaboration apps. Note that these activities often tend to be the ones where you are doing more than one thing at once. That's because a classic signature of the middle gear is constantly switching between tasks. Though much of this sort of cognitive work is ultimately important, most of our middle-gear time is spent doing work that makes us feel busy but isn't actually work.

Too often, our entire schedule is filled with middle-gear activities. We check our email when we're meant to be doing more focused work like formulating a strategic plan or studying for an exam. We let app notifications drag our attention away from an important document that we're supposed to be writing. Or, when we're supposed to be relaxing, we start switching our attention across multiple devices and unnecessarily adding cognitive load—checking our phones while talking to friends or scrolling through social media while (supposedly) watching a TV show with our partner. As a result, *everything* becomes a middle-gear activity—we're less focused and productive when we want to be in high gear, and low gear is far less restorative than it should be.

Spending all day in the cognitive middle gear is a bit like the amateur athlete in chapter 12 ignoring their total allostatic load. They push too hard in training sessions that are supposed to be for recovery, but then they also find that they're not fresh enough for the really hard sessions and have to pull back. As a result, everything becomes hardish, and they might try to do even *more* because they feel like they're not progressing. In runners, this type of training would likely result in an injury like a stress fracture in the foot. In cognitive athletes, however, it increases the risk of burnout. But just as a professional athlete learns how to balance hard training sessions and recovery, one of the simplest ways to balance the load as a cognitive athlete is to structure and plan types of work based on their cognitive gear.

It's helpful to think about these gears in terms of a typical workday. It might start with some emails or other communications, followed by an attempt to get into that day's main piece of focused work. But, as other colleagues get started on their days, you receive more emails and messages. When these notifications pop up, you feel drawn to check them. That distracts you from the research you need to accomplish for an important presentation next week. All of a sudden, you notice it's 11:00 A.M. and you have three one-hour meetings over the next few hours, with only a thirty-minute break between each one. Those breaks aren't enough time to allow you to get back to your research, but they may provide just enough time to reply to a few more messages.

As with (almost) all meetings, a lot is said but no productive work is done. You also feel distracted because, even though you should be paying attention to the people in the room, you are actually checking your email (or TikTok, Instagram, or Facebook) whenever you can. You then leave the meeting with a list of action items to add to your already overwhelming to-do list.

Back at your desk, you look at your watch and it's 3:00 P.M. You find yourself in a weird afternoon slump. You listlessly return to your research for a bit before going back to some emails and admin tasks until it's time to go home. You were *busy* all day, and you're tired after all that constant cognitive running, but you didn't accomplish the one thing you really needed to do, the thing that was actually the most important (and perhaps meaningful) task of your professional day. Because you know how important stimulus is for the brain, you might even feel a bit disappointed that you didn't get to really test your capacity with any meaningful, focused work. The fact that you haven't done the research

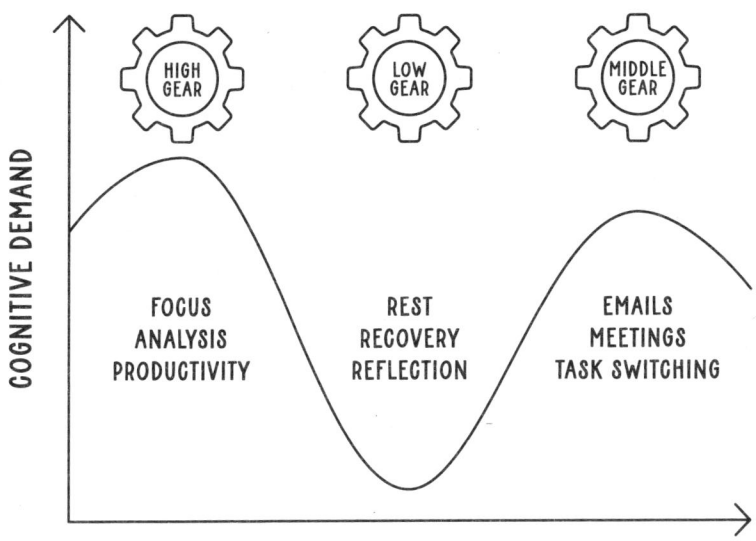

FIGURE 1. Like a well-balanced training programme for your body, the way we use our brains day in and day out should have a balance of different intensities. This includes prioritising high-gear, focused work when we can learn or feel productive, as well as recovery periods when we truly switch off. We still need to spend time doing more menial tasks in the middle gear, but by structuring those into defined periods we can push harder when we need to and also relax harder afterwards. Adapted from *Exponential* by Hewitt and Hintsa.

you needed to do also plays on your mind for the rest of the evening. Even though you're mentally exhausted, it takes you longer to fall asleep because you're worrying about how you'll manage that research when you have *another* full slate of meetings tomorrow.

While this scenario is a bit of a caricature, I bet a lot of it feels familiar. It could describe any one of countless days I've experienced myself. Alas, completely eliminating meetings and emails is an unrealistic utopian fantasy. But some simple planning can help to increase the number of days when you feel like you did more of your best work without as much cognitive load. The goal isn't necessarily to completely change your job or the work you do but to restructure the work so that you experience a balance of cognitive gears—high-gear, focused work where you feel challenged and productive, recovery breaks to replenish and reflect, and then more dedicated time to emails and administrative work (figure 1).

FEEL THE RHYTHM

On any given day, you probably have one or two tasks that need your undivided attention. You'll also no doubt have some meetings and a few administrative tasks, not to mention all those emails and messages to deal with. If you have the luxury of having complete control over your calendar, you might be able to plan these tasks over a week or month rather than over a single day. But either way, the ideal place to start is blocking out time for high- and middle-gear tasks in advance—ideally, penciling a break in between them, like a quick walk or an extended lunch with a friend or colleague. The goal is to undulate between tasks with varying intensity—one or two peaks of high-gear work, followed by a break when possible, with alternating periods of middle-gear work so you can stay on top of your meetings and emails.

An added layer that we might consider here is the natural fluctuations in energy that we all feel throughout the day. Due to the circadian rhythms that run our biology on a twenty-four-hour cycle, our hormones, body temperature, and metabolism all wax and wane across the morning, afternoon, and evening. Because of this, performance in certain tasks tends to fluctuate in a similar manner. For example, it's thought that, on average, mental alertness peaks a couple of hours after waking, with physical performance (e.g., strength) peaking in the mid- to-late afternoon when body temperature is highest.[3] However, these average effects don't necessarily map to our individual daily rhythms when it comes to work performance.

Our own experience of energy and performance fluctuations throughout the day are at least partly driven by our *chronotype*—a component of circadian rhythm that influences when we're most alert. Chronotype has a genetic component but is also influenced by your environment (especially light and dark exposure), as well as your typical work and activity patterns. This last point is important because it means that most of us can adjust the time we work or feel best, if we need to. For example, several studies of exercise training show that you can change the time of day you perform at your best, because you tend to perform best at the time of day that you regularly work out.[4]

The strength of our individual chronotypes and how that affects our focus and energy across the day differs a lot from person to person. At one end of the spectrum are the definite morning larks—wide-awake and raring to go when they get up—and at the other end are the night owls, who are sleepy and grumpy (and maybe dopey too) first thing in the morning. But there are also plenty of people in the middle who feel pretty much the same regardless of the time of day.

The strongest evidence for daily fluctuations in cognitive performance comes from looking at people who have a strong lark- or owl-type chronotype. When you average across all people, chronotype and time of day don't influence cognitive function themselves.[5] However, people who have a strong preference for the morning or afternoon/evening tend to do slightly better on tasks that require effortful focus during their time of peak alertness—known as the *synchrony effect*.[6] What's really interesting, though, is that there is also evidence for *asynchrony*—meaning that we do better on tasks that require creative insight or unconscious thought at the time of day when we are less alert. That may be because when our focus and attentional control is weaker, our brains are more likely to bring novel and divergent ideas to the surface.[7]

It's important to note that any differences in function across the day could be very minor. And even if you aren't doing high-gear work in your preferred time block, it doesn't mean that you'll automatically perform *badly*. The idea is simply to think about how you can best break up the workday to maximise the likelihood of success—and minimise potential distractions and friction.

CONSIDER YOUR CHRONOTYPE

A recently validated questionnaire called the Caen Chronotype Questionnaire considers both the timing of your alertness peak and how much your energy level changes across the day. This can be useful when considering how you want to schedule different types of activities.[8] Think about (or write down) a number from one (totally disagree) to five (totally agree). You don't need to create a final score, but the answers to the questions can help you discover the times when you feel at your best, which provides guidance on how to best structure your day.

1. I can work efficiently at any time of the day.
2. I feel I can think the best in the morning.
3. There are moments during the day when I would prefer to avoid any work.

4. I feel drowsy for a long time after awakening.
5. If I were to study anything by myself, I would rather do it in the evening.
6. My mood stays the same throughout the day.
7. I like to get up earlier than necessary, e.g., in order to prepare things for the whole day.
8. I can focus at any time of the day.
9. My work goes better in the afternoon than before noon.
10. At any time of the day, my motivation is the same.
11. I am usually in an excellent mood in the morning.
12. If I need to, I'm able to concentrate at any time of the day.
13. I am in my best form in the morning; in the course of the day my energy runs out.
14. There are moments during the day when I feel unable to do anything.
15. There are moments during the day when it is harder for me to think.
16. I feel sluggish in the morning, and I warm up slowly during the day.

After getting a feel for your chronotype, consider the times of day when you find you are the most alert or motivated. Then block off those times for focused work on your calendar. It could be as little as thirty to sixty minutes to get high-priority stuff done, or a course of several hours that you break up with shorter periods of rest. If you can, schedule some time for low-gear processes to help you reset and recover after these high-intensity work periods. Just as if you had to do multiple physical workouts in a day, your brain will be able to go longer and harder when you let it rest between each effort. Low-gear periods could be anything that feels like a real break from work—some light physical activity like a walk outside, a meal or a conversation with a friend, or maybe even a quick rerun of a nostalgic TV show on your favourite streaming service.

After this low-gear period, you'll be better primed to accomplish whatever block of work you have planned next. If you're like me (definitely a morning-type person), you'll have done a good session of work, taken a break (I usually have a snack and take the puppies for a spin outside), and then be ready for another focused work session before noon. Early afternoon is usually when I switch to dealing with emails and other messages, or schedule most of my meetings. My energy levels are a little lower then, which I find is fine for discussions around work, or for more creative thinking. I also personally prefer to schedule meetings back-to-back if I can, because otherwise all those thirty-minute gaps in the day consume the time that could otherwise be used on a defined period of focused work.

It is important to understand that there's no one way to apply cognitive gears to your own workday. If you're the kind of person who likes fifteen-minute breaks between meetings to knock out a few emails—do that. If your best time for focused work is 8 to 10 P.M. and working at that time still allows you to get enough sleep to feel restored the next day—great. If you don't have full control of your own calendar, try to prioritise some small blocks of time that will allow you to feel good at the end of the day. For most of us, that means either taking a few minutes to recharge between long chunks of time in the middle gear or ensuring we have an opportunity to do some focused work without being interrupted. Or both. The key is to focus on blocking off time in the calendar to get what you need. This will increase your ability to deal with whatever comes your way.

As you think back on some of the material from previous chapters about what our brains need in order to benefit from (and engage with) stimulus, you may notice that a common theme is control. Control is a central part of autonomy, which we discussed in chapter 8, and is integral to self-determination theory. We also saw in chapter 9 that people with hard or stressful jobs can have a lower risk of dementia and depression—but only as long as they have control over their work. When you consider that one of the biggest reasons we experience overwhelm or burnout is because we feel a loss of control—constantly having to respond to and do work on somebody else's timeline—this makes sense.[9]

Though it won't always be possible, a combination of some planning and calendar management can help you regain some footing and control in your day. As much as possible, schedule your calendar according to your personal preferences and work style so you can map your different work gears onto your daily energy levels like the example in figure 1. But also know that it might be enough just to carve out small chunks of time for you to do what you need to do—focus and recover—so that you'll ultimately be able to accomplish whatever you need to at any time of day.

If I'm honest, it feels a bit strange writing about the importance of calendars and schedules. A younger Tommy would have found these ideas completely alien—I didn't maintain a calendar and just assumed that I'd remember the important things I needed to do or be reminded of them by somebody else. While you can usually get away with that when you're younger and have fewer tasks to juggle, this gets harder over time as the responsibilities stack up.

A lot of the ideas covered here stem from some of the downsides I experienced with a less structured approach—missed deadlines, endless days feeling exhausted by middle-gear work with no time to focus and think, and then sleepless nights being worried about all the tasks I still had left to do. One reason for highlighting this impact of working styles on our brains is the insidious accumulation of stress that occurs when we don't regain control over our tasks and commitments.

For me, finding some balance in my workday required heavy trial and error, as well as learning from true experts like James Hewitt and my wife, who has scheduling down to an artform. While it might feel strange to add even more structure into the workday, in many ways it can be quite freeing. We don't need to decide when to do something and can get on with the business of actual work. A good schedule can also ensure that we have time for what we really care about—which usually is the stuff that happens outside of work—and show up to that with more headroom and mental energy. As Shane Parrish, former spy and author of the book *Clear Thinking*, says: "Don't tell me your priorities; show me your calendar."

PLANNING A DAY

Depending on your typical workweek, the days might look quite similar or very different. I tend to keep Mondays and Fridays clear of meetings so that I can do focused work, like doing experiments in the lab. The middle of the week then provides me with a lot of time for middle-gear work, although I do try to leave some of the mornings free for high-gear activities. Regardless of what your workday looks like, a little bit of planning can make a big difference. If this requires an overhaul, worry less about what you're doing today and start the calendar management a few weeks out, at a time when your days aren't already full. Then schedule in blocks of work based on their gear and your preferred timing. I recommend (and use) this approach, but the order will be a little different for everybody:

1. Start by scheduling non-negotiable activities (e.g., family time) or headroom-building activities you want to start doing more of (e.g., going to the gym). If it's on the calendar, it's more likely to happen.
2. Next, block time for high-gear work when energy levels are highest or when you know you can take time for focused work.
3. Schedule some low-gear time between longer or more intense work blocks, even if you can only manage ten or fifteen minutes.
4. Protect numbers 1–3 at all costs. If the time is blocked off, you're less likely to squeeze in a quick meeting when you need to be focused elsewhere.
5. Schedule meetings and other administrative tasks around high-gear and low-gear periods. Alternatively, leave open blocks in your schedule where you're happy for middle-gear work to accumulate.
6. Know when your workday will end to avoid ambiguity and maintain some control. Even better, schedule something that forces you to head home or step away from your desk.

Just as a good plan for how to start the day can help you make the most of it without feeling overwhelmed, having a plan for how to end your day is also important. It can create a natural break between work and homelife, even when you work from home. Computer scientist and productivity expert Cal Newport calls this a *shutdown ritual*.[10] He reviews his task list and calendar to make sure he's up to date on everything before going home. This way, he knows where to pick up the next day so he can let go and not worry about work once he leaves the office. My own shut-down ritual involves a physical break. At 4:00 P.M. every day, I work out and then cook dinner immediately afterwards. Finding a way to create a natural break, if you can, will allow you to come back feeling more refreshed the next day.

THE MYTH OF MULTITASKING

One of the most fascinating enigmas in neuroscience is the vast gulf between the phenomenal speed with which the human nervous system can gather information from the environment and the (by comparison) relatively slow speed and direction of human thought and action. This was recently detailed in a paper written by neurobiologists at Caltech called "The Unbearable Slowness of Being."[11] When looking at record-breaking performances of human cognitive function—tasks like speed memorization, actions per minute in video games like Tetris, and even blindfolded speedcubing (where individuals study a Rubik's Cube and then solve it as fast as they can while blindfolded)—the maximum speed of human thought is around ten bits per second. One "bit" is the equivalent of a computer storing a single 1 or 0, so the sequence 0110111001 is ten bits of information. Our processing speed is similar for both thought (memorising the pattern on a Rubik's Cube) and action (moving the cube to solve it), and the limit of ten bits per second seems to be driven by the average firing rate of neurons in the human cortex.

To put ten bits per second into proper context, your internet connection likely runs at about one hundred *mega*bits per second (Mbps). That is a whopping ten million times faster. Despite the fact that thoughts and actions are so surprisingly slow, our nervous system does have the capacity to take in large amounts of information in record time. For example, the cells in our eyes collect information at a rate about ten times faster than your internet—more than one gigabit per second. But all that information is filtered down, so you only ever experience one ten-billionth of it. In fact, 90 percent of that information never even leaves the eye. The authors of the paper compare the fraction of information that we experience relative to what our body collects to the amount of water that one person could drink relative to all the water passing through the Hoover Dam.

I bring up this paper not because of these mind-boggling numbers but because it nicely frames the processes of human cognition. All of our brain's immense computing power ends up directing relatively slow and deliberate processes when it comes to thought and movement. This occurs largely because the brain spends a lot of its power filtering out most of the information coming at us. And we're not even aware of it happening.

One upshot of these filtering processes is that humans can only *really* focus on doing one thing at a time. Even the best performers in any given field, such as memory specialists or chess players, think through objects or moves one after the other. This is because humans *can't* multitask.

Let me clarify what I mean by that. Decades of research in both work environments and neuroscience labs have found that humans can't fully pay attention to and perform two complex cognitive tasks at the same time. I've heard people say that *of course* humans can multitask, because they can eat and watch TV at the same time, or talk and drive at the same time. But in both of those scenarios, at least one activity has become automatic enough that you can do it without a huge amount of focus or conscious thought. As a result, the brain is running automatic subroutines instead of consciously focusing on the task.

A good example of the difference between what happens when we multitask and what happens if we do one task at a time is eating while doing something else. While I'm absolutely no stranger to a TV dinner, it's clear from multiple studies that if we're distracted while eating—for instance, by the television—we end up eating more, and we're more likely to overeat.[12] This is, at least partly, because we are completely unaware of how much we've actually eaten. So, yes, while it's technically true that adult humans can successfully transfer food into their mouths while watching TV, critical information can be lost in that process, because we're only able to fully attend to one thing at a time. And the TV will win out every time.

By comparison, one thing that humans *are* good at is performing multiple complementary complex skills at once, especially if they are learned and practised together. Singing and playing a musical instrument at the same time is a good example. I would argue that this isn't multitasking because, with practice, these parallel processes become automatic so that it's all essentially one bigger and more complex skill rather than two different tasks occurring simultaneously. Therefore, when I talk about issues with multitasking, I mean splitting our attention between two unrelated processes that both require focused attention.

When it comes to future-proofing the brain, the multitasking that we really care about is the kind that occurs all the time at work. Trying to answer emails while on a Zoom call. Or opening up social media while you're working on a spreadsheet. We might call this multitasking, but we're never really doing both things at the same time. Instead, we're going back and forth between one and the other—a process known as *task-switching*. While we can probably get away with this kind of back-and-forth and ultimately finish the job we are being paid to do, more often than not, we do so at the cost of less efficiency and higher cognitive load.

Gloria Mark is a psychologist at the University of California, Irvine, whom we met briefly in chapter 12. She has spent decades trying to understand patterns of attention and focus, as well as the ways that task-switching and cognitive load at work can affect an individual's well-being and performance. In her book *Attention Span,* she shows that the days of knowledge workers have become increasingly fractured. By asking people to log their activities as they work, Dr. Mark and her colleagues found that even twenty years ago people spent an average of two and a half minutes on a work task before switching to another. Now that's down to less than fifty seconds, a decrease of more than two-thirds.[13]

We often switch between tasks that are both directed at the same goal—for example, after writing this sentence I might look over at my other screen to check the reference and re-read the section of the book or paper I'm writing about. That is technically a task switch, yet it is moving me toward the goal of my current period of focused work. Because of this, it might be more useful to think about moving between what Mark calls *spheres of work*—bigger overarching goals or projects that require multiple small tasks to accomplish.

We may switch tasks every fortyish seconds, but on average we spend around twelve minutes on one sphere of work before switching to another. And one study found that people tended to cycle through two other spheres of work—taking just over twenty-five minutes on average—before they returned to what they were originally working on.[14] With the ever-increasing burden of email and collaboration app messages, it's likely that the frequency of switches has only increased since the study was originally published a few years ago. It's this type of switching—going back and forth between different projects or completely unrelated tasks—that takes a real toll on our cognitive resources over time.

One of the biggest problems with switching between unrelated tasks is the time it takes to fire up the right set of cognitive processes associated with each particular activity. You've likely experienced this yourself. It's that feeling you get when you're in a conversation with somebody and you start doing or thinking about something else. When you snap back into the conversation, it will take you a minute or two to catch up. This sort of downtime occurs every time we switch our attention between unrelated tasks.

Cognitive downtime between tasks is partly driven by what is known as the *psychological refractory period*, which is a way of saying that the slow nature of our thought processes means it takes our brain a moment after finishing one task before we can initiate the next one.[15] As you switch from one task to another, you also experience *attentional residue*, which you can think of as the ghost of your thought processes from the previous task. Going back to the conversation example, even as you are *trying* to tune back into what your friend is saying, you're probably still thinking about the thing you were distracted by, and as a result, you're still not listening fully to what they're saying.

Depending on what you were doing and the task you switch to, the downtime associated with a task-switch could last several seconds or even several minutes. That adds up to significant losses every time you switch between tasks. Gloria Mark has shown that over the day, this increases cognitive load while also making people feel more stressed and less productive.[16]

FOCUS AS A SKILL

As we find our attention increasingly fractured both at work and through the various technologies we interact with every day, our brains respond accordingly. Just as with any stimulus, our brain adapts and becomes accustomed to the tasks we expose it to. Unfortunately, if we spend most of our time flitting back and forth between multiple tasks, apps, and screens, that means we can lose our ability to focus in certain ways. It's not that we *can't* focus, just that we've trained ourselves away from being able to centre our attention on individual cognitively challenging activities for prolonged periods. But just as we train ourselves to get stronger in the gym, we can also build up our focus with a little bit of effort and training. Modern technology hasn't made us incapable of high-gear cognitive work, but all the time spent task-switching in middle gear means we might need to build up and maintain our capacity to focus. In reality, learning how to focus means spending time doing just *one* thing, and there are a whole host of ways to do that.

Learning to Focus

In chapter 9, we said that the effect of formal education on headroom and cognitive function might be because it provides an opportunity for *learning to learn*. This same rule applies to focus. In order to study or perform well in exams, you will have to regularly spend long periods of time focused on the material, which, over time, increases your ability to pay attention and stay on task. As a result, it's likely that the simple act of doing *any* kind of focused attention work will improve your ability to focus overall. That's good news. It means that anytime you are fully engaged with learning a skill, you are also building the skill of focus. Start small if you need to—a few minutes a few times a week—and build up your focusing capacity from there.

Structure High-Gear Work

Given that the modern work environment can make it harder for us to maintain our focus muscles, it's not a surprise that many of us have difficulty focusing for longer periods. One way to overcome this is by building some structure into our high-gear work. A great example is the Pomodoro technique, where twenty-five-minute periods of focused work are interspersed with five-minute breaks. If you do multiple sessions in a row, you then take a longer break before continuing the cycle. There are a number of free Pomodoro apps and websites available, and many let you change the designated time frames for work and rest. Twenty-five minutes of focus seems to be a nice middle ground that most people should be able to do, though others might need to start with shorter periods of focus while they build that skill.

Microbreaks

One of the fundamental rules of Pomodoro is that your five-minute rest period should be spent doing something *other* than work. No emails or anything related to the task you were just doing. Instead, use your break to make a cup of tea, or maybe even fit in an exercise snack to get your brain back in the zone for the next focus period. This idea fits very nicely with recent studies looking at breaks during work. Perhaps surprisingly, evidence suggests that people can feel cognitively restored with very short planned microbreaks scattered across the workday.[17] One study found that a defined five-to-ten-minute break decreased fatigue and restored vigour when participants either did a relaxing activity (meditation) or completely disengaged from work by watching short comedy clips. Similar results have been found with very short periods of looking at nature through a window.[18] If, by comparison, people spent their break doing a cognitively challenging task, this increased fatigue.[19] Therefore, a short five-to-ten-minute break between focused bouts of work can help restore cognitive resources as long as you are taking a true mental break.

Be Mindful

Just as active engagement with skill learning can sharpen our ability to focus, the process of learning to sit with, or control, our thoughts also

> helps. In a study by Wendy Suzuki at NYU, participants who did guided mindfulness meditation involving breathing exercises and body scans for thirteen minutes a day for eight weeks saw improvement in some measures of attention and working memory. They also reported lower anxiety responses to a stressful test compared to a control group that instead listened to podcasts for thirteen minutes a day.[20] As breathing exercises and body scans require you to focus internally, it makes sense that any activities like this would strengthen our ability to pay attention.

It's important to point out that task-switching isn't inherently bad. When studies in the lab let people choose the number of tasks to complete at once, or let people switch between tasks at will, it's clear there is no one-size-fits-all approach to work. We all have our own preferences that help us with productivity. For instance, some people like to engage in multiple tasks at once because it makes them feel challenged or because they feel like they are being more efficient.[21] And some people switch between tasks because they're frustrated with the lack of progress in one area and switching provides them with a break or a change of approach.[22] The issue is less with our personal approach to task-switching and more to do with being distracted from our task—or being *forced* to do multiple things at once. Our brains can, over time, also become so accustomed to task-switching and distractions that it's harder for us to stay focused even when there isn't anything interrupting us.[23]

If somebody tries to (or is forced to) juggle multiple challenging tasks simultaneously, you'll often see either a performance decline or an increase in stress.[24] When this is happening regularly as part of our jobs, it increases allostatic load and cognitive load, which decreases our headroom. It can also increase the likelihood that we'll make mistakes. For example, one study followed emergency medicine physicians over dozens of shifts. The researchers found that both interruptions (an external stimulus that changed the physician's task) and multitasking (e.g., talking while typing on the computer) increased the number of prescribing errors a doctor made.[25] Some of this can be offset—for instance, those who had slept well scored better in a working memory test (perhaps evidence that they had more headroom?) and made fewer errors. But regardless of the scenario, if we want to do high-quality work while minimising unnecessary stress and errors, we should do what we can to focus on one thing at a time rather than "multitasking," or task-switching.

One final—and fascinating—piece of the multitasking puzzle is that it is possible we can expand our ability to do multiple activities at once. But, as with any specific adaptation in the brain, there will probably be some trade-offs as a result. A classic paper by a group from Stanford looked at cognitive function in those who performed a lot of multi-tasking across multiple platforms (print media, television, videos, computer games, email, apps, etc.).[26] During cognitive function tests, the heavy media multitaskers were more distractible and *less* able to reliably task-switch, largely because of their decreased ability to filter out irrelevant information.

This finding is particularly interesting in light of a more recent study looking at media multitasking and ability to perform two cognitive tasks at the same time.[27] The researchers found that people who performed more multitasking were *better* at maintaining function in a cognitive task (like searching for a specific shape in a jumble of shapes) when a second task was layered on top (counting the number of circles on the periphery of the screen). Though everybody lost some accuracy on the main task, the cost of multitasking was lower in people who were accustomed to multitasking. This makes perfect sense when we think about how the brain adapts to stimulus. If we multitask a lot, we might get better at multitasking, but this comes at the expense of increased distractibility. To multitask, our brains learn to filter out less information so we can be on the lookout for all the different things we might need to pay attention to.

So, as ever, when you think about how to accomplish tasks (and whether it makes sense to have your smartphone next to you while you work on them), we must consider what skills we ultimately want our brains to be good at. Some of the relationship between different types of media and multitasking are driven by personal preference. Therefore, it's possible that there are some inherent differences between people who multitask or task-switch heavily and those who don't.[28] However, in the Stanford study, multitasking didn't seem to be related to other elements of personality or cognitive function. Multitasking is also clearly influenced by the environment. For example, in another study by Gloria Mark, when knowledge workers turned off email for a week, they decreased task-switching, increased the time spent on individual tasks, and had lower levels of stress.[29]

It's clear that the pace and direction of human thought makes us better suited to doing one thing at a time. There's also a cognitive and physiological cost associated with the kind of frequent task switching seen in the modern work and multimedia environments. When we're interrupted or distracted, it increases errors while also upping stress responses. This not only can make us feel less productive over time but also takes a cumulative toll if we feel like we're not in control of our workloads.

In many ways, modern work and technology can end up doing exactly the *opposite* of what we want for our brains based on the 3-S model—the type of stimulus we receive makes us more distractible and less able to focus. At the same time, as we juggle tasks, we often feel a chronic level of stress (decreased support) from spending all day in the middle gear. One of the best ways to combat this is to take some time to learn to focus—and structure your calendar to include periods of focused work and recovery. Doing so can decrease errors and stress across the day while improving cognitive function today and in the long term.

MINIMISING DISTRACTION

A critical part of our ability to stay focused on a specific task is how we manage the everyday distractions that enter our consciousness and pull our attention in different directions. Studies suggest that somewhere between one-third and half of task-switches are due to something that interrupts or distracts us.[30] In addition to instigating a task-switch, distractions that are not relevant to our current goal, or that make it harder for us to focus on the task at hand, increase cognitive load. They either slow us down or increase our rate of errors.[31] Finding ways to minimise these external distractions is therefore important, as we know their effects can build up over time.

Interestingly, though, at least half of task-switches happen when we interrupt *ourselves*. Some of this is part of normal attention switching during the completion of a specific work sphere (e.g., alternating between research and writing when working on a book), but some of it is because we get conditioned to a certain pattern or frequency of distractions. As a result, we become primed to go looking for a new task or input at regular intervals, even when nothing external interrupts us.[32] If you find interruption or task-switching is problematic for you, some of these tweaks can help you better manage your time. Not only will you be interrupted less often, but over time, it could help reduce the cadence of self-interruption.

Eliminate (Nonessential) Notifications

At first, it was just emails and texts, but these days it seems that every app and widget you interact with wants to send you notifications. Almost none of these are necessary, and even fewer are essential. Even worse, if you have a smartwatch, these notifications are being beamed directly onto your body through what can quickly transform into your own personalised interruption device. Unless you make your living as a professional influencer, it's unlikely that you need to know that somebody commented on your social media post at exactly 10:13 A.M. on a Tuesday. And we all have those apps we only use once in a while that are programmed to intermittently pop up and remind us they exist because they feel lonely. Think about all the notifications you receive that you don't *need* but that interrupt you while you're trying to work. Silence or remove as many of them as possible.

Pace Your Email and Communication Apps

For most people, I would venture that email notifications aren't necessary, even during the workday. Though it often doesn't feel like it, most emails are not urgent (no matter what the sender happens to say). The same can be said for the more intrusive notifications that can pop up on your computer screen from collaboration and productivity apps. One study found that email and messaging apps interrupt people around four times per hour on average, and if you respond to them, it takes ten to fifteen minutes to return to the original task.[33] A recent meta-analysis explored more than two decades of research examining how to improve your relationship with email, suggesting that setting clear boundaries and dealing with email on your own schedule were two of the best ways to support both well-being and performance.[34] Most apps allow for notifications to be muted for specific periods during the day, so if you can't turn them off entirely, consider silencing them during high-gear work. But as with everything discussed so far in this chapter, your approach to work-related notifications requires some personalization. Some people will tell you to never start your day by opening your email. Others recommend only checking email a couple of times a day (or even less) to maximise productivity. These ideas can be helpful for some, but not for those who will feel stress knowing that there are unattended messages building up and would prefer to stay on top of emails throughout the day. Depending on your job—and your stress level—your mileage may vary. The main idea is to prevent emails from intruding on periods of focused work. Find your own approach to managing email that gives you back control and maintains your ability to focus—and recover—when you need to.

Tune Out Distractions

In addition to all those pesky notifications, noise from the environment can also be distracting. Our own internal thoughts can distract us too. Both of these can be improved through sound. For example, one study found that a low level of white noise—loud enough to mask other background sounds but not loud enough to be stressful—improved sustained attention when compared to ambient office noise.[35] The evidence is even stronger for music. Several studies show that self-selected music improves sustained attention and focus.[36] This increase in focus appears to be caused by a music-driven increase in arousal. Grab some headphones and then play the tunes that keep you in the mood to focus (but avoid songs that might be distracting in their own right). In case you were wondering, this entire book was written to a background of melodic drum and bass, with the occasional dash of house and techno.

Manage Your Project List

Just as with emails, having a long mental list of tasks or projects to complete can become a source of low-level stress and additional cognitive load, for different reasons. One reason is the Zeigarnik effect mentioned in chapter 11—the mental friction and stress that simmers under the surface as we think about unfinished tasks. Another reason is the cognitive load of trying to remember all the things we have to do while trying to focus on the most important task at hand. Many of these issues can be managed with a well-constructed to-do list. Cal Newport suggests actually having *two* to-do lists. The first consists of just two or three projects to be prioritised while others are actively ignored. This gives you the ability to switch between projects based on your mood or if you need some variety, but it also means that you aren't constantly having to switch around so often that your productivity suffers. The second list is one that you ignore on most days, documenting future tasks so you don't have to worry about forgetting something (similar to the mental offloading we saw in chapter 11). Dividing current and future projects into two separate lists also prevents scenarios where you're unable to prioritise because you're overwhelmed by the volume of tasks you need to accomplish. This way, when one project is done, you can move something from the future-project list to the current to-do list and have a much higher likelihood of completing it.

RISE TO THE OCCASION

When we think about what our brains need in order to perform at their best *today*, a clear pattern emerges. Whatever we're trying to use our brains for in the moment will require an appropriate level of mental energy, with intense focus requiring matched periods of recovery to help us restore our cognitive resources. Greater peaks and troughs of attention allow for better performance and productivity and less overall stress. In addition to following our natural rhythms of energy throughout the day to create a schedule for focused work, our engagement with a task is a critical determinant of whether we're able to deliver. Engagement could simply be getting in the right frame of mind for focused-work blocks each day, or it could be an event, like a big presentation, where you have to perform or focus for a certain period of time. Because of this, you probably won't be surprised to learn that I'm bringing back the arousal curve.

As we discussed extensively in chapter 11, with every complex cognitive activity there is a range of arousal that maximises the likelihood of a good performance. The target range of arousal is one where you aren't so stressed that you feel anxious and jittery, but also not so relaxed that you are disengaged and apathetic. When I work with Formula 1 drivers and their coaches to think about how to manage arousal to enhance performance, we usually break it down into two periods: a baseline period and the period leading up to the performance. You may not be a Formula 1 driver, but the same principles apply to athletic and cognitive performances of any kind, even the day-to-day ones we do at work or when we're learning new skills.

Baseline performance management is built around the day-to-day factors that build headroom and provide a foundation for future performance. These are the topics covered in part 2. For example, though nutrient status may not necessarily be the main factor that gets in the way of performance on the day, it helps to attend to nutrition in the run-up to any event because it might be harder to do once you're in the thick of it. We also know that our nutrient demands can increase when we ask for more performance. For example, high levels of physical and cognitive stress can increase the need for B vitamins as well as micronutrients like zinc, magnesium, and iron.[37] And as we saw in chapter 8, several other nutrients are required for cognitive function in general. Therefore, eating a nutrient-rich diet can provide a buffer if performance is required over a long period of time, or if our work or our environment involves prolonged exposure to stress.

For both day-to-day performance and big events, it can also be critical to attend to overall allostatic load as well as sleep—both to ensure that you have adequate cognitive resources on the day and to avoid illness. Decreasing our risk of severe illness is particularly important as we get older, so we don't lose cognitive and physical function due to loss of stimulus, but acute illness is also a concern when we need to perform at a specific time.

Poor sleep and chronic stress are two common and interrelated risk factors for acute illness—especially viral illnesses—as well as decreased performance. In athletes, international travel across multiple time zones increases the risk of illness, at least partly due to the effect of jet lag on sleep.[38] Illness is also more likely during periods of heightened or prolonged stress.[39] Stress over a period of several days can also increase fatigue (decreasing baseline levels of arousal) since stress impairs sleep (making you more tired the next day).[40] And we already know that increased stress and cognitive load can decrease headroom over time. Therefore, paying attention to your allostatic load and focusing on sleep can help to reduce the risk of sudden losses in performance (due to illness) as well as providing a better baseline level for you to perform from. This is where a good sleep routine can come into its own—having a specific way to wind down and ensure quality sleep is one of the best ways to help you achieve the necessary level of performance the next day.

WHAT IF I DIDN'T SLEEP WELL?

Knowing that sleep is such a critical component of cognitive function can sometimes be a double-edged sword. On one hand, it helps us to appreciate the importance of sleep. On the other hand, it can become a source of stress when we need to sleep and can't, or if the anticipation of an event prevents us from being able to sleep as well as we'd like.[41] Luckily, our brains can be quite good at adapting to a loss of sleep in the short term. In fact, some of the problems we experience when we don't sleep well are due more to expectation than physiology.

You Perform Based on How You *Think* You Slept

Steven Lockley is a neuroscientist at Harvard who studies sleep. He also helped to develop the travel and jet lag plans used by Hintsa Formula 1 drivers. In a classic study by the Lockley group, some participants were brought in to sleep in the lab overnight. They were randomised to two lengths of sleep: one group slept five hours; the other slept for eight. The participants did not know which group they were in, and the clocks in the room were manipulated so they were not aware of how long they'd actually slept. Some participants slept for five hours, but the clocks made them think they had slept for eight. Other participants slept for eight hours but thought they had slept for five. When their cognitive performance was tested the next day, cognitive function and fatigue was only affected by how long people *thought* they had slept, rather than how long they had truly slept.[42] A similar study by a group at Oxford gave participants a wearable device to track their sleep. Regardless of how well they slept, participants were randomised to be given either positive or negative feedback about their sleep. Those told they hadn't slept well reported feeling more fatigued and cognitively impaired, regardless of how many hours of sleep they really got.[43] This means that it's our *expectation* of poor performance after a night of poor sleep that influences our function more than the lack of sleep itself. Obviously, things will change if sleep is impaired for several nights, but if you have one bad night, remember that your brain is capable of performing just fine the next day. And if you check your wearable data every morning, you might want to consider just not wearing it if you know you are likely to have a restless night.

Slower (and Grumpier) but Not Less Accurate

While we tend to assume that sleep loss is universally detrimental for our cognitive function the next day, it's not all bad news. Some studies suggest that the brain adapts by altering what networks are activated the next day in order to maintain function.[44] As a result, our thought processes might change, but they don't necessarily get *worse*. For instance, one study from The Norwegian Defence Leadership Institute looked at the effect of sleep deprivation on the performance of naval cadets going through ranger training. This required them to read maps, plan rescues, and decipher coded messages.[45] When sleep-deprived, cadets were slower but acted more deliberately. They were also less likely to overestimate the level of their performance compared to the grade given to them by their instructors. These findings align with meta-analyses exploring the effect of sleep loss on cognitive function, which have consistently found that speed is impaired more than accuracy after poor sleep. Mood also tends to be affected more than performance is.[46] This means that we're probably able to maintain our performance after some sleep loss, but we might rate our efforts less highly. Of course, this doesn't continue indefinitely, and other meta-analyses have found that performance losses increase based on both the number of nights of poor sleep and how many hours of sleep are lost, as you might expect.[47] But I think studies like these can help us realise that we're still able to perform even if we tossed and turned the night before an important event.

Caffeine Comes into Its Own?

For those of us who regularly consume caffeine, that first jolt of the day seems to bring magical restorative properties. It's almost like we can feel the lights suddenly switching on in our brains. Over the past few decades, we've learned that at least part of this improvement can be explained by the placebo effect, and some of it is thanks to a reversal of the cognitive deficit caused by caffeine withdrawal.[48] Though caffeine does improve athletic performance as well as mood in regular consumers,[49] it can easily push people too far up the arousal curve. As a result, caffeine reliably boosts simple cognitive functions like reaction time but can impair more complex cognitive functions because all that stimulant makes people feel more jittery.[50] Similar results have also been found for other stimulants like methylphenidate and modafinil (Ritalin and Provigil) in people without ADHD.[51] However, caffeine seems to be particularly good at maintaining or improving performance in low-arousal states, especially after sleep deprivation.[52] In addition to its effects directly blocking adenosine that creates sleep pressure and impairs cognitive function after a long day of cognitive activity, caffeine also boosts dopamine signaling by increasing the availability of dopamine receptors that are downregulated with sleep deprivation.[53] Therefore, targeted caffeine use can help to improve both arousal and focus when we haven't slept enough.

Think about baseline performance management as the key to building headroom, which will hopefully now become a lifelong pursuit. By building headroom you have a higher baseline—as well as a better ability to manage stress or a lost night of sleep around an event—but also high capacity to tap into when your moment to shine arrives. Tapping into this capacity relies on arousal management in the moment. The same is true even if you're just sitting down to some high-gear work that you need to focus on to complete a project.

When it comes to high-gear work, one of the main reasons increased arousal helps us maintain focus is that we become better at filtering out distractions. In that way, a little bit of cognitive load and a small increase in stress response helps you to narrow your attention and concentrate on the task at hand.[54] This means that when focus is required but we're in a low-arousal state, increasing arousal can improve our cognitive function and help us engage with—and perform better at—the work in progress.

Increasing your arousal before engaging in a cognitive task is just as important as it is for an athlete to warm up for a race or before they lift something heavy in the gym. You wouldn't step into the gym and immediately try to lift a personal record or sprint as fast as you can. It takes the body some time to warm up so it can direct the necessary resources to get your muscles ready to perform. The brain is the same. Anytime we want to engage with a new task, we need to fire up the necessary networks and orient ourselves with the information or environment required to get the job done.

Engaging in a mental warm-up can also help you create a routine that primes you for work or performance. Just like your warm-up in the gym gets you feeling more confident and ready to move, taking the time to get ready also improves performance during a period of focused work. *How* you do your warm-up is up to you. There are a number of different ways to increase arousal; just be sure you don't push yourself too far over the arousal curve.

Exercise is probably one of the best-studied ways to immediately boost cognitive function and focus. In addition to the long-term effects of movement on the brain, brief periods of exercise can improve aspects of processing speed and executive function as well as improving energy and mood.[55] In general, studies suggest that around twenty minutes (and up to sixty minutes) of moderate-intensity physical activity like brisk walking, jogging, or resistance training consistently improves cognitive function, with the effects often lasting for multiple hours afterwards.[56] This is thought to be due to release of norepinephrine and dopamine as arousal increases. However, we also know from chapter 7 that even very short sprints of a few seconds can be enough to immediately improve cognitive function. This means that you have a fair amount of latitude in terms of what kind of exercise you could do as your mental warm-up. If it fits into your schedule, doing a workout before or during work can help to set you up well for any upcoming bouts of focused high-gear work. However, it's probably best to plan your most intense workouts for times when you don't need all your brain power immediately afterwards. This is because prolonged or exhausting exercise can momentarily *decrease* cognitive function.[57] The key to getting yourself in the right zone for focus and performance is making it intense enough to get your heart rate up while leaving you feeling energised rather than fatigued.

There are a number of ways we can increase arousal by activating similar pathways to the ones activated by exercise. Though the evidence often isn't as good in terms of improvement to acute cognitive function, these warm-ups can benefit mood in ways that mirror the effects of exercise and, as such, are likely to translate to improved focus. One example is cold exposure. Not chisel-the-ice-off-the-top-of-a-frozen-lake kind of cold exposure—just like with exhausting exercise, very cold or prolonged cold exposure can decrease cognitive function for a period of time afterwards.[58] More like jumping-in-a-slightly-chilly-swimming-pool kind of cold exposure. A quick trip into a cold shower or even just splashing your face with cold water can have a similar effect. One study had individuals spend five minutes immersed in water at 20°C (68°F).[59] When the researchers compared their reported mood and their brain connectivity, as seen on a brain scan, before and after the plunge, they found that even this short period of mild cold exposure made people feel more attentive and alert and created changes in brain networks related to attention.[60]

Light is another way to acutely boost arousal. We know that light is an important biological input that helps to coordinate a whole host of our biological functions, including alertness. One reason we have different peaks of arousal during the day is because of our habitual light exposure—and that's a variable we can manipulate in moments when we need to increase focus. In one study, researchers exposed participants to either standard indoor lighting (two hundred lux of light intensity) or one thousand lux (about the same as being outside on a cloudy day) using a bright lamp. Those exposed to the bright light felt less sleepy and showed faster reaction times compared to those who were in the standard-lighting group.[61]

In reality, any brief exposure or activity that makes you feel more alert will probably do the trick here. Music is another way to increase arousal and performance,[62] as well as the fast-paced breathing techniques mentioned in chapter 11. Assuming you're in a safe and accepting space (or alone), even swearing has been found to increase arousal and improve performance, at least in the physical realm (not recommended when trying to psych yourself up in front of the company board before your presentation on the quarterly report).[63] Pick something you can build into a routine that signals to your brain that it's time to get to work. With practice, you'll know that once your phone or any other connected device is put to the side, notifications are switched off, and you've done your preferred mental warm-up, you'll be raring to go when it's time for high-gear work.

Of course, when it comes to focus and performance, the goal isn't necessarily to develop some complex set of "perfect" conditions every time. In fact, I would argue that if you consistently have to rely on the same routines, supplements, and hacks to get you in the perfect zone for cognitive performance, that would imply that you need to build some resilience and that your headroom isn't where it needs to be. Whether it's focused periods of deep work every day or one-off moments when you need your brain at its best, often the conditions will be less than ideal, but you have to show up and get the work done anyway. Having a set of tools to get you in the right frame of mind can help to make sure you can perform whenever you need to.

DON'T (ALWAYS) GO WITH THE FLOW

One idea that has become very popular in the world of productivity and work performance is flow. This concept, developed by psychologist Mihály Csíkszentmihályi, describes a state when both skill level and challenge level are high. Many people liken flow to being *in the zone,* a state where you're completely immersed in an activity and your performance is at the highest possible level.

A classic example of flow in the world of Formula 1 comes from Ayrton Senna—regarded by many as the greatest driver of all time—describing his experience during the 1988 Monaco Grand Prix:

> One lap after the other, quicker, and quicker, and quicker... Suddenly, I was nearly two seconds faster than anybody else, including

my teammate with the same car. And I realised that I was no longer driving the car consciously.... I was just going, going—more, and more, and more, and more. I was way over the limit but still able to find even more.... I realised I was well beyond my conscious understanding. [Lightly edited for clarity.]

If we think about the arousal curve, flow is one of the states that you can enter when you reach the peak—when everything aligns perfectly, and you can perform at a high level automatically. In this way, flow is the maximal expression of a learned complex skill. Senna was such a good driver that he was able to enter a state where it could happen without conscious thought. When we're locked into something we're really good at or are part of a well-oiled group or team, flow is possible.

However, a problem arises when we think that flow is always the best possible state for performance at optimal levels of arousal. Though being in flow feels fantastic, this is *not* how most knowledge-work—or even most high-level performance—feels. For example, alongside flow states, high-level sports performance often includes something known as *clutch* states.[64] Arousal is heightened, focus is complete, but the athlete must engage in intense effort in order to perform. Even when an athlete is performing to the best of their abilities, clutch states can feel like extremely hard work. Similarly, athletes will often talk about the rule of thirds. A third of workouts will feel great, where you imagine yourself as unstoppable. A third will be just average—nothing remarkable, but you feel fine. The last third will suck, and you'll have to grind through it, even if you did everything right beforehand. This is how a lot of high-gear work feels for cognitive athletes, and that's OK.

When it comes down to it, we can't always be in a state of flow. In fact, we often don't *want* to be. Flow is one possible outcome when we've learned to train our focus, but if flow is the maximal expression of what we've already learned, then we know that any time we're pushing against the edge of our abilities, failing, or learning something new, we can't be in flow. When we are challenging ourselves in that way, it *should* feel a little uncomfortable. And even if we're locked in and focused, sometimes whatever we are doing will feel like hard work. All of this to say that even when it doesn't feel easy, that doesn't mean you're not doing it right.

HOW TO NOT FORGET

If there's one cognitive function that is most closely tied to our desire to future-proof our brains, it's memory. While whole books have been written just on memory, there are some ideas in this chapter we can apply to learning and memory on a day-to-day basis to better support our overall cognitive function right now. But before we talk about improving memory, perhaps the most important thing to mention is that the brain's default state is to *not* remember something. Given the (relatively) ponderous speed of human thought compared to all the information it is exposed to, the brain is better off never even fully registering information in the first place, let alone investing time and effort in remembering it.

This is exemplified by a classic experiment by German psychologist Hermann Ebbinghaus in 1884. Ebbinghaus learned and relearned lists of new words to see how long he could remember them. What he found was that around one-third of new information is forgotten within twenty minutes, and more than half is forgotten within an hour (figure 2). Though his study involved just one highly motivated participant (himself), the results have generally been replicated time and time again in the decades since.[65] This means that even when we actively *try* to remember something, we forget most of it fairly quickly.

One particularly excellent book on memory is *Why We Remember* by psychologist and neuroscientist Charan Ranganath. He has a framework for how memories are constructed that can help us to learn and remember better. It also offers some tools we can leverage to support those processes. His framework postulates that five things are required for a memory to be stored (encoded and consolidated) and then retrieved. These are importance, distinctiveness, meaning, context, and error.

The importance of a given memory is perhaps the most closely linked to the other topics covered in this chapter so far. For your brain to perceive something and attempt to remember it, it needs to know that this piece of information is meaningful. Therefore, the more important something feels to us—personally, emotionally, or socially—the more likely it is to be stored and retrieved later. This also requires attention, and some level of arousal. Attention and memory are intricately

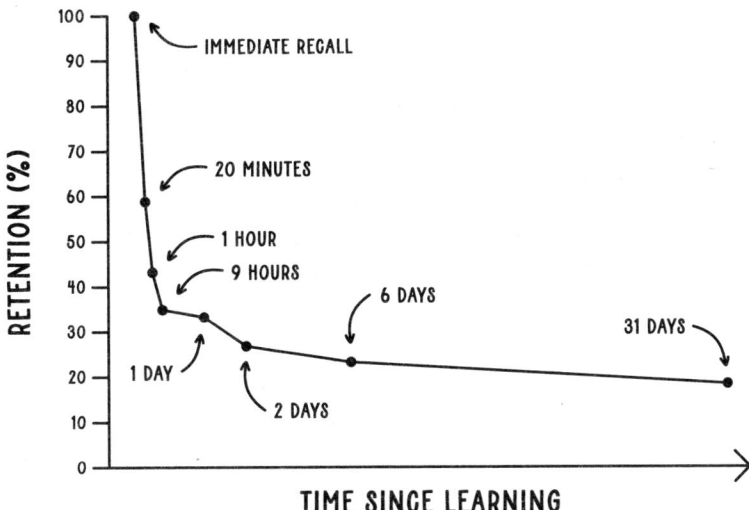

FIGURE 2. The forgetting curve. Ebbinghaus learned lists of nonsense syllables (to prevent the influence of previous knowledge) like DAX, BOK, and YAT and determined how well he retained the information over time. The graph shows time since learning in days along the bottom, and the percentage of information retained is on the side. Retention drops rapidly over the first 9 hours and then remains relatively stable. Modified from Yue, *International Journal of Emerging Technologies in Learning (iJET)*, 2017.

linked, first as part of our ability to consciously detect the information and then to activate the necessary brain networks so that information can be stored.[66] The importance of arousal for memory is one reason emotional information is more likely to be remembered.

When an experience itself causes arousal, that is often enough to up the likelihood that you will remember it. But if you need an arousal boost, exercise is one of the best-studied ways to support memory. Meta-analyses have shown that exercise either before or after learning improves recall, and the same has been found when learning motor skills.[67] Around twenty minutes of moderately intense exercise, once again, seems to be the most consistent way to boost memory, though, as with performance in general, the level of arousal is more important than the exact way you achieved it.[68] When you're in the process of learning and want to remember a new skill or piece of information, moving yourself up the arousal curve using your preferred method—either before or after the learning period—is going to help you support that process by getting the brain's attention and neuroplasticity machinery in gear.

Next up is distinctiveness. This refers to how novel a particular piece of information is, or how much it deviates from expectation. Remember that our brains are constantly working to predict what will happen next, and strong signals for neuroplasticity and learning are generally driven by the unexpected. So, if a stimulus breaks the pattern of expectation, it gets flagged for storage. If we want to remember something, it helps to find a way to make it distinctive from other similar pieces of information that we've encountered before. Meaning and context (critical areas three and four) help fit the information into the bigger picture of how we understand the world and the place where we happened to learn it. Contextual binding is a process performed by the hippocampus that ties information to the context where it was learned—like pairing a name with a face or a person with a place.[69] This aids with encoding and retrieval. Contextual binding is one reason certain smells can evoke such strong memories and also help us retain information.[70]

As you consider the different ways we construct and store memories, some of our daily experiences become more understandable. When we can't remember something that we feel like we should be able to, it is probably because we weren't paying enough attention. Maybe we were not aroused enough (bored or sleep-deprived) or were experiencing a high cognitive or allostatic load or thinking about something else. Unless your brain has a reason to think that something is important, is novel, or has meaning or context to be assigned to it, the information is likely to just flow in and out, even if we briefly become aware of it.

Think, for a minute, about the last time you couldn't remember where you'd put your car keys or your wallet. Maybe you worried for a brief second that this was the beginning of the end of your cognitive faculties. But was there anything about the experience of setting down your car keys that fulfilled Dr. Ranganath's criteria? Probably not. In the grand scheme of things, where you put your car keys isn't that important. You know they're in the house somewhere, and I bet you were distracted by or thinking about something else when you set them down. Distinctiveness, meaning, and context were probably all missing, because the location of your keys is not emotional information, nor is it critical for your survival. So, while this kind of forgetting is decidedly annoying, it's usually not proof that your memory isn't working like it's supposed to.

When you really need to remember something that lacks some of the other factors above, the best place to focus is the last memory criterion—error. As we discussed in chapter 11, one of the most important triggers for learning is making errors. Your mistakes trigger signals for neuroplasticity and learning in a similar way to distinctiveness. One of the ways errors can be leveraged for learning, and memory specifically, is by testing yourself. In fact, several studies show that trying to recall the information you've learned is better for memory than reading the same material again.

In one classic study, students studied two passages from a test-preparation book for the Test of English as a Foreign Language (TOEFL). They were then allowed to either restudy the material several times or test themselves by trying to recall what they had read, without getting any feedback on how they did. A week later, those who tested themselves outperformed those who had studied the material several times.[71] A later study from Charan Ranganath's lab suggested that the benefit of self-testing comes from increased activity of the hippocampus when trying to remember information.[72] So it's not just error that triggers learning—challenging yourself to remember the information works too. This same process—in addition to cementing connections between brain regions required for the activity—is probably why visualization can help enhance skill learning and athletic performance, as well as a range of other areas, from maths to decision-making.[73]

Part of the trade-off between studying and self-testing may be that relearning too soon is an inefficient way to improve what you retain. In fact, several studies suggest that the most efficient way to go back over material you want to learn is to re-expose yourself to it two or three days later.[74] Regardless of the scenario, whether you are trying to remember where you left your car keys or all that biochemistry material you've just read, step away from your notes (or the keys) for a while. Then test yourself on what you remember. That will maximise the likelihood that the information is encoded and stored.

I should mention one final critical aspect of memory. While it's not included in Raganath's framework, recovery after the stimulus is something that he speaks about frequently. We've covered extensively why sleep is critical for both storing and accessing memories, which is probably why it's better to revisit information after a couple of nights of sleep if you want to remember it. Just as with any stimulus, encoding information in our memory requires a period of recovery and adaptation.

FUTURE-PROOFING YOUR BRAIN TODAY HELPS BUILD HEADROOM FOR TOMORROW

A practical approach to building and maintaining the kind of cognitive function you can rely on day-to-day requires thoughtful application of all the tools we've covered in this book so far. The goal is to balance stimulus with recovery while minimising the factors that interfere with those processes. Over weeks or months, anything we do that increases headroom—either through improved stimulus, support, supply, or, ideally, all three—will provide a foundation for focused work or performance. We can then leverage that foundation in the moment by using tools to optimise arousal, boost focus, and minimise distractions. Embracing these brain-healthy activities can also make us more confident that we've built up the headroom needed to get the job done even when we face suboptimal conditions.

At the same time, as we tend to spend at least half of our waking hours at work, the way we engage with stimuli and tasks during the workday plays a huge role in how our brains function in the long term. When we can structure our day so that we get true peaks and troughs of activity, we stack the deck in favour of maximising our brain's performance. Creating defined periods of high-gear work and recovery, and matching cognitive gears to the natural fluctuations in energy that we all experience throughout the day, result in better overall productivity. This also keeps us from feeling like we slogged through the day—or getting so behind on work that we are stressed, adding to our allostatic load. When we balance stimulus and recovery in our day-to-day work, we can minimise the daily drain we place on our headroom, perform our best when we need to, and free up some headspace and time for other activities (like sleep or connecting with loved ones). As a result, we feel better today while also working toward future-proofing our brains over the long haul.

HOW LONG SHOULD I FOCUS (OR LEARN) FOR?

There are a number of schools of thought as to how long our periods of learning or focus should be, but there's no strong evidence that any one particular formula or recommendation is best.

In the early 1960s, physiologist Nathaniel Kleitman proposed that the brain operated on ninety-minute cycles (often called *ultradian rhythms*) during the day, similar to the cycles seen during sleep.[75] He hypothesised that alertness would increase to a peak during that time period and then decline again over the final twenty to thirty minutes before a lull. Based on this, you'll often see productivity recommendations that include cycles of work or focused activity for ninety minutes before a break.

This idea is at least partly supported by research in attention and skill learning, with the most frequently cited study in this area being a classic paper by Anders Ericsson, who studied the habits of violinists and pianists at a music academy in Berlin.[76] If you've ever heard that it takes ten thousand hours of practice to become an expert in a skill, that statistic comes from a misinterpretation of Ericsson's study. Ten thousand hours was actually the average amount of practice that the best violinists and pianists had accrued by the age of twenty, well before they were considered true experts.

When Ericsson looked at the practice habits of the best musicians, he saw that they tended to do two or three sessions of practice per day, each lasting an average of eighty or ninety minutes. Most had one session in the mid-to-late morning, with the rest spread throughout the afternoon and evening. These observations lend themselves to the idea that highly skilled individuals spending time doing deliberate, focused work and learning naturally do so in chunks of time that average somewhere around ninety minutes.

If you go looking for biological ninety-minute cycles of alertness or cognitive function, however, the evidence becomes a bit murky. One study that tracked the eye movements of a small group of young adults in the late 1970s found that their pupils constricted and dilated on a roughly ninety-minute cycle throughout the day. As pupils tend to dilate when we're aroused—due to the action of noradrenaline released by the sympathetic nervous system—it was suggested that this was evidence of a ninety-minute ultradian rhythm of arousal. However, the dilation of pupils didn't correlate with how awake the participants reported they felt.[77]

Other studies have found no evidence that cognitive function fluctuates on ninety-minute cycles.[78] Instead, when looking at patterns of electrical activity in the brain, scientists have found multiple different cycles of activity that are all happening at the same time—some that happen every hour and others that occur up to every twelve hours.[79] It's also worth mentioning that arousal and cognitive function will be strongly influenced by multiple factors besides ultradian rhythms, including how well we slept and how interested and engaged in (or aroused by) a given activity we are.[80]

All this to say that there's no hard-and-fast rule when it comes to how long you should focus on your high-gear work. Remember that focus is a skill that needs to be built up over time. Ericsson's expert musicians didn't start out practicing for ninety minutes at a time—they got there through years of training their focus muscles along with their musical skills. The best advice is to start with a period of time for which you can reliably focus or work, take a break, and then build up from there.

FUTURE-PROOFING YOUR BRAIN FOR TOMORROW

The fact that brain function is underpinned by the same core principles that determine the health of every other bodily system—in humans as well as in numerous other species—reassures me that the 3-S model and the tools described in this book will continue to be useful in future-proofing the brain, even as we learn more about its inner complexities in the coming years. Thinking about the brain in terms of the three S's can also provide some guiding principles when our reductionist tendencies want to take over because we are suddenly enamored with a new mechanism, pathway, or drug linked to dementia. While I hope that the burden of dementia will be dramatically reduced, regardless of how that happens, I strongly believe that's most likely to occur by considering our brains at the level of the whole body, the environment, and society rather than at the level of individual biochemical pathways.

Wherever you are on your life trajectory, it's not too early (or too late) to start building headroom. Even if retirement is far in the distance, be mindful that this is when we are at the greatest risk of losing elements of the 3-S model—not just cognitive stimulus but also social connection and other important factors like physical activity. You should think about pushing back against those potential losses *now*, before the transition occurs. But even if retirement is already behind you, there's still plenty of time to get started and plenty of benefit to be gained. Across all the topics covered in part 2, the risk factors most consistently associated with the diseases of aging—including cognitive decline—are those related to mismatch caused by either the absence of critical inputs, like physical and social activity, or exposures that our bodies aren't accustomed to (e.g., smoking and a calorie-dense, nutrient-poor diet). This means that retirement is an ideal time to put a greater focus on those factors—not to give up but to continue to minimise mismatch in whatever ways you can.

The main message I hope you take away from this book is that the brain is capable of neuroplasticity, growth, and change at any age. By zooming out and thinking about the bigger picture—and understanding how small actions can synergise to have big effects—each of us has the capacity to build headroom and future-proof our brains no matter who we are or what point we might be starting from. And better yet, because of the way the core components of brain function interact and feed off one another, there are billions of different combinations of activities and lifestyle changes that can help us start improving our brains today.

As I consider the different factors that help maintain a stimulated mind, I'm reminded of a visit I made to my mother in Iceland a few years ago. She is a professor with expertise in multiple fields including geology and economics, a former university dean, and an advisor to several governments around the world. She's also what I lovingly think of as an old-school hippie. She's a political and environmental activist. She meditates, does yoga, and has always been interested in the ways nutrition can affect our health and well-being. My mum's flat has bookshelves on almost every available wall, and many of the books they contain also lined the walls of the house I grew up in—sitting in my direct eyeline for nearly two decades.

Though I largely ignored those books for the better part of my early life, during my last visit to Iceland I took the opportunity to finally read some. The contents were immediately familiar, detailing the critical importance of sleep, movement, stress management, and nutrition to overall well-being. While it took two decades of my own research and experience for these ideas to coalesce into a workable model of brain health and function, they've clearly been percolating somewhere in my subconscious for even longer. They've also been out in the world and part of the human experience for millennia before that. This is why I have so much hope about our ability to improve and protect our cognitive function as we age—both individually and as a society. The same core aspects of biology will always be important to our brain health, no matter what happens in the future. While this book contains details on some of the mechanisms of these—exercise, diet, social connection, and more—and how they affect our brains, I continue to believe those mechanisms matter much less than the fact that we know these things work through the common pathways of stimulus, supply, and support.

That last point is critical. Because it means that we *already* have the knowledge and ability to make a huge impact on the health of our brains. We are empowered to act—and find ways to incorporate the three S's to help future-proof our brains, both today and well into the future. The time to start is right now. Not just to help prevent dementia and cognitive decline later on in life, but because you never know when you might need more headroom. It will help provide a buffer against the twists and turns of life, preserving cognitive reserve and function—putting you in the best possible place to enjoy a good life for decades to come.

You may recall my father's advice when I first went off to university: "Remember, this doesn't mean you actually know anything." I certainly haven't forgotten it. But while there are still many questions to be answered regarding the complexities and function of the brain, even in its healthiest state, I feel like there is one thing I can now say for sure: all of our brains have remarkable promise and capability. Not only that, but *your* brain is perfectly adapted to help you navigate the world around you. And with a little care and *stimulus,* you can be sure it will continue to do so for decades to come.

REFERENCES

When I first set out to write this book, I made a commitment to making sure that readers would be able to follow up on the sources and scientific papers I used as evidence for the recommendations and ideas I presented. My list of references ended up being so long that it was impossible to include them all within the book itself. Instead, a full list of all my sources—sorted by chapter and the superscript numbers you see throughout the text—can be found at thestimulatedmind.com.

ACKNOWLEDGMENTS

It turns out that thinking you might one day like to write a book is relatively easy. Actually making that book come to fruition is a whole other matter entirely. Honestly, I'm still surprised that it did. The fact that this book exists at all is thanks entirely to a huge number of people who have mentored me, supported me, and contributed along the way. I am more grateful for having them in my life than I am able to adequately describe.

Perhaps the biggest group of contributors is the most important, even though they were unwitting participants. These are the scientists whose research I have relied upon to build the ideas presented in this book. Only a very small number of these scientists are actually mentioned by name in the text, but I am indebted to anybody whose work I have cited. In the reference list, you'll find more than 1,700 scientific papers, and though I didn't count them all, this likely represents the toil of more than ten thousand people. Each small piece and idea requires years of dedication to a process that is often difficult and discouraging, and their research will become even more important as the population—and our brains—continue to age.

The story of this book as a physical entity starts with Anya Hayes, my editor in the UK. It was Anya who really got this whole ball rolling by suggesting I write a book in the first place, and I'm incredibly glad and grateful that she did. Not having had any idea what writing a book would entail, I have to thank Gabrielle Lyon for her advice and contacts, as well as her endless support and encouragement through the whole process. Which brings me to my agent, Joy Tutela. I learned early on that Joy is right about pretty much everything when it comes to the world of books, and a lot of this process was just me doing what she told me to. I later learned that Joy is also pretty picky when it comes to clients, so I'm very grateful that I made the cut.

A huge thanks to the team at Harmony for everything it took to get this book into print. The process started with Diana Baroni, whom I have to thank for investing in me and the book, as well as for her guidance as I made several false starts getting it off the ground. It was Matthew Benjamin who shepherded the project across the finish line, and I am very grateful for his thoughtful expertise. Though he's a man of few words, they were usually the right ones, and he always knew what I needed in order to get the most out of my writing. Speaking of words, I have to thank Greg White for reading every word in this book multiple times and providing critical insights from the view of both a writer and a reader. He volunteered before really knowing what he was getting into and helped me maintain the confidence that I would figure it all out. The final piece to the puzzle was Kayt Sukel—another masterstroke of advice from Joy—who was the critical eye, sounding board, amateur therapist, and "ray of sunshine" I needed to wrestle this book into its final form. Though I know she'll chide me for abdicating credit, I really couldn't have done this without her. Thank you to Mark Birkey and the copyediting team for their incredible attention to detail and help making every sentence as good as it could be. And a huge thanks also to Ash Sandberg, SL Keenan, and the team at Triple 7 for their help spreading the word about the book and getting it into as many hands and ears as possible.

Before the proposal was even written or the idea fully formed, there were a number of people who were willing to vouch for me as somebody who could write a book and then maybe sell a few copies afterwards. Without their kind words, it would have been much harder for me to get my foot in the door of this world, and I am incredibly grateful for their years of support, friendship, and mentorship—in particular, Peter Attia, Robb Wolf, Joshua Fields Millburn, Lesley Paterson, and Thomas DeLauer. With their own considerable success in publishing and media, I know their full-throated support—as well as some conversations in the background—absolutely tipped the balance in my favour. Thomas even offered to show up topless to the book launch, which pretty much anybody would agree should be quite a draw. A big thank-you also to

Juliet and Kelly Starrett, Nick Stenson, and Michael Easter, who have been incredible resources and supporters as I tried to figure out what you're supposed to do with a book after you've written it.

I am particularly indebted to the people whose expertise, stories, and input I received or borrowed as I wrote. This includes Greg Bennett, James Hewitt, and Pauly DiTuro at the bleeding edges of human performance, the neuroscience nerdery of Chantel Prat and Andrea Stocco, the jungle rescue of my *bróðir* from another mother Ben House, the joy of movement of Darryl Edwards, and the nuanced and compassionate clinical expertise of Deborah Gordon, Rangan Chatterjee, and Simon Marshall. My life and this book are so much richer for having them all in it, and it's an honour to call them all friends and colleagues. Though I am sad that I never quite got to tell him this in person, Simon completely changed the way I think about the brain and human behaviour, and this book would have been very different without his considerable influence. And an additional huge and special thank-you to Rangan, who has supported me and my career in ways that would be too numerous to count since we first met a decade ago. Thanks also to everybody who read a chapter or section of the book to make sure I was heading in the right direction, especially Kristi, Megan, Candy, and Ben.

Then there are the two people whose influence is clearest across multiple chapters and pages of the book—Alex Stewart and Josh Turknett. Alex has been there for pretty much every formative event in my life, from science classes and band practice in secondary school to best man at my wedding (though we disagree slightly on whether I asked him to do that job months or twenty-four hours in advance), to the illustrations you see on these pages. Though it was a little different from the work he's now accustomed to as founder and creative partner of a renowned and award-winning design agency, Alex somehow managed to turn my increasingly esoteric and complex illustration requests into figures that are a joy to look at. For more than twenty years I hoped that one day we would find a way to work together despite very different careers, and I'm incredibly happy and proud that we managed it in the end.

At this point, my and Josh's work is often so intertwined that I'm sure there are moments in the book where I accidentally took credit for an idea that was originally his. If that's the case, I can only wholeheartedly apologise. Josh is my cohost on our podcast, *Better Brain Fitness,* and co-conspirator on the demand-driven theory of age-related cognitive decline (DDToARCD for short), and many of the core ideas presented in *The Stimulated Mind* were a result of his influence and expertise as a neurologist as well as his considerable abilities as a thinker, educator, and banjo enthusiast. There's a lot more for us to do in this area, but I'm incredibly grateful for all of Josh's input and support—both big and small—as this book came together.

Outside of the writing itself, I wouldn't have been in the position I find myself today without the mentors that have helped shaped my career. This includes Sandra Fulton, Marianne Thoresen, and Sunny Juul—each of whom encouraged and supported me at different stages of my academic career, even as I became pulled in increasingly disparate directions as an undergraduate who spent most of his time in a rowing boat; a PhD student with a burgeoning interest in health, sport performance, and podcasting; and eventually a neonatal neuroscientist who spent his spare time working with F1 drivers. It is thanks to them that I have been able to have the eclectic career and experiences that informed the work I do.

The fact that I had the time to write this book is solely because of the amazing people working in the lab, keeping our research going. Thank you, Daniel, Kylie, Olivia B., Olivia M., and all our students. It's an honour to work with such a dedicated team, and I am thankful for you every day. Special thanks to OM for helping to arrange the final references—it was a pretty monumental task in the end, but the book is much better for it. Thanks also to my other colleagues at the University of Washington and elsewhere who patiently waited while I paused meetings and let papers and projects gather dust on my desk so that I could get the writing done—especially Ulrike, for taking up the slack on multiple projects as the deadlines piled up. Thank you to Bob Hansen, Dan Pardi, Mike T. Nelson, and Ken Ford for the advice, friendship, and guidance over the years, as well as to my colleagues, past and present, at Hintsa Performance—Luke Bennett, Pete McKnight, Antti Kontsas, and Andy Harrison—and the drivers and coaches I've had the pleasure of working with in F1. I am excited for all the work forthcoming through Hintsa and via planned projects with Josh, Pauly, Andrea, Chantel, Kevin Gluck, Ben, Andy Galpin, Cody Burkhart, Vince Bryan, Miguel Zeran, Federica Conti, Patrick Holford and the team at Food for the Brain, as well as many others, which will help people better understand how to keep their brains as healthy as possible for as long as possible.

Of course, I am who I am and can do what I do only because of my friends and family. Thanks to Jim, Jill, and Andy for the dinners and laughs before this book-writing endeavour began and during the few breaks I took over the months of getting it written. Thanks to Sanj for the intermittent but always enthusiastic support from afar (YUH!). Thanks to Magga for being the best auntie and cheerleader that anybody could ask for. And to my sister, Katie, who over the years has been my protector, friend, and counselor, even when things get difficult and we're thousands of miles apart. A special thank-you to my mum and dad for instilling in me a desire to learn and give back, and for supporting me every time I decide to move to a different country, start another degree, or embark on a whole new career.

And lastly but mostly, none of this would be worthwhile or possible without my family in Seattle—Elizabeth, Bowen, and Morgan. And before Morgan, Parker. Thanks to the puppies for the endless companionship, love, laughs, kisses, and snuggles. While I often joke that getting a dog is the best possible biohack, in reality, they're usually the best part of my day. Something that I didn't know I needed until I met Elizabeth—one of the countless things that she has taught me. Elizabeth, my love, I think we both know that I have found my place in the world—both as an academic and a man—because of you. Thank you for always seeing opportunities and promise in me that I don't, for loving me and pushing me in equal measure, for being an incredible scientific collaborator and life partner, and for making sure that this book remained true to my values and my love of the Oxford comma. You are my best friend and the best thing that ever happened to me, and I can't wait to see what the years ahead have in store.

INDEX

Abel, Julian, 205, 209
acetylcholine, 304–5, 313
adaptation
   chronic stress and, 222–24
   finding, 257–60
   finding right levels of, 231–37
   impact of, 227–31
   managing arousal and, 237–44
   stress and, 225–30, 229*fig*, 244–57
adaptation energy, 244
adenosine, 282, 283, 405
Adolescent Brain Cognitive Development study, 296
adolescents, 379–80
adrenaline, 179, 223, 225–26, 227, 231, 232, 236
adrenomedullin, 207
Adult Changes in Thought study, 195–96, 322
Advanced Cognitive Training for Independent and Vital Elderly (ACTIVE) study, 186–87
aerobic exercise, 95
aging
   behaviour's impact on, 52
   brain development and, 40–43
   brain function and, 6
   perceptions of, 202–3
   as state of mind, 48–50
Aging Adult Brain Connectome (AABC), 314
air pollution, 334
air quality, sleep and, 294
alarm phase, 225
albumin, 267

alcohol use, 57, 60–61, 60*fig*, 300–301
allostasis, 228
allostatic load, 230–31, 236–37, 244–45, 251, 257, 264–67, 337, 341, 397, 403
altruism, 211
Alzheimer, Alois, 17–18, 20
Alzheimer Cohorts Consortium, 55
Alzheimer's disease. *See also* dementia
   ApoE and, 355
   early-onset, 18, 22
   gut microbiome and, 332
   heart health/disease and, 55–56, 306–7
   hippocampus and, 36, 150
   history of, 17–23
   as human disease, 42
   late-onset, 18, 22
   microglia and, 30
   MIND diet and, 146
   neuroplasticity loss and, 42
   oral health and, 331
   potential blood tests for, 356–58
   preclinical, 21
   racial differences in rates of, 338
   rates of in women versus in men, 313, 315
   smoking and, 304
   sporadic, 18
   statins and, 310
Alzheimer's Disease Neuroimaging Initiative (ADNI), 22
Ames, Bruce, 118, 119, 126, 127–28
amino acids, 124
amygdala, 247, 254, 280
amyloid beta, 19

INDEX

amyloid cascade hypothesis (ACH), 19, 21–22
amyloid/amyloid plaques, 19, 20, 21, 22–23, 24, 82, 283–84, 330, 356–57
anaerobic exercise, 105
anger, 265
Angry Birds analogy, 58–59
animal moves, 113
anthocyanins, 336
antidepressants, increased use of, 5
anti-frailty toolkit, 324–26
antihistamines, 313
antihypertensives, 308, 311
antioxidants, 119–20, 124, 127, 153
antipsychotics, 313
Anyone Can Play Music (Turknett), 162
apolipoprotein B (ApoB), 309–10, 311
apolipoprotein E (ApoE), 355–56
arousal
   flow and, 409
   increasing, 406–8
   managing, 405–6
   memory and, 410–12
   performance and, 231–34, 233*fig*, 402
   procrastination and, 234–36
   stress response and, 231–32
artificial intelligence (AI), 190–92
aspartate, 282
assistive technologies, 370
astaxanthin, 127
astroglia/astrocytes, 27, 28, 32, 137, 283, 285, 355
asynchrony, 387
atherosclerosis, 133, 306, 309–10
Atherosclerosis Risk in Communities (ARIC) study, 338
athletes, 46–47, 69, 188–89, 261–62, 287–88, 381
ATP, 282
Attention Span (Mark), 272, 394
attentional narrowing, 223–24
attentional residue, 395
automaticity, 393
autonomy, 141–43, 389
autophagy, 25, 84, 136
axons, 19, 26, 28–29

B vitamins, 119–20, 124, 125–26, 129, 147, 312, 334, 378
bacteria, oral hygiene and, 329–30
baseline performance management, 402–3, 405
Beers, Mark, 313
Beers Criteria, 312–13
belonging, social stress and, 337–38
Bennett, Greg, 263–64
Bennett, Laura, 263–64
Bennett, Luke, 374–75
benzodiazepines, 313
beta-blockers, 232
beta-carotene, 127
ß-glucan, 336
biking, 94
bilingualism, 175–76
biotin, 124
blood pressure
   high, 56
   improving, 307
   medications for, 308–9, 311
   sitting less and, 87
blood sugar
   cardiovascular health and, 307, 308
   GLP-1 drugs and, 137
   nutrition/diet and, 150
   resistance training and, 100
   testing, 138–39
blood tests, development efforts for, 356–58
blood vessels/supply, 31–32, 55–56, 163, 285, 305–7
blood-brain barrier (BBB), 106
blood-flow restriction (BFR) training, 325
body mass index (BMI), 138
body measurements, 138
boredom, 272
brain
   building model of, 354–56, 359–62
   challenges of studying, 13–16
   components of, 26–28
   regions of, 122*fig*
   as reticulum, 27
   variability in, 354
brain age, 179–80
brain development
   aging and, 40–43
   nutrients and, 121–22, 122*fig*
   overview of, 37–38
   timing of, 42–43
brain fog, 340–41

brain health
 activity and, 25–26
 definition of, 4–5
 game of, 53–62
 as long game, 72–73
brain imaging, 32
brain processing speed, 44, 45*fig*, 47–48
brain reserve (brain maintenance), 7, 8
brain size/volume
 alcohol use and, 302
 decreasing, 131
 energy availability and, 132–35, 133*fig*
brain training, 199
brain trauma, 21, 28, 30, 57
brain-computer interfaces, 370
brain-derived neurotrophic factor (BDNF), 83–84, 94, 105–6, 107, 112, 227
BrainHQ, 187
Brave Athlete, The (Marshall and Paterson), 258–59
bravery, 256–57
breaks, 396
breathing
 sleep and, 296
 stress and, 238–40
breathwork, 254, 272, 295, 318, 408
Bredesen, Dale, 321
Brenner, Charles, 135
British Cohort Study, 216
BROAD trial, 143, 146, 151
Brooks, Arthur C., 200–201
burnout, 264–65, 267, 384

Caen Chronotype Questionnaire, 387–88
caffeine, 158, 294–95, 405
Cajal, Santiago Ramón y, 17, 27, 183
calcium, 120–21, 124, 326
calendars/planning, 389–91
caloric restriction, 135, 136
camaraderie, 72–73
Campbell, Simon, 367
Cannon, Walter Bradford, 227–28
capillaries, 31–32
cardiovascular health. *See* heart health/disease
carotenoids, 127, 129–30
carrying, 101
cataract surgery, 196

causal loop diagrams, 347–50, 348*fig*, 349*fig*
ChatGPT, 191
Chatterjee, Rangan, 302–4
Chicago Health and Ageing Project, 60–61, 60*fig*, 68–69, 306, 338
chlorpheniramine, 313
cholesterol, 308, 309–10, 311, 355
choline, 119, 124–25, 130
chronic inflammation, 25, 323–24, 341
chronic stress, 223, 267, 403
chronic traumatic encephalopathy (CTE), 19
chronotypes, 386–88
Cialis, 367
circadian rhythm, 290–92, 293, 296, 298, 339, 386–87
Clear Thinking (Parrish), 390
closed-skill movements, 111
clutch states, 409
coaching, xvi, xx–xxi
cobalamin, 124
coding, 185–86
coenzyme Q10 (CoQ10), 312
cognitive activity, impact of, 60–61, 60*fig*
cognitive behavioural therapy for insomnia (CBT-I), 297
cognitive decline
 demand-driven, 163
 education and, 171–72, 171*fig*
 expectations of, 11
 loneliness and, 206
 nutrients and, 125–26
 protein and, 153
 retirement and, 192, 200
 subjective, 340–41
cognitive efficiency, 177, 187
cognitive function
 aging and, 6
 band of potential, 352–53, 353*fig*
 changes in over time, 6, 7*fig*
 crystallised intelligence and, 46–47
 dancing and, 182
 decreasing mismatch and, 11
 education and, 170, 175
 enhancing, 173–77
 exercise and, 81*fig*, 84, 176, 364, 406–7
 headroom and, 65–67
 perceptions of, 76

cognitive function (cont'd):
  rates of worsening, 5
  resistance training and, 100
  sleep and, 404
  SLS and, 164–65
  social environment and, 210–11
  as stimulus-driven process, 163, 171*fig*, 205
  task-switching and, 397–98
  technology and, 186
  tests for, 369
  ultradian rhythms and, 415–16
cognitive gears, 382–86, 385*fig*, 388–89, 396, 405–6
cognitive orthotics, 191
cognitive reserve, 7–8
cognitive resilience, 7, 8
cognitive training, 186–88
cold exposure, 407
cold sores, 328
Cole, Steven, 206
communication apps, pacing, 400–401
community. *See* social environment
compartment syndrome, 194
compassion, 204, 205, 211, 268–74
competence, 141–43, 200
complex environments, 165–66
component-based approach, 16
conscientiousness, 212
contextual binding, 412
control, 389–90
coordinative physical activity, 109–14, 162, 176, 188, 199, 377
cortisol, 208, 223, 225–26, 227, 243–44, 245, 273
COSMOS (Cocoa Supplement and Multivitamin Outcomes Study), 126
Counterclockwise study, 49–50
Covid-19 pandemic, 215–16, 219
C-reactive protein (CRP), 100, 207, 266
creatine, 148–49
creativity, 236, 273, 279, 348
CrossFit, 210
cross-stressor adaptation, 246
Crum, Alia, 248–49
crystallised intelligence, 46–47, 201, 319
Csíkszentmihályi, Mihály, 408
Cutting Alzheimer's Risk through Endocrinology (CARE), 314, 317

cytokines, 83–84, 282–83, 323

dancing, 181–84, 198
Darwin, Charles, 204
DASH (Dietary Approaches to Stop Hypertension) diet, 145–46
De Vany, Art, 6
Deci, Edward, 141
deep sleep, 277–78, 278*fig*, 284–85
default mode network (DMN), 41–42
dehydroepiandrosterone (DHEA), 244
deliberative prefrontal cortex, 37
dementia. *See also* Alzheimer's disease
  aerobic exercise and, 95
  alcohol use and, 301–2
  allostatic load and, 237, 257
  among Tsimané, 54–55
  ApoE and, 355
  being sedentary and, 86
  blood pressure and, 308–9
  burnout and, 267
  dancing and, 182
  decreasing mismatch and, 11
  decreasing rates of, 55–56
  depression and, 208
  description of, 17
  early-onset, 18
  education and, 169–70
  energy availability and, 133, 134–35
  exercise and, 82, 84
  GLP-1 drugs and, 137
  gut microbiome and, 332
  interventions for, 370–74, 373*fig*
  isolation and, 212
  lifestyle factors and, 60–61, 60*fig*, 68–69
  light exposure and, 291–92
  loneliness and, 206
  loss of sensory input and, 196–97
  Mediterranean diet and, 146
  neuroplasticity loss and, 42
  omega-3 fatty acids and, 122
  overload and, 265
  presenile, 18
  as preventable, 56–57, 67–68, 299, 351–52
  protein and, 153
  rates of, 5
  red meat and, 120

reductionism and, 21
risk and protective factors for, 299–300
sleep and, 283, 284–85
smoking and, 304
statins and, 310–11
stress and, 245–46
testing for risk of, 356–59
Viagra and, 367–68
dendrites, 26
depression
  creatine and, 148
  dancing and, 182
  isolation and loneliness and, 208
  omega-3 fatty acids and, 122, 147
  periodontal disease and, 330
  red meat and, 120
  resistance training and, 98–99
  risk and protective factors for, 299–300
  sense of purpose and, 201
  SMILES trial and, 155
  social media and, 216
  stress and, 246
  vitamin D and, 148
Descent of Man, The (Darwin), 204
Deter, Auguste, 18, 20
DHA (docosahexaenoic acid), 122, 124–25, 126, 127–28, 147, 326
diabetes, 56, 125, 132, 134, 137, 312, 326
dietary patterns, 139–47, 151–52, 155–58. *See also* nutrition/diet
dieting, 139–40
digit symbol substitution test (DSST), 43–45, 44*fig*, 47–48
digital amnesia, 185
digital dementia, 186, 190
digital twins, 368–69
diphenhydramine, 313
DIRECT PLUS (the Dietary Intervention Randomised Controlled Trial Polyphenols Unprocessed Study), 138
disconnection, social stress and, 337–38. *See also* isolation
distraction
  minimising, 399–401
  task-switching and, 397–98
  tuning out, 401, 406
  while eating, 393

DiTuro, Pauly, 237–38, 241, 243, 244
DNA damage, 25
Dodson, John, 232–33
dopamine, 217–18, 220, 405, 406
dorsolateral prefrontal cortex, 37
drug treatments, false optimism regarding, 35
dual-task training, 188

Ebbinghaus, Hermann, 410, 411*fig*
e-cigarettes, 305
ED medications, 367–68
education. *See also* learning
  cognitive decline and, 171–72, 171*fig*
  cognitive function and, 175
  dementia and, 169–70
  impact of, 57
  sex differences in access to, 336
Edwards, Darryl, 109–11, 113, 114, 162
email, pacing, 400–401
emotional lability, 266
emotions
  senses and, 242
  sleep and, 280
endothelial cells, 32
endothelial dysfunction, 306
energy, nutrition and, 130–39
energy availability, 132–39, 133*fig*
energy metabolism, 29
energy production, impaired, 25
engagement, 402
English Longitudinal Study of Aging, 134
environment. *See also* social environment
  adaptation to, 37–38
  as determinative, 38–40
  dominance of, 34–52
  impact of, 336–39
  mismatch in, 162
  restructuring, 303–4
EPA (eicosapentaenoic acid), 122, 147, 326
epilepsy, 19, 21
ergothioneine, 127
Ericsson, Anders, 415
esomeprazole, 312
oestrogen, 315–17, 319
ethanolamine, 125, 130
evolution, 204
executive function, overload and, 266
exenatide, 137

exercise/physical activity
  aerobic, 95
  anaerobic, 105
  BDNF and, 105–6
  brain health and, 25, 82–83
  brain processing speed and, 48
  cognitive function and, 81*fig*, 84, 176, 406–7
  complexity of effects of, 59
  coordinate/coordinative, 109–14, 162, 176, 188, 199, 377
  as core requirement, 83, 84
  disengagement and, 51
  framework for, 84–86
  group, 377
  heart disease and, 89–90
  impact of, 57, 60–61, 60*fig*, 83
  intensity of, 104–6
  loneliness and, 209–10
  medicalization of, 80
  memory and, 411
  menopause and, 318
  microglia and, 30
  moderate-to-vigourous, 94
  neuroplasticity and, 43
  peak performance times and, 386
  perceptions of, 75–76
  propel, 89–95
  recommendations regarding, 81*fig*
  resist, 95–104
  rules of the game and, 80–81
  sleep and, 363–66
  snacks of, 86–89
  society's views of, 79
  sprints and, 104–9
  stress and, 246–47
  white matter and, 29
  at work, 89–90
exerkines, 83–84
exhaustion, 265
exhaustion phase, 227
expectations
  of cognitive decline, 11, 50
  cognitive function and, 178–79
  impact of, 50
  lowering, 268–69
  sleep and performance and, 404
  unrealistic, 77
Exponential (Hewitt and Hintsa), 382
expressive writing, 250

Facebook, 214, 215
failure
  discomfort of, 166–67
  learning from, 178–79
falls, 322, 324–25
familiar, re-experiencing, 272–73
family history, 358–59
far transfer, 175, 177
fasting, 135–36
fast-twitch muscle fibres, 324–25
fermented foods, 333
fibre, 310, 332, 333
fibromyalgia, 330
fight or flight response, 227–28, 231
FINGER (Finnish Geriatric Intervention Study to Prevent Cognitive Impairment and Disability), 61, 371–72, 373*fig*
first-night effect, 287
fish, 121
flavonoids, 127
flossing, 329
flow, state of, 408–9
flu, 327
focus
  improving, 272
  as skill, 395–97
  ultradian rhythms and, 415–16
folate, 124, 125–26
FOMO (fear of missing out), 216
forest bathing, 273
forever chemicals, 335
forgetfulness, minimising, 410–14
Formula I racing, xx–xxi, 374–75, 382, 404, 408–9
4-6-8 ramp, 240
4-7-8 breathing, 239
frailty, 322, 324–26
Framingham Heart Study, 133–34, 284
friends, spending time with, 377–78
From Strength to Strength (Brooks), 200
frustration, 272
functional magnetic resonance imaging (fMRI), 32

gardening, 273
gears, cognitive, 382–86, 385*fig*, 388–89, 396, 405–6
Gebrselassie, Haile, 382
general adaptation syndrome, 225–27

genetic tests, 358
genetics, 354–56, 358–59
glia/glial cells, 27–31, 283, 355
glial fibrillary acidic protein (GFAP), 357, 358
GLP-1 drugs, 136–37, 308
glucose, 124, 139, 225, 315, 316
glutamate, 281–82
glutathione, 153
glymphatic system, 283–85, 290–91, 292, 298, 306
Golgi, Camilo, 17, 27
Google effect, 185
Gordon, Deborah, 321, 322, 324–25, 326, 327
grandparent hypothesis, 201
gratitude practices, 254, 255
grey matter, 29, 42–43
grip strength, 98
growth factor IGF-1, 99–100, 227
growth mindset, 248
gum disease, 329–30
gut health, 331–34
gut-brain axis, 332

habits
  changing, 302–4
  starting new, 140–41
Häkkinen, Mika, 382
Hall, Jeffrey, 290
Hall, Kevin, 151–52
haloperidol, 313
Hartley, Howard, 86
Harvard Study of Adult Development, 211
Haspel, Tamar, 144
headroom
  diagram of, 9fig
  importance of, 65–67
  as lifelong pursuit, 170–71
  overview of, 6–9
  starting process of building, 375–77
healthspan, 202
hearing loss, 196–97
heart health/disease
  alcohol use and, 300–301
  cognitive function and, 165
  dementia and, 55–56, 305–11
  exercise/physical activity and, 89–90
  oral health and, 330

heart rate variability, 212, 273
Haemoglobin, 318
herpes simplex virus 1 (HSV-1), 328
Hertzog, Christopher, 352
Hewitt, James, 382, 390
high blood pressure, 56
high-intensity interval training (HIIT), 105, 106–7
high-ventilation breathwork, 240
hinging movements, 101
Hintsa, Aki, 381–82
Hintsa Performance, xx–xxi, 374–75, 381–82, 404
hippocampus
  blood vessels/supply and, 307
  coordinative physical activity and, 112
  dancing and, 182, 198
  oestrogen and, 316
  memory and, 36, 412, 413
  menopause and, 317
  mindfulness and, 256
  nutrition/diet and, 150
  size of, 94, 107, 209
  stress and, 245
  video games and, 189
Holt-Lunstad, Julianne, 206
homeostasis, 227
homocysteine, 126, 147, 334, 378
hormesis, 228–29, 301
hormones
  disruptions to, 119
  oestrogen, 315–17
  sex differences and, 315
  stress response and, 227
  testosterone, 319–20
hospitalization, impact of, 195–96
House, Ben, 226
Human Nutrition Unit, 151
hydration, 158–59
hypostress, 229
hypoxic-ischemic encephalopathy (HIE), 14–15

IGF-1, 99–100, 227
Iliff, Jeff, 283, 285
Illinois Brain Ageing Study, 119
illness/infections, 195–96, 327–28. *See also individual illnesses/conditions*
immune system, 206, 225–26, 323

implementation intentions, 140
incretin system, 136
indecision, 240
indifference, 265
Indigenous Northern Americans, 355
inflammation
   allostatic load and, 237, 266–67
   ApoE and, 355
   chronic, 25, 323–24, 341
   cytokine interleukin-6 (IL-6) and, 83–84
   frailty and, 322
   isolation and, 207
   microglia and, 30
   periodontal disease and, 329–30
   resistance training and, 100
   sleep and, 283, 365–66
   smoking and, 304
information overload, 74–75
insomnia, 317–18
insulin resistance, 125, 137, 150, 310, 322, 324
interleukin-6 (IL-6), 83–84
intermediate transfer, 175
intermittent fasting (IF), 135–36
interval training, 105, 106–9
interventions, effect of, 61
iodine, 120
iron, 120, 121–22, 124, 128, 318
ironman triathlon, off-road, 69–71
irritability, 265
Isaacson, Richard, 358
isolation
   disconnection and, 337–38
   exercise and, 365–66
   loneliness versus, 207–9

John, Dan, 101
journaling/therapeutic writing, 251–52, 270
juggling, as stimulus, 198
juggling study, 168
jumping, 324–25
Juul, Sunny, 39

Keltner, Dacher, 204
ketones, 124
Kleitman, Nathaniel, ultradian rhythms and, 415
Knowledge of London exam, 36

knowledge workers, 262, 382, 394, 399
Kraepelin, Emil, 17, 20
Kross, Ethan, 242, 249–50

laboratory testing, 138–39
lactate, 105–6, 107, 282
Lagakos, Bill, 84
Lancet commission, 169, 299, 300, 351
Langer, Ellen, 48–50, 52, 76, 97
language learning, 176, 198
large-language models (LLMs), 191–92
last-in first-out hypothesis, 41–42
lateral parietal lobe, 37
lateral temporal lobe, 37
Lazebnik, Yuri, 15–16
LDL cholesterol (LDL-C), 309–10, 311
lead, in water, 335
learning. *See also* stimulation/cognitive challenge
   in classes, 377–78
   dopamine and, 217–18
   errors and, 413
   from failure, 178–79
   focus and, 395–96
   human development and, 50–52
   impact of, 57, 166–73, 175
   languages and, 176–77, 198
   music and, 178
   sleep and, 278–79
leg strength, 48, 97, 106, 324
Levi-Montalcini, Rita, 170–71
Levine, Benjamin, 107
libraries, 213
Lieberman, Daniel, 80, 145, 152
life expectancy, increases in, 55
lifestyle factors, 60*fig*, 68–69
Lifetime Fitness Series, 263
light exposure, 291–92, 293, 296, 407
Livingston, Gill, 56–57, 169, 299
Lockley, Steven, 404
locus coeruleus, 236
loneliness, 206–12
longevity, focus on, 202
longevity vitamins, 126–27
loving-kindness meditation, 253–54, 255, 270
low energy availability, 119, 131
lutein, 119, 127, 129–30
lycopene, 127

macronutrients, 145, 156*fig*
magnesium, 120–21, 125, 129, 148, 312, 326
Maintain Your Brain study, 372, 373*fig*
Malawi, 329–30
Manson, Mark, 263
Mark, Gloria, 75, 272, 394, 395, 398–99
MARS-500, 208
Marshall, Simon, 258–60
maternal education, impact of, 39–40
McEwan, Bruce, 230
medial parietal cortex, 41
medical school, author's experience in, 345–46
medicalization of exercise, 80
meditation, 253–55, 270, 272, 295
Mediterranean diet, 145–46, 150
Mediterranean-DASH Intervention for Neurodegenerative Delay (MIND) diet, 120, 145–46
melatonin, 293
memory
  aerobic exercise and, 95
  forgetting curve and, 411*fig*
  functioning of, 410–11
  Google effect and, 185
  improving, 410–14
  isolation and, 209
  pets and, 212
  sleep and, 278–80
  spatial, 36
  stress and, 245
  training, 187
menopausal hormone therapy (MHT), 316–17, 318, 319
menopause, 314, 315, 318–19
mental fatigue, 281–82
mental health. *See also* depression
  resistance training and, 98–99
  strength and, 98
mental offloading, 250, 252–53
mental toughness, 257, 271
Merzenich, Michael, 187
metabolic syndrome/disease, 55, 138, 139, 143, 307, 318, 326
metabolites, 281–83, 297
metformin, 312
methylation, 125, 126, 147
microbreaks, 396
microglia, 27, 30–31, 137, 324

microplastics, 335–36
miliary foci, 18–19
Millennium Cohort Study, 216
mindfulness, 253, 255, 256, 269, 270, 318, 396–97
mismatch
  decreasing mismatch and, 50–52
  environmental, 162
  retirement as, 9–10, 11, 26
Mithridates VI, King, 228
mitochondria, 124, 135–36, 312
modern stimuli, 184–90
monotony, work-related, 172
mood
  exercise and, 406
  sleep and, 404–5
Morris, Jeremy, 90
Morris, Martha Clare, 146
Mosconi, Lisa, 314, 316, 317
Mosetén people, 132, 134
Mosso, Angelo, 32
motivation
  lack of, 265
  redirecting, 270
Mounjaro, 136–37, 308
movement funnel
  context for, 84–86
  coordinate, 109–14
  diagram of, 85*fig*
  propel, 89–95
  resist, 95–104
  snack, 86–89
  sprint, 104–9
multiple sclerosis (MS), 346–47, 350
multitasking, myth of, 391–95, 397–99
multivitamins, 126, 128, 149
muscle mass, 97–101, 102, 104, 153, 196, 320, 322–23, 325, 326
music, 177–81, 198, 242, 401, 408
myelin, 28–29, 30, 346
myokines, 83, 112

Nagelhus, Erlend, 283
Naiman, Ted, 154
napping, 273–74
nasal breathing, 239
National Child Development Study, 216
National Health and Nutrition Examination Survey (NHANES), 47–48

naturalistic fallacy, 145
nature, 241, 242, 273, 349, 377, 396
near transfer, 174–75
Nederaard, Maiken, 283
Neff, Kristin, 269–70
negative, focus on, 54, 67
neurofilament light chain (NfL), 306, 357, 358
neurons, 17, 19, 26–29, 30, 32, 105, 123–24, 137, 278, 281
neuroplasticity
  brain-derived neurotrophic factor (BDNF) and, 83, 94
  capacity for, 42, 43
  cognitive training and, 187
  errors and, 178–79
  learning and, 166–68
  music and, 180
  stress response and, 231
neuroscience
  field of, xviii–xix
  history of, 17
neuroticism, 212
neurotransmitters, 124–25, 179, 281–82, 304. *See also individual neurotransmitters*
neurovascular coupling, 32
neurovascular unit, 32
Newport, Cal, 236, 391, 401
Nexium, 312
Next Steps, 216
niacin, 124
nicotine, 304–5
Niotis, Kellyann, 358
nitrate, 309
nitric oxide (NO), 309
noise, sleep and, 294
non-REM (NREM) sleep, 277–78, 278*fig*, 281, 282, 289, 291, 292, 298
non-sleep deep rest (NSDR), 272
noradrenaline, 236, 415
norepinephrine, 179, 406
Norwegian 4 x 4 protocol, 107
notifications, reducing, 400
nutrition/diet
  blood pressure and, 309
  calorie-dense, nutrient-poor foods, 149–51
  cholesterol and, 310
  components of, 116*fig*, 117–18
  differing opinions on, 115–16
  energy, 116*fig*, 130–39
  gut health and, 333
  impact of, 60–61, 60*fig*
  judgment surrounding, 116
  menopause and, 318
  nutrients, 116*fig*, 117–30
  pattern, 116*fig*, 139–49
  performance and, 402–3
  protein and, 326
  sleep and, 294
  supplements and, 147–49

obesity, 132, 134, 137, 138, 143
offloading, 250, 252–53
Ohio Longitudinal Study of Ageing and Retirement, 202
olanzapine, 313
older people, role of in society, 10–11
oligodendroglia/oligodendrocytes, 27, 28–29, 30
omega-3 fatty acids, 119–20, 121, 122–23, 125–26, 128, 147, 148, 326, 371, 378
omeprazole, 312
On the Origin of Species (Darwin), 204
online support groups, 214
open-skill movements, 111–12, 113
oral health/hygiene, 329–31
orthosomnia, 295
Osler, Sir William, 10, 165
osteoarthritis, 104
osteoporosis, 100
Our Epidemic of Loneliness and Isolation, 206
overload, 264–67
overtraining, 263–64
oxidative stress, 124, 131, 150, 276, 300–301, 304, 306, 315, 334, 361
Ozempic, 136–37, 308

pantothenic acid, 124
parasympathetic nervous system, 206
parietal lobe, 37, 41
Parker, Gordon, 265
Parrish, Shane, 390
passion, lack of, 265
Paterson, Lesley, 259
Pennebaker, James, 251–52
perfect, as enemy of good, 74

perfectionism-related stress, 268–69
performance, reduced, 266
pericytes, 32
perimenopause, 314, 315–16, 317–18
periodontal disease, 329–30
pets, 212, 213, 348–50, 349*fig*
phone calls, 213
phosphodiesterase 5 (PDE5) inhibitors, 367–68
physical activity. *See* exercise/physical activity
physiological sigh, 239–40, 254
pianists, study involving, 43–46, 51
Pilates, 113
placebo effect, 405
pneumonia, 327
POINTER (Protect Brain Health Through Lifestyle Intervention to Reduce Risk), 371–72
pollutants, 334–36
polyfluoroalkyl substances (PFAS), 335, 336
polygenic risk scores, 358
polyphenols, 124, 127–28, 130, 150, 300–301, 333
Pomodoro technique, 396
Pontzer, Herman, 100
posterior hippocampus, 36
potassium, 124, 309
Potter, Greg, 293
Prat, Chantel, 175–76, 185–86
prefrontal cortex, 37, 41, 234, 280, 281–82
preterm births, 38–40, 329–30
Preterm Erythropoietin Neuroprotection Trial (PENUT), 39–40
Prilosec, 312
Primal Play, 110–11
PRIME (Prestigious, Ingroup, Moral, or Emotional) information, 217, 218
prioritization, 240–41
problem-solving, 345–46
processing-speed training, 187
procrastination, 234–36
progress, as goal, 73–78
project list, managing, 401
protein, 152–54, 155–57, 326, 378
protein bars/powders, 150, 153
proton pump inhibitors (PPIs), 312

psychological refractory period, 395
Pugh, Emerson, 13–14, 33
pulling movements, 101
purpose, having sense of, 73, 201
pursed lips, breathing through, 239
pushing movements, 101
pyridoxine, 124

quetiapine, 313
quiet eye, 243

race analogy, 69–72
racial differences in Alzheimer's rates, 338
Ranganath, Charan, 410, 413
reading, 201
reasoning training, 187
Reasons for Geographic and Racial Differences in Stroke (REGARDS) study, 200
recovery
  brain-focused, 271–74
  compassion and, 268–74
  importance of, 261–64
  inadequate, 264–67
  making room for, 269–70
  resets and, 281–86
  sleep and, 274–81, 286–98
red meat, 120
reductionism, 14–16, 18, 122–23
reflection, 250
relatedness, 141–43
relationship structures, complexity of, 34
relationships, importance of, 72–73. *See also* social environment
relaxation, 295
REM (rapid eye movement) sleep, 277–81, 278*fig*, 285, 288, 289, 290, 291, 292, 298
reminiscing, 49
resilience, 246–47, 271
resistance phase, 225
resistance training, 80, 96–104, 153, 324–25
resolve, 8
retirement
  cognitive decline and, 192, 200, 321
  as example of mismatch, 9–10, 11, 26
  new stimuli during, 201–2
riboflavin, 124, 125–26

risk, 256
risperidone, 313
Robinson, Sir Ken, 169
Rodin, Judith, 49
Rosbash, Michael, 290
rote activities/attention, 272
rowing, xv, xvi–xvii, 173–74
Roy, Charles, 32
rule of thirds, 409
rules of the game, 65–78
Rush Memory and Ageing Project, 146, 322, 354
Ryan, Richard, 141
Rybelsus, 308

San-Millán, Iñigo, 83
sarcopenia, 97, 98, 100, 322–23, 324, 326
sarcopenic obesity, 322
Satiety per Calorie (Naiman), 154
Sato, Yoshiaki, 325
Schaie, Warner, 164–65, 352, 360
Seattle Longitudinal Study (SLS), 90, 164–65, 337, 352, 360
selenium, 121
self-compassion, 268–74
self-determination theory, 141–43, 200, 389
self-talk, 250
self-testing, 413
Selye, Hans, 225, 226–27, 229, 244
semaglutide, 137, 308
Senna, Ayrton, 408–9
senses, leveraging, 242–43
sensory loss, 196–97, 199
serotonin, 124, 319
sex differences
    brain markers and, 358
    at cellular level, 315
    HIE and, 15
    nutrient deficits and, 120
    in rates of dementia, 313
    studies on, 314
Sherrington, Charles, 32
Shift (Kross), 249
shingles, 327–28
shock phase, 225
shutdown rituals, 391
sildenafil, 367–68
Singh, Sanjula, 376

sitting, 86–87
16S sequencing, 332
Slavich, George, 206
sleep
    assessing amount needed, 286–87
    astroglia/astrocytes and, 28
    basics of, 286–98
    brain function and, 281–84
    deep, 277–78, 278*fig*, 284–85
    exercise and, 363–66
    improving, 292–97
    light exposure and, 292, 293
    main components of, 288–91
    memory and, 414
    microglia and, 30
    napping, 273–74
    omega-3 fatty acids and, 147
    overload and, 265
    performance and, 403–5
    perimenopause and, 317–18
    problems with, 403–5
    procrastination and, 236
    recovery and, 274–81
    routine for, 296–97
    social media and, 220
    stages of, 277, 278*fig*
    as starting place, 378
sleep aids, 290
sleep apnea, 296, 318
"Sleep Inspires Insight," 279
sleep opportunity, increasing, 289, 296, 366, 378
sleep pressure, 281
sleep trackers, 295
Sleepmore in Seattle study, 287, 289
slow-wave sleep, 277, 278*fig*
SMART (Study of Mental and Resistance Training), 100–101
smells
    emotions and, 242
    novel, 199
SMILES (Supporting the Modification of lifestyle in Lowered Emotional States) trial, 155
Smith, David, 125–26
smoking, 56–57, 60–61, 60*fig*, 300, 304–5, 351–52
snacks, exercise, 86–89
snakebite incident, 193–95, 226
social environment

in digital age, 214–20
finding connections within, 213, 220–21
impact of, 205–7
importance of, 204
isolation and, 207–9
loneliness and, 207–13
social headroom, 205–7
social media, 214, 215–20
social rejection, 216–17
social stress, 216–17
Social Vulnerability Index, 338
socioeconomic environment, impact of, 338–39
sodium, 124, 309
Soft-Wired (Merzenich), 187
Sparrow, Betsy, 185
spatial memory, 36
spheres of work, 394
Spitzer, Manfred, 186
squats, 87–88, 101
statins, 308, 310–11, 312
stereotype-embodiment theory, 50, 97
stimulants, 405
stimulation/cognitive challenge
    choosing skills and, 167–68
    environment and, 165–66
    importance of, 160–63
    intensity of, 165–66
    learning and, 166–73
    recovery after, 413–14
    suggestions for, 198–99
    work-related, 172–73
Stocco, Andrea, 175–76
stopping, importance of, 274
storm analogy, 71
Storoschuk, Kristi, 136
stress
    building tolerance for, 244–57
    chronic, 223, 267, 403
    downregulation of, 238–44
    overload and, 265
    perfectionism-related, 268–69
    procrastination and, 234–36
    reframing, 243–44, 247–50
    as requirement for adaptation, 225–30, 229*fig*
    sleep and, 365
stress fractures, 261
Stress Mindset Measure, 249

stress optimization, 247–48
stress response, 206–7, 231–32
striver's curse, 200
stroke, 3, 299–300
strongman competitions, 96, 97–98
Study of Women's Health across the Nation (SWAN), 318, 319
subjective cognitive decline, 340–41
sugar consumption, 151–52
suicide, increased rates of, 5
Super Mario, 189
superagers, 360
supplements, 147–49
support groups, online, 214
survival of the kindest, 204–5
Suzuki, Wendy, 397
synapses, 17, 26, 30, 124–25
synchrony effect, 387
syncing, 253–56
syphilis, 20, 21
Systematic Multi-Domain Alzheimer Risk Reduction Trial (SMARRT), 373–74
systems dynamics, 347–52
Szasz, Thomas, 166–67

tai chi, 112
task-switching, 393–95, 397–98, 399–400
taste, emotions and, 242
tau, 19, 21, 82, 356–57
tauopathies, 19
taxi driver studies, 35–36
technological advancements, 368–70
technology use, 184–92
temperature, sleep and, 293–94
temporal lobe, 37, 41
testosterone, 319–20
therapeutic writing/journaling, 251–52, 270
thiamine, 124
third-person self-talk, 250
thoughts/thinking
    impact of, 48–50, 75
    speed of, 391–92
3:7 breathing, 239
3-F framework, 302–4
3-S model of brain health
    beginner's guide to, 377–78
    diagram of, 363*fig*

3-S model of brain health (cont'd):
  impact of, 381
  overview of, 360–62
  in practice, 362–66
thrombolysis (clot busting), 3
time travel, mental, 250
time-restricted eating (TRE), 135, 136
tirzepatide, 308
to-do lists, 401
touch, emotions and, 242
toxins, 334–36
trackers, focus on, 369
tracking how you feel, 340
traffic light system, 258–60
transcendental meditation, 254, 255
transfer, concept of, 174–75, 177
traumatic brain injury/brain trauma, 21, 28, 30, 57
triage theory, 118–19
Tsimané people, 54–55, 132, 134, 152–53, 355
Turknett, Josh, 58–59, 162, 176, 181, 205, 214
two-photon microscopy, 283
Tyson, Mike, 258

ultradian rhythms, 415–16
ultraprocessed foods, 150, 152
uncertainty, 240
under-recovery, 264–67

vaccinations, 327–28
vagus nerve, 206, 212, 273
Valentine, Greg, 329–30
vapes, 305
vascular dementia, 306, 310
VEGF (vascular endothelial growth factor), 112
Viagra, 367–68
video games, 189, 199
virtual reality (VR), 188–89, 273, 370
vision, stress and, 241, 243
vision loss, 196–97
visualization, 413
VITACOG study, 125–26
vital exhaustion, 264–65
vitamin C, 120, 124
vitamin D, 119, 124, 129, 148, 266, 326, 378
vitamin E, 119–20, 124

vitamin K2, 326
vitamins, B, 119–20, 124, 125–26, 129, 147, 312, 334, 378
volunteering, 211, 213, 377

waist-to-height ratio, 138
waist-to-hip ratio, 138
Walker, Matthew, 276, 282, 284
walking, 90–92, 91*fig*, 94, 95, 273
water quality, 335
water requirements, 158–59
Wegovy, 308
weight lifting, 80, 96–104. *See also* resistance training
white matter, 29, 100, 122
white noise, 401
Why We Remember (Ranganath), 410
Why We Sleep (Walker), 276
Willis, Sherry, 165, 186–87
wisdom, 46–47, 201
withdrawal, 266
Women's Health Initiative Memory Study (WHIMS), 316
Wood, Sidney, 89–90
WOOP (wish, outcome, obstacle, and plan) framework, 140–41
work, spheres of, 394
work opportunities
  sex differences in access to, 336–37
  socioeconomic environment and, 339
workday/work environment, 380–81, 382, 384–86, 388–90, 399, 414
World Happiness Report, 209
Wright, Kenneth, Jr., 291
writing, stress tolerance and, 250–52

xylitol gum, 330, 331

Yerkes, Robert, 232–33
yoga, 113
yoga nidra, 272, 295
Yoruba, 355
Young, Michael, 290

zeaxanthin, 119, 127, 129–30
Zeigarnik, Bluma, 235
Zeigarnik effect, 235, 401
Zepbound, 308
zinc, 120, 125, 129
Zostavax, 328

ABOUT THE AUTHOR

Tommy Wood, BM BCh, PhD, is a neuroscientist, performance coach, and elite-level professional nerd. He is currently an associate professor of paediatrics and neuroscience at the University of Washington, where his research focuses on brain health across the lifespan. This includes therapies for newborn brain injury, prevention and treatment of adult brain trauma, and factors that contribute to long-term cognitive function and decline. He received a bachelor's degree in biochemistry from the University of Cambridge, a medical degree from the University of Oxford, and a PhD in physiology and neuroscience from the University of Oslo. Alongside his academic training, Dr. Wood has worked as a performance consultant to elite athletes in numerous sports, including multiple Formula 1 drivers. He is a founding Trustee of the British Society of Lifestyle Medicine, Head of Research for the dementia prevention charity Food for the Brain, and co-host of the *Better Brain Fitness* podcast. He lives in Seattle, Washington, with his wife, Elizabeth, and their two boxers, Bowen and Morgan.